Communication Disorders in Spanish Speakers

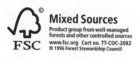

Communication Disorders Across Languages

Series Editors: Dr Nicole Müller and Dr Martin Ball, *University of Louisiana at Lafayette, USA*

While the majority of work in communication disorders has focused on English, there has been a growing trend in recent years for the publication of information on languages other than English. However, much of this is scattered through a large number of journals in the field of speech pathology/communication disorders, and therefore, not always readily available to the practioner, researcher and student. It is the aim of this series to bring together into book form surveys of existing studies on specific languages, together with new materials for the language(s) in question. We also envisage a series of companion volumes dedicated to issues related to the crosslinguistic study of communication disorders. The series will not include English (as so much work is readily available), but will cover a wide number of other languages (usually separately, though sometimes two or more similar languages may be grouped together where warranted by the amount of published work currently available). We envisage being able to solicit volumes on languages such as Norwegian, Swedish, Finnish, German, Dutch, French, Italian, Spanish, Russian, Croatian, Japanese, Cantonese, Mandarin, Thai, North Indian languages in the UK context, Celtic languages, Arabic and Hebrew among others.

Other Books of Interest
Bilingual Children's Language and Literacy Development
  Roger Barnard and Ted Glynn (eds)
Bilingual Minds: Emotional Experience, Expression and Representation
  Aneta Pavlenko (ed.)
Culture-Specific Language Styles: The Development of Oral Narrative and Literacy
  Masahiko Minami
Developing in Two Languages: Korean Children in America
  Sarah J. Shin
Language and Aging in Multilingual Contexts
  Kees de Bot and Sinfree Makoni
Language Acquisition: The Age Factor (2nd ed)
  David Singleton and Lisa Ryan
Making Sense in Sign: A Lifeline for a Deaf Child
  Jenny Froude
Phonological Development in Specific Contexts: Studies of Chinese-Speaking Children
  Zhu Hua
Phonological Development and Disorders in Children: A Multilingual Perspective
  Zhu Hua and Barbara Dodd (eds)
Understanding Deaf Culture: In Search of Deafhood
  Paddy Ladd

For more details of these or any other of our publications, please contact:
Multilingual Matters, Frankfurt Lodge, Clevedon Hall,
Victoria Road, Clevedon, BS21 7HH, England
http://www.multilingual-matters.com

Communication Disorders Across Languages
Series Editors: Nicole Müller and Martin Ball

Communication Disorders in Spanish Speakers
Theoretical, Research and Clinical Aspects

Edited by
José G. Centeno, Raquel T. Anderson
and Loraine K. Obler

MULTILINGUAL MATTERS LTD
Clevedon • Buffalo • Toronto

Library of Congress Cataloging in Publication Data
Communication Disorders in Spanish Speakers: Theoretical, Research and Clinical
Aspects/Edited by José G. Centeno, Raquel T. Anderson and Loraine K. Obler.
Communication Disorders Across Languages
Includes bibliographical references and index.
1. Communicative disorders–Treatment–United States. 2. Communicative disorders
in children–Treatment–United States. 3. Bilingualism–United States. 4. Bilingualism in
children–United States. 5. English language–Acquisition. 6. Spanish
language–Acquisition. 7. Hispanic Americans–Language. 8. Hispanic American
children–Language. 9. Bilingualism–Physiological aspects.
I. Centeno, José G. II. Anderson, Raquel Teresa. III. Obler, Loraine K. IV. Series.
[DNLM: 1. Communication Disorders–ethnology–United States. 2. Hispanic
Americans–United States. 3. Multilingualism–United States. WL 340.2 C73378 2007]
RC423.C6427 2007
362.196' 855–dc22   2007006872

British Library Cataloguing in Publication Data
A catalogue entry for this book is available from the British Library.

ISBN-13: 978-1-85359-972-9 (hbk)
ISBN-13: 978-1-85359-971-2 (pbk)

Multilingual Matters Ltd
UK: Frankfurt Lodge, Clevedon Hall, Victoria Road, Clevedon BS21 7HH.
USA: UTP, 2250 Military Road, Tonawanda, NY 14150, USA.
Canada: UTP, 5201 Dufferin Street, North York, Ontario M3H 5T8, Canada.

The policy of Multilingual Matters/Channel View Publications is to use papers that
are natural, renewable and recyclable products, made from wood grown in
sustainable forests. In the manufacturing process of our books, and to further support
our policy, preference is given to printers that have FSC and PEFC Chain of Custody
certification. The FSC and/or PEFC logos will appear on those books where full
certification has been granted to the printer concerned.

Typeset by Datapage Ltd.
Printed and bound in Great Britain by the Cromwell Press Ltd.

Contents

Contributors

Raquel T. Anderson, Ph.D., Department of Speech and Hearing Sciences, Indiana University, Bloomington, IN, USA

Ana Inés Ansaldo, Ph.D., Faculté de Médecine, Université de Montréal, Québec, Canada

Alfredo Ardila, Ph.D., Department of Communication Sciences and Disorders, Florida International University, Miami, FL, USA

Fredericka Bell-Berti, Ph.D., Department of Speech, Communication Sciences, and Theatre, St. John's University, Jamaica, NY, USA

Alizah Z. Brozgold, Ph.D., Department of Rehabilitation Medicine, St. Vincent's Hospital, New York, NY, USA

Anny Patricia Castilla, ABD, Department of Speech-Language Pathology, University of Toronto, Toronto, Ontario, Canada

José G. Centeno, Ph.D., Department of Speech, Communication Sciences, and Theatre, St. John's University, Jamaica, NY, USA

Barbara T. Conboy, Ph.D., Institute for Learning and Brain Sciences, University of Washington, Seattle, WA, USA

Hia Datta, M.S., Department of Speech and Hearing Sciences, The Graduate Center, City University of New York, New York, NY, USA

Willard Gingerich, Ph.D., Office of the Provost, Fairleigh Dickinson University, Teaneck, NJ, USA

Martin Gitterman, Ph.D., Department of Speech-Language-Hearing Sciences, Lehman College, and Department of Speech and Hearing Sciences, The Graduate Center, City University of New York, New York, NY, USA

Brian Goldstein, Ph.D., Department of Communication Sciences, Temple University, Philadelphia, PA, USA

Elizabeth Ijalba, M.Phil., Department of Speech and Hearing Sciences, The Graduate Center, City University of New York, New York, NY, USA

I. Carolina Iribarren, Ph.D., Postgrado en Lingüística Aplicada, Universidad Simón Bolívar, Caracas, DF, Venezuela

Donna Jackson-Maldonado, Ph.D., Universidad Autónoma de Querétaro, Querétaro, México

Pui Fong Kan, M.A., Department of Speech-Language-Hearing Sciences, University of Minnesota, Minneapolis, MN, USA

Hortencia Kayser, Ph.D., Department of Communication Sciences and Disorders, St. Louis University, St. Louis, MO, USA

Kathryn Kohnert, Ph.D., Department of Speech-Language-Hearing Sciences, University of Minnesota, Minneapolis, MN, USA

Azucena Lozano, Lic., Facultad de Psicología, Universidad Nacional Autónoma de México, México, DF, México

Karine Marcotte, M.S., Centre de Recherche, Institut Universitaire de Gériatrie de Montréal, Université de Montréal, Québec, Canada

Loraine K. Obler, Ph.D., Department of Speech and Hearing Sciences, The Graduate Center, City University of New York, New York, NY, USA

Feggy Ostrosky-Solís, Ph.D., Facultad de Psicología, Universidad Nacional Autónoma de México, México, DF, México

Lourdes G. Pietrosemoli, Ph.D., Centro de Investigación y Atención Lingüística, Universidad de Los Andes, Mérida, Venezuela

Maura J. Ramírez, Lic., Facultad de Psicología, Universidad Nacional Autónoma de México, México, DF, México

M. Adelaida Restrepo, Ph.D., Department of Speech and Hearing Sciences, Arizona State University, Tempe, AZ, USA

Belinda A. Reyes, Ph.D., Department of Communication Disorders, Our Lady of the Lake University, San Antonio, TX, USA

Brendan Weekes, Ph.D., CPsychol, Department of Psychology, School of Life Sciences, University of Sussex, Brighton, UK

Acknowledgments

Publication of this volume would not have been possible without the enormous amount of patience and careful work from a group of people. We are indebted to all of our contributors who supported this project since its planning stages and throughout its various evolutionary phases. Our deepest thanks to the energetic and supportive Multilingual Matters family, starting with Mike Grover, former head publisher and currently enjoying his semi-retirement, who, in conjunction with his editorial advisors, Nicole Müller and Martin Ball, welcomed our proposal. Thanks Nicole for the long hours reading the manuscripts and all of your challenging comments. Marjukka and Tommy Grover answered our many questions and Marjukka patiently led us through the initial developmental processes before Ken Hall guided the production phases with meticulous care and encouraging emails, and Kathryn King shaped the wide marketing efforts. José thanks Jeffrey Fagen, his College Dean, and his colleagues on the faculty for allowing him the teaching reduction to give attention to this volume and his many other projects. Raquel thanks her colleagues in the Department of Speech and Hearing Sciences, especially Karen Forrest and Laura Murray for their continued support and their belief that working with diverse populations is a necessary endeavor for our field. She also thanks her family for tolerating her long days working on this book. Loraine thanks José and Raquel for engaging her in working on this book, and for all the thoughtful, careful work they have put in on it. We all thank Bonnie Lorenzen at Indiana University for assisting with the author index.

Introduction

JOSÉ G. CENTENO, LORAINE K. OBLER and RAQUEL T. ANDERSON

There are approximately 330 million Spanish speakers in the world today (Gordon, 2005). Besides being spoken in Spain, Spanish is the official language in Mexico, of most of South America and Central America, and of several Caribbean islands. Spanish also is spoken in Equatorial Guinea, the West coast of Africa, the Philippines, and parts of Morocco. A variety of Spanish known as Ladino is spoken in Israel and Turkey (Katzner, 1995). Additionally, Spanish is used by about 21 million people in the USA, hence representing the second most frequently spoken language after English (US Census Bureau, 2003).

Spanish coexists with other languages in bilingual contexts as a majority or minority language. As a majority language, Spanish is found in several Latin American countries along with indigenous languages, as in Ecuador, Peru, and Colombia; with Portuguese, as in Uruguay; and with English, as in Puerto Rico. As a minority language, it coexists with English in the USA, with Basque in the Basque sections of Spain and France, with Arabic, French, and indigenous languages in Africa, and with indigenous languages in the Philippines (Centeno & Obler, 2001; Silva-Corvalán, 1995).

Thus Spanish speakers, whether in monolingual or bilingual situations, or in majority or minority contexts, represent a considerable population worldwide. Such a prominent demographic presence underscores the need to understand the different variables that impact clinical service delivery with communicatively impaired Spanish users. Spanish speakers in the USA, most often individuals of Hispanic ancestry, represent an illustrative context to discuss both theoretical and clinical variables relevant to monolingual and bilingual Spanish speakers. Hispanic individuals in the USA, also identified as Latinos(as), constitute a vibrant and diverse community. Although it has a minority presence relative to English in most parts of the USA, Spanish has a great vitality resulting from the constant influx of new Spanish monolingual speakers and growing institutional support by newspapers, magazines, television and radio programs (Centeno & Obler, 2001; Torres, 1997). Hispanics represent both the largest minority group and the group with the strongest demographic growth in the country (National Alliance for

Hispanic Health, 2004; US Census Bureau, 2002; also see Centeno & Gingerich, ch. 8, this volume for a related discussion). They constitute about 42 million people (14%) of the total US population, exceeding the size of other minority groups, such as African–American, Asian American, or Native American groups. They also are projected to be one of every four persons (25%) of the US population by the year 2050 (National Alliance for Hispanic Health, 2004; US Census Bureau, 2002).

Latinos(as) in the USA are a heterogeneous group. In terms of ancestry, Mexican–Americans (66.9%) constitute the largest group of Hispanics followed by Central Americans and South Americans (14.3%), Puerto Ricans (8.6%), Cubans (3.7%), and other Hispanics (6.5%) (US Census Bureau, 2002). Like other culturally and linguistically diverse (CLD) groups, Hispanics represent varied levels of schooling, life experiences, and socioeconomic circumstances that have an impact on their communication performance (Centeno, 2005, 2007). Hispanics' language skills also reflect different dialectal varieties of Spanish consistent with their countries of ancestry, and, like all bilingual populations in the USA and elsewhere, exhibit varying degrees of bilingualism with a wide range of receptive and expressive skills in their first (L1) and second (L2) languages (Spanish and English, respectively) (Centeno, 2007; Centeno & Obler, 2001; Iglesias, 2002).

Steady increases in the Latino(a) population in the USA have had an impact on speech-language clinics throughout the country. Hispanics have been the most common ethnic group in US speech-language caseloads after Asians for the past 15 years, as suggested by pediatric caseloads (Roseberry-McKibbin *et al.*, 2005). This trend has resulted in the publication of several important works largely focusing on service delivery with Hispanic children in the USA (Brice, 2002; Goldstein, 2004; Kayser, 1995; Langdon & Cheng, 1992; Oller & Eilers, 2002).

Because demographic estimates suggest a steady growth in Hispanics' presence in speech-language clinics, it is imperative for speech-language pathologists to have access to clinically relevant research and publications. However, there is still considerable paucity in the amount of literature on Hispanic individuals available for student clinicians and licensed professionals. Particularly lacking are works that would link both empirical and theoretical bases to evidence-based practices for child and adult Spanish users. Additionally, given that communication performance depends on multiple phenomena in addition to strictly linguistic ones, speech-language students and practitioners must avail themselves of interdisciplinary research and discussions to gain a realistic understanding of each Spanish-speaking client's communication skills (Miccio *et al.*, 2000; also see Ball, 2005).

This book attempts to address those gaps. Developed as a team effort, this volume brings together papers by a number of researchers and practitioners with extensive expertise on Hispanic individuals. All have been invited to bring their expertise in order to apply advancements in clinical communication research on Spanish speakers to clinical practice with this population, to disseminate research and clinical procedures on the under-researched adult Spanish speakers, and to bring cross-disciplinary input into the clinical and research problem-solving process for Spanish speakers.

Planning for this book started at the annual convention of the American Speech-Language-Hearing Association in Washington, DC, November, 2000. At that time, two seminars on Spanish speakers were conducted: one on young children and the other on older children and adult speakers, organized by Raquel Anderson and José G. Centeno, respectively. Presenters at the seminars were invited to participate in this book. Loraine K. Obler, one of the presenters, graciously accepted our invitation to additionally offer her vast research and publication experience, as part of the editorial team. Later, other investigators and practitioners, particularly those from allied fields, were invited to contribute in order to make the content of the publication broad and interdisciplinary.

In this book, we provide conceptual and empirical information on Spanish speakers that can be employed in the training of future clinicians and as part of continuing education resources available to licensed professionals. This book differs from earlier speech-language pathology (SLP) volumes on Spanish speakers in that these prior publications focused largely on service-delivery issues and descriptions of various aspects of the Spanish language (i.e. syntax, phonology, etc.) as they applied to clinical procedures with Spanish-speaking children in the USA (e.g. Brice, 2002; Goldstein, 2004; Kayser, 1995; Langdon & Cheng, 1992). In contrast, this publication targets typical and atypical communication skills in both monolingual and bilingual children and adults who speak Spanish within the context of research-based discussions and clinical implications. Additionally, we take an interdisciplinary approach because, as mentioned earlier, addressing the needs of communicatively impaired Hispanic individuals often requires collaborative input and/or empirical evidence from other disciplines to gain a broader range of insights on the client. To this effect, this book includes pertinent information from allied fields, such as Neurolinguistics, Neuropsychology, Education, and Clinical Psychology, to assist in the understanding of additional important aspects of the communication performance of Spanish speakers, such as neurocognitive accounts of literacy skills, the interaction between immigrant resettlement and psychoemotional variables, and neuroanatomical bases of language processing.

Although this book focuses on Spanish speakers in the USA, it also includes discussions on monolingual Spanish speakers in other countries, such as Mexico and Venezuela, for their theoretical and clinical implications in the management of the monolingual Spanish speakers we treat in the USA. Material discussed in this book similarly has clinical implications for Spanish speakers in other countries. Moreover, in this era of globalization, many Spanish speakers who are today in monolingual Spanish-speaking countries may find themselves at some periods of their life in the USA or in a similar bilingual context such as that of another country, like Australia, England, and so forth, where English is the majority language.

The content of the book has been structured into three sections. In Part 1, 'Preliminary Considerations', introductory chapters set the scene for subsequent chapters in the book. Chapters discuss the theoretical, methodological, and ethical principles essential to conduct and interpret clinical communication research in both monolingual and bilingual Spanish-speaking individuals. In Part 2, 'Research in Children: Conceptual, Methodological, Empirical, and Clinical Considerations', chapters focus on three key areas, namely, morphosyntactic impairments in specific language impairment (SLI), cognitive development in bilingual children, and speech differences/disorders in young bilingual children. These areas, prominently covered in the literature on monolingual Spanish-speaking and bilingual Spanish–English-speaking children, often present challenges to the SLP clinician working with young Hispanic clients. Finally, in Part 3, 'Research in Adults: Empirical Evidence and Clinical Implications', authors address important topics relevant to adult monolingual and/or bilingual Spanish speakers. Because a large number of the clinical profiles exhibited by Hispanic adults involve neurogenic communicative deficits, some of the chapters in this section discuss research and evidence-based diagnostic and therapy methods directed at this population. Also, as many of these adult clients similarly have had educational experiences different from the mainstream population and, in addition, started acquiring English later in life, issues concerning differing levels of literacy skills and late acquisition of speech patterns in a second language (i.e. English, in this case) are also presented in this section. In particular, chapters describe studies leading to evidence-based clinical procedures in neurogenic linguistic disorders; development, use, and acquired disruption of literacy skills, and the clinical analysis of speech patterns. We conclude with an 'Epilogue', which will summarize the main arguments presented earlier in the book as a backdrop to future directions in clinical communication research in Spanish speakers and CLD populations.

This volume primarily aims to provide useful information to an audience interested in clinical communication research on monolingual Spanish or bilingual Spanish–English speakers, particularly SLP graduate and doctoral students, and licensed professionals. In addition, the book's interdisciplinary content will similarly be valuable to readers in allied fields, namely, Linguistics, Education, and Psychology, interested in similar topics on Hispanic individuals for research purposes or further professional growth. Furthermore, because the conceptual principles and findings treated here should be relevant to the understanding of similar communication aspects in other languages, this volume will be useful to those professionals and researchers interested in cross-linguistic discussions in applied/clinical linguistics.

As Hispanics in the USA are the main focus of our discussions, this publication supports current professional mandates in the USA. Cognizant of the impact of demographic changes in the country on speech-language service delivery, the American Speech-Language-Hearing Association's (ASHA) Executive Board requires the inclusion of specific information and course content to address the communication needs of individuals from 'socially, economically, and linguistically diverse populations' (Resolution LC 50-85) (Cole, 1990: 35). Further, stressing the need to use evidence-based clinical procedures and responding to the shortage of doctoral-level professionals, ASHA recommends that professional training and continuing-education programs implement teaching approaches that connect research and clinical work to stimulate the implementation of evidence-based clinical practice and to interest master's-level students in pursuing doctoral studies (Bernthal, 2001; Logemann, 2000).

Thus, one of our goals, was to assist faculty in complying with ASHA's mandate to ensure the incorporation of information on CLD populations in training curricula, and to provide students and teachers alike with examples of the connection between research and clinical training (Cole, 1990). Specifically, we developed this book to be relevant to both theoretical and research courses covering language and speech issues on children and/or adults from CLD groups.

Because, according to ASHA, SLP programs may follow either the 'infusion' or the 'course' curriculum approach to impart knowledge on multicultural populations (Cole, 1990: 35), we envisioned that, in accord with the first approach, content from this book may be 'infused' into the corresponding language or speech units concerning CLD clients in each course. In accord with the second approach, we hope that training programs will use this book in a single course devoted to CLD populations or, even more specifically, to Spanish speakers.

In sum, it is hoped that this book serves to amplify the call to increase clinical research on Spanish speakers and other under-researched CLD populations of all ages, to link research and clinical procedures, and to study and interpret clinical communication profiles in CLD groups within an interdisciplinary framework.

References

Ball, M. (ed.) (2005) *Clinical Sociolinguistics*. Malden, MA: Blackwell.

Bernthal, J.F. (2001) Discipline and professions face critical shortage of research doctorates. *The ASHA Leader* 6, 23.

Brice, A.E. (2002) *The Hispanic Child*. Boston: Allyn and Bacon.

Centeno, J.G. (2005) Working with bilingual individuals with aphasia: The case of a Spanish–English bilingual client. *American Speech-Language-Hearing Association Division 14-Perspectives on Communication Disorders and Sciences in Culturally and Linguistically Diverse Populations* 12, 2–7.

Centeno, J.G. (2007) From theory to realistic praxis: Service-learning as a teaching method to enhance speech-language pathology services with minority populations. In A.J. Wurr and J. Hellebrandt (eds) *Learning the Language of Global Citizenship: Service-learning in Applied Linguistics*. Bolton, MA: Anker.

Centeno, J.G. and Obler, L.K. (2001) Principles of bilingualism. In M. Pontón and J.L. Carrión (eds) *Neuropsychology and the Hispanic Patient: A Clinical Handbook* (pp. 75–86). Mahwah, NJ: Lawrence Erlbaum.

Cole, L. (1990) *Multicultural Professional Education in Communication Disorders: Curriculum Approaches*. Rockville, MD: American Speech-Language-Hearing Association.

Goldstein, B. (2004) *Bilingual Language Development and Disorders in Spanish–English Speakers*. Baltimore: Paul H. Brookes.

Gordon, R. (ed.) (2005) *Ethnologue: Languages of the World* (15th edn). Dallas, TX: SIL International.

Iglesias, A. (2002) Latino culture. In D. Battle (ed.) *Communication Disorders in Multicultural Populations* (3rd edn, pp. 179–202). Boston: Butterworth-Heinemann.

Katzner, K. (1995) *The Languages of the World*. London: Routledge.

Kayser, H. (ed.) (1995) *Bilingual Speech-Language Pathology: An Hispanic Focus*. San Diego: Singular.

Langdon, H. and Cheng, L.R. (eds) (1992) *Hispanic Children and Adults with Communication Disorders: Assessment and Intervention*. Gaithersburg, MD: Aspen.

Logemann, J.A. (2000) Are clinicians and researchers different? *The ASHA Leader* 5, 28.

Miccio, A.W., Hammer, C.S. and Toribio, A.J. (2002) Linguistics and speech-language pathology: Combining research efforts toward improved interventions for bilingual children. In J.E. Alatis, H. Hamilton and A-H. Tan (eds) *Georgetown University Round Table on Languages and Linguistics 2000 – Linguistics, Language, and the Professions: Education, Journalism, Law, Medicine, and Technology* (pp. 234–250). Washington, DC: Georgetown University Press.

National Alliance for Hispanic Health (2004) *Delivering Health Care to Hispanics: A Manual for Providers*. Washington, DC: Estrella Press.

Oller, D.K. and Eilers, R.E. (eds) (2002) *Language and Literacy in Bilingual Children*. Clevedon, UK: Multingual Matters.

Roseberry-McKibbin, C., Brice, A. and O'Hanlon, L. (2005) Serving English language learners in school settings: A national survey. *Language, Speech, and Hearing Services in Schools* 36, 48–61.

Silva-Corvalán, C. (ed.) (1995) *Spanish in Four Continents: Studies in Language in Contact and Bilingualism*. Washington: Georgetown University.

Torres, L. (1997) *Puerto Rican Discourse: A Sociolinguistic Study of a New York Suburb*. Mahwah, NJ: Lawrence Erlbaum.

US Census Bureau (2002) *Annual Demographic Supplement to the March 2002 Current Population Survey*. Washington, DC: US Census Bureau.

US Census Bureau (2003) Nearly 1-in-5 speak a foreign language at home. *US Census Bureau News, Report CB03-157*. Washington, DC: US Census Bureau.

Part 1
Preliminary Considerations

Chapter 1
Contrastive Analysis between Spanish and English

RAQUEL T. ANDERSON and JOSÉ G. CENTENO

Knowledge of typical and disordered communication profiles in speakers of different languages is imperative in linguistically diverse clinical contexts. Particularly, in the multilingual scenario of the USA, in which English is the majority language, cross-linguistic comparison of communication skills in speakers of languages other than English has both theoretical and clinical value in monolingual and bilingual situations. Theoretically speaking, because theoretical accounts have largely been based on English speakers, cross-linguistic data allow speech-language investigators and practitioners to assess the suitability of English-based proposals as explanatory accounts of communication performance in speakers of other languages (Leonard, 1996; Paradis, 2001; see Anderson, Ch. 6, this volume). Clinically, cross-linguistic knowledge enhances the accuracy of both diagnostic interpretation and intervention design. Yet, realistic cross-linguistic analysis and interpretation will not be possible without understanding pertinent linguistic features of the languages being discussed.

The purpose of the present chapter is to provide the reader with an overview of the linguistic features of the Spanish language, focusing mainly on its phonological, morphological, and syntactic aspects. Because we assume that the reader will be familiar with the linguistic descriptions of English, in order to enhance the understanding of data from Spanish monolingual and Spanish–English bilingual populations reported in this book, Spanish will be discussed as it compares to English.

The chapter will be divided into three main sections: phonology, morphology, and syntax. Each section will discuss how the particular features of the Spanish language differ from or are similar to those of English. The first section will describe the Spanish phonological system in terms of the general consonant inventory, the vowel system, and syllable structure. The second section will discuss Spanish morphology, particularly focusing on inflectional properties of nouns, verbs, and pronouns. The third section will focus on Spanish syntactic structure to describe word order structure and its variability, and structural aspects of wh- questions, negative formation, and use of complex sentences in Spanish.

Throughout the chapter, our discussions will summarize important descriptive features of the three target areas and will provide additional sources for more theory-driven accounts of the relevant aspects. Our discussions assume the reader has basic knowledge of the terminology used, as an introduction to phonological, morphological, and syntactic theory is beyond the scope of this chapter. Finally, because Spanish speakers in the USA primarily are of Latin American ancestry, dialectal examples provided in this chapter will be based on Latin American Spanish varieties. In particular, we will survey dialectal differences in pronunciation because this is the area of most variation, among the most frequently cited linguistic areas of Spanish dialectal variation, namely, vocabulary, grammar, and pronunciation (see Zentella, 1997).

Phonology

This section discusses the main characteristics of Spanish phonology, namely, the general consonant inventory, the vowel system, and syllable structure. A summary of the Spanish consonant system is presented in Table 1.1. Regarding dialectal variation, it is important for the reader to be aware that Spanish dialects mainly differ with respect to consonant production, thus not all sounds represented in the table are produced by all speakers, or produced in similar ways across syllabic contexts. In this section, particular production patterns of Spanish consonants and vowels will also be discussed, as they contrast to English.

Plosives

Like English, Spanish has three voiceless – /p, t, k/ – and three voiced – /b, d, g/ – plosives. Although these appear to parallel the stops in English, there are three major differences in how they are produced. The first difference concerns the distinction between voiced–voiceless phonemes, as signaled by differences in voice onset time (VOT). Plosive consonants are produced by having complete blockage of the airstream, followed by a small burst of sound when the articulators are separated (Mackenzie, 2001). The moment when the voicing starts in the following voiced segment is referred to as VOT. Three VOTs have been described in the literature. Stops can be prevoiced, meaning that voicing (i.e. vocal fold vibration) occurs prior to the release of the articulators (e.g. [g]). They can also be produced with voicing initiated at the moment the burst of sound occurs (e.g. unaspirated stop – [k]). Finally, voicing can occur after the articulators are released (e.g. aspirated plosive – [k^h]). This difference in VOT impacts how phonemes are identified in the language. In English, the difference between voiced and voiceless plosives is established between aspirated plosive and unaspirated plosive. Spanish, on the other hand, identifies a voiceless plosive as one that is unaspirated and a voiced plosive

Table 1.1 Spanish consonants

	Bilabial		Labiodental		Interdental		Alveolar-Dental		Post-Alveolar		Palatal		Velar		Glottal	
	V+	V-	V+	V-	V+	V-	V+	V-	V+	V-	V+	V-	V+	V-	V+	V-
Plosive	b	p					d	t					g	k		
Fricative	β			f	ð	θ		s	ʒ	ʃ			ɣ	x		h
Affricate									dʒ	tʃ						
Nasal	m		ɱ				n				ɲ		ŋ			
Lateral									l		ʎ					
Tap							ɾ									
Trill							r									
Glide	w										j					

Note. Not all sounds presented in the table are present in all Spanish dialects. V+ refers to voiced consonants, V- to voiceless consonants as one that is pre-voiced. Aspirated plosives are not part of its consonant inventory.

A second difference in the production of plosives pertains to place of articulation of the phonemes /d, t/. In English, tongue placement for the production of these sounds is alveolar, while in Spanish, it is dental. The final difference concerns the production of the Spanish voiced plosives /b, d, g/. By a process referred to as *spirantization* (Ortega-Llebaria, 2004), these sounds are produced as voiced fricatives in the same place of articulation when they occur in intervocalic position. Thus, each voiced plosive has a voiced fricative allophone, [β, ð, ɣ], respectively. For example, the word *cubo* 'bucket' would be produced as [kuβo], the word *todo* 'all' as [toðo], and the word *soga* 'rope' as [soɣa].

Fricatives

Spanish and English differ significantly with respect to their fricative consonantal inventory. They share the following fricative sounds: /f, ð, s, h/. In addition, some peninsular Spanish dialects also have /θ/ as part of their fricative inventory (Mackenzie, 2001), a sound also present in English. Within these shared sounds, some differences are worth noting. First, /ð/, while phonemic in English, is an allophonic variant of /d/ in Spanish. In addition, /h/, while used in many dialects of Spanish, especially in the Americas, is not present in some peninsular dialects, as well as others in Latin America (e.g. some Mexican dialects) (Canfield, 1981). Instead, the velar fricative /x/ is used. Thus, the word *caja* 'box' may be realized as either [kaha] or [kaxa], depending on the speaker.

Other cross-language differences are worth noting. First, English presents with a larger number of fricative sounds that are phonemic, as for example /v, z, ʃ, ʒ/. Some of these sounds do occur in some Spanish dialects, but as allophonic variants of Spanish phonemes. For example, in some Latin American dialects (e.g. El Salvador) and in central dialects of Spain, /s/ may be realized as [z] when it precedes a voiced consonant, as in the word *mismo* 'same' (Canfield, 1981; Mackenzie, 2001). As mentioned in the discussion of plosives, the Spanish sound inventory includes two fricative sounds that are not part of the English system, [β, ɣ].

Nasals

Spanish has three nasal phonemes: /m/ (*m̠adre* 'mother', *cam̠a* 'bed'), /n/ (*n̠ido* 'nest', *can̠a* 'gray hair'), and /ɲ/ (*cañ̠a* 'cane', *sueñ̠o* 'dream'), the latter occurring mainly in intervocalic position. When nasals occur before consonants, they undergo a process of neutralization, where the place of articulation of the following sound influences how the nasal sound is produced (Mackenzie, 2001). As a result, the pattern is one of assimilation, where the nasal becomes more similar to the following consonant. In these contexts, the place of articulation of the nasal sound

is the same as that of the consonant that follows it. For example, the word
énfasis 'emphasis' in Spanish is realized as [eɱfasis], and the word *pongo*
'I put' as [poŋgo].

Affricates

Like English, Spanish has the affricate sound /tʃ/ (e.g. *chispa* 'spark',
coche 'car'). Some Spanish varieties, such as those spoken in the
Caribbean (Canfield, 1981) also have the palato-alveolar voiced affricate
/dʒ/ as part of their sound systems. In these dialects, this sound mainly
occurs in word initial position (though it can be produced in intervocalic
position, as well), while the palatal glide /j/ is used mainly in
intervocalic position. Other Latin American dialects, such as in Uruguay
and Argentina, also include the palatal voiced fricative /ʒ/ where other
dialects use /dʒ/ or /j/. Furthermore, other Spanish dialects, especially
those in Latin America, as in Bolivia, use the lateral palatal /ʎ/. For
example, a word such as *lluvia* 'rain' can be realized, depending on the
speaker, as [dʒuβja], [ʒuβja], [juβja], or [ʎuβja].

Liquids

Liquid phonemes in Spanish consist of three alveolar sounds: the lateral
/l/, the flap (tap) /ɾ/, and the trill /r/. The lateral phoneme occurs in any
syllable position, as for example [loβo] (*lobo* 'wolf'), [kola] (*cola* 'tail'), and
[asul] (*azul* 'blue'). The flap appears in both intervocalic (e.g. [kaɾa] – *cara*
'face'), and postvocalic or syllable final position (e.g. [aɾbol] – *árbol* 'tree',
[maɾ] – *mar* 'sea'). Although this sound is not considered to be part of the
English sound system, it does occur as a variant of /t/ in intervocalic
position in some American English dialects, as in the words 'butter' and
'letter' or in the homophonous 'writer' and 'rider'. The trill /r/ is
produced in syllable-initial and in intervocalic position, as in the words
[ropa] (*ropa* 'clothes') and [karo] (*carro* 'car').

Vowels

In contrast to English, the Spanish vowel inventory is small, consisting
of five primary vowels. These include two front vowels, /i, e/, and three
back vowels /a, o, u/. All vowels in Spanish are described as tense. This
pattern also contrasts with English, where both tense and lax vowels are
present. As mentioned previously, most of the dialectal differences in
Spanish occur in the production of consonants. Nevertheless, some
differences have been reported in the use of vowels by different Spanish
speakers, sometimes even within a broad dialectal group, as for example
Puerto Rican Spanish (Navarro Tomás, 1974). Finally, Spanish has a
considerable number of diphthongs. Some of them also are found in
English, such as /aɪ/ (*baile* 'dance', eye), /eɪ/ (*ley* 'law', lay), and /ɔɪ/

(*hoy* 'today', boy), whereas others are not /ɪo/ (*labio* 'lip'), /ɪa/ (*sucia* 'dirty'), /eu/ (*deuda* 'debt') (Qüilis & Fernández, 1985).

Syllable structure

A summary of the various Spanish syllable types is presented in Table 1.2. Various patterns are worth noting. The most frequent syllable structure in Spanish is that of a consonant (C) and a vowel (V); thus, most syllables are considered open (i.e. ending in a vowel with no coda). Groups of consonants occurring within a syllable consist of a plosive (i.e. /p, b, t, d, k, g/) or a fricative (i.e. /f, β, ð, ɣ/) and a liquid sound. These occur in prevocalic and in intervocalic position, as in words such as *grande* 'big', *letra* 'letter', *cofre* 'treasure chest', and *sable* 'sable'. Unlike in English, three-consonant sequences are not permitted within the same syllable, nor is [s]+ consonant sequence within the same syllable (e.g. *escuela* 'school'). Other combinations occurring in Spanish consist of a glide+vowel (e.g. *suave* 'soft', *miel* 'honey') or a vowel+glide (e.g. *jaula* 'cage', *vaina* 'pod'). These have traditionally been described in Spanish as diphthongs, as described above.

Morphology

This section discusses inflectional features pertinent to noun phrase (NP), verb phrase (VP) morphology, and pronominal morphology in Spanish. Unlike English, Spanish is a highly inflected language. English has eight *inflectional affixes* (bound grammatical morphemes): plural (boys), possessive (boy's), comparative (bigger), superlative (biggest), present (closes), past (closed), past participle (closed), and present participle (closing) (Parker & Riley, 2000; Tserdanelis & Wong, 2004); and a limited set for pronouns (he, him, his, etc.). In contrast, Spanish has multiple inflectional affixes to indicate a variety of syntactic and semantic functions at both NP and VP levels, and for pronoun cases.

Noun phrase

Spanish has a number of inflectional features at the NP level beyond those in English. While English nouns do not receive gender markings (except for some rare circumstances: prior/prioress, actor/actress) but have plural markers, Spanish nouns are marked for both grammatical gender and number. Spanish nouns typically include feminine {a} or masculine {o} markers. However, there are exceptions to this pattern (e.g. *flor* [feminine] 'flower', *mano* [feminine] 'hand', *guardia* [masculine] 'guard'). Regarding number, the plural marker {-s} has two context-determined allomorphs. The morpheme {-s} is attached to nouns that end in a vowel (*casa* 'house', *casas* 'houses'), and the morpheme {-es} is appended to nouns ending in a consonant (*camión* 'truck', *camiones* 'trucks').

Table 1.2 Syllable types in Spanish* (based on Qüilis & Hernández Alonso, 1990)

Syllable type	Example**	English translation
CV	ca-sa /casa gran-de/grande	house big
CVC	cam-bio/cambio ár-bol/árbol	change tree
V	a-gua/agua san-di-a/sandía	water watermelon
VC	en-trar/entrar an-cla/ancla	to enter/come in anchor
CVV	cie-lo/cielo sa-bue-so/sabueso	sky hound
CCV	an-cla/ancla pre-so/preso	anchor prisoner
CVVC	dien-te/diente duer-me/duerme	tooth s/he sleeps
VV	hie-lo/hielo hue-co/hueco	ice hole
CCVV	true-que/trueque plie-gue/pliegue	exchange seam
CCVC	an-clar/anclar plan-cha/plancha	to anchor flatiron
CCVVC	trein-ta/treinta cruel/cruel	thirty cruel

*These are ordered in terms of frequency, from most to least. There are some instances where a CC coda occurs, as in the word instante, where [ins] is one syllable, but these are highly infrequent in the language.
**All words are divided into syllables. Those underlined represent the examples of the target syllable type.

In contrast to English, all NP constituents modifying the noun, that is, most determiners and adjectives, must agree with the noun in both gender and number. Within the Spanish determiner system, both articles (e.g. *un* 'a', *el* 'the') and demonstratives (e.g. *este* 'this', *ese* 'that') follow this rule while other determiners, such as possessives (e.g. *mi* 'my', *tu* 'your') and numerals (e.g. *cuatro* 'four', *ocho* 'eight'), do not. Further, unlike English, Spanish has a neutral determiner form, *'lo'*, which expresses a nominalized attribute of an event, idea, or object (see Anderson, 1995) (e.g. *lo bueno del café es que te da energía* 'the good [attribute] of coffee is that it gives you energy'). Table 1.3 summarizes the preceding agreement features for both articles and demonstratives in the Spanish determiner system.

Finally, while most adjectives are typically assigned gender and number markings to correspond to the noun, there are some exceptions. For instance, those adjectives that end in a consonant or in a vowel other than {o} (masculine) or {a} (feminine) only receive number markings (*la camisa marrón* 'the brown shirt'/*las camisas marrones* 'the brown shirts', *el carro grande* 'the big car'/*los carros grandes* 'the big cars').

Verb phrase

The Spanish verb system, unlike that of English, is highly inflected. English only has five inflectionally distinct verb forms (i.e. base form 'walk', third person singular 'walks', past tense 'walked', past participle 'walked', and imperfective [present] participle 'walking'). In contrast, Spanish verbs represent a complex inflectional system because each inflectional affix is required to encode a number of morphological specifications for thematic vowel, tense, mood, aspect, person, and number. Based on the morphological descriptions by Stockwell *et al.* (1965) and Qüilis and Hernández-Alonso (1990), the structural paradigm of a Spanish verb can be summarized as stem + thematic vowel + morpheme I + morpheme II, in which morpheme I stands for tense, mood, and aspect, and morpheme II represents the person and the number encoded by the particular verb. Table 1.4 shows the different syntactic and semantic features encoded in Spanish verb inflections.

Each Spanish verb includes a thematic vowel, *a*, *e*, and *i*, easily recognized in the infinitive (e.g. habl<u>ar</u> 'to speak', beb<u>er</u> 'to drink', compart<u>ir</u> 'to share'). According to their thematic vowel, Spanish verbs can be classified into first, second, and third conjugation classes depending on whether their inflectional endings for tense, mood, aspect, person, and number follow the *-ar*, *-er*, or *-ir* inflectional patterns. Conjugational inflectional features are marked in the finite, personal forms of the verbs and not on their nonfinite, impersonal counterparts (e.g., infinitive, present participle [-ing form], and past participle). For example, personal forms of the verb include simple verb forms (e.g., *hablo* 'I speak') and the auxiliary in auxiliary–past participle compound verb forms (e.g. *he hablado* 'I have spoken'). There is great overlap among the finite morphological markers for both second (*-er*) and third (*-ir*) conjugational classes within the Spanish verb paradigm. They differ from each other in very minor ways and are not distinguished at all in two tenses, preterite and imperfect (Schnitzer, 1993).

Table 1.3 Agreement features for both articles and demonstratives in the Spanish determiner system (adapted from Anderson, 1995, and Bedore, 1999)

| | | Articles | | Demonstratives | | |
		Indefinite	Definite	Near	Middle	Far
Singular	Feminine	una una casa	la la casa	esta esta casa	esa esa casa	aquella aquella casa
	Masculine	un un carro	el el carro	este este carro	ese ese carro	aquel aquel carro
	Neutral		lo lo bueno	esto esto es bueno	eso eso es bueno	aquello aquello es bueno
Plural	Feminine	unas unas casas	las las casa	estas estas casas	esas esas casas	aquellas aquellas casas
	Masculine	unos unos carros	los los carros	estos estos carros	esos esos carros	aquellos aquellos carros

Table 1.4 Syntactic and semantic features in the inflectional system of Spanish verbs (based on Centeno, 1996)

Feature	*Types*
Theme	-ar -er -ir
Tense	Present Past Future
Mood	Indicative Subjunctive Imperative
Aspect	Imperfective Perfective
Person	First Second Third
Number	Singular Plural

Mood refers to verbal meanings communicating the speaker's attitude to the proposition or to its reality (Alarcos Llorach, 1999; Gili-Gaya, 1981). Three moods can be identified in Spanish: indicative, subjunctive, or imperative. The indicative mood expresses actions considered real or certain (e.g. *tomo vino* 'I drink wine'), the subjunctive mood refers to possible, wished, or uncertain actions (e.g. *dudo que yo tome vino* 'I doubt that I would drink wine'), and the imperative mood expresses commanded actions (e.g. *¡Toma!* 'Drink!'). In English, there is only a vestigial subjunctive in the high-register phrase 'if it were'.

Three tenses can be communicated by Spanish verbs; present, past, and future, depending on when the action described by the verb occurs. However, the action expressed by the verb can involve temporal shades of meaning unrelated to tense. These result from the ways in which sentential context contributes to the action's duration or completion. These temporal specifications are identified as aspectual features. Comrie's (1976) terminology illustrates these fine temporal descriptions by referring to tense as situation-external time and aspect as situation-internal time. To Comrie, aspect is not concerned with relating time of the situation to any other time-point (as tense does), but rather with the internal temporal consistency of the one situation. For instance, consider the aspectual differences in these examples of past-tense sentences: *when she called, I was having dinner* and *when she called, I had dinner*. In the first sentence, the two actions, *calling* and *having dinner* occur within the same time frame, whereas in the second sentence *calling* precedes *having dinner*. Both sentences denote past tense situations yet differ in their internal temporal dynamics.

Stockwell *et al.* (1965) identifies aspect as imperfective or perfective depending on whether we conceptualize an event in terms of the course of its occurrence (imperfective) or its termination (perfective). Perfective forms in Spanish are necessarily past tense, and imperfective forms can be either past or non-past. The Real Academia Española (REA) (1985) calls perfect tenses the *pretérito perfecto simple* (*tomé* 'I drank') and all the compound tenses, such as *pretérito perfecto compuesto* and *pretérito pluscuamperfecto* (*he tomado* 'I have drunk'; *había tomado* 'I had drunk'), as the past participle (*tomado* 'drunk') gives the auxiliary a perfective meaning. In contrast, excluding the *pretérito perfecto simple* (*tomé* 'drank'), REA identifies as imperfect tenses all of the simple tenses: *presente* (*tomo* 'I drink'), *pretérito imperfecto* (*tomaba* 'I was drinking'), *futuro* (*tomaré* 'I will drink'), and *condicional* (*tomaría* 'I would drink') in the indicative mood; and *presente* (*tome*), *pretérito imperfecto* (*tomara, tomase*), and *futuro* (*tomare*) in the subjunctive.

Verb forms have different frequency of use in spoken Spanish. Sociolinguistic discourse studies support that verb tenses in the indicative mood are the most frequently used in conversational Spanish. Those tenses are the *presente* and *pretérito perfecto simple*, the most frequently used tenses, followed by the *pretérito imperfecto*, *condicional*, *pretérito perfecto compuesto*, and *pretérito pluscuamperfecto* (Centeno, 1996; Centeno & Obler, 2001; Silva-Corvalán, 1983). Regarding the future tense, although it figures prominently in conversational discourse, its periphrastic form (*ir a* 'to be going to + infinitive', *voy a comer* 'I'm going to eat') is more frequently employed than its inflected form (*comeré* 'I will eat') (Centeno, 1996; Schnitzer, 1989). Table 1.5 illustrates the inflectional features of the Spanish verb system, as exemplified by the verb forms used in conversational Spanish.

The Spanish verb system does not have a different morphological marker to indicate aspect, as do Greek, Russian, and Arabic (Marcos-Marín, 1975). The only exception in which the perfective–imperfective aspectual opposition is morphologically distinguished in Spanish, independent of sentential or discourse context, is in the *pretérito perfecto simple* (*tomé* 'I drank') and the *pretérito imperfecto* (*tomaba café cuando él llegó* 'I was drinking coffee when he arrived'). Otherwise, tense, mood, and aspect meanings in Spanish coalesce at the morphological level (Morpheme I in the above paradigm) thus being identified as

Table 1.5 Examples of verb conjugations in the indicative mood for the most frequently used verb tenses in spoken discourse (adapted from Centeno, 1996)

	Conjugational class					
	-ar *Tomar* (to drink)		*-er* *Comer* (to eat)		*-ir* *Subir* (to move up)	
Simple tenses						
Presente[a]						
Yo/I	TOM	o	COM	o	SUB	o
Tú/you		as		es		es
El/he Ella/she		a		e		e
Nosotros(as)/we		amos		emos		imos
Ustedes/you		an		en		en
Ellos(as)/they		an		en		en
Example:	Yo tomo agua todos los dias/I drink water everyday					
Pretérito perfecto simple						
Yo/I	TOM	é	COM	í	SUB	í
Tú/you		aste		iste		iste

(Continued)

Table 1.5 (*Continued*)

	TOM		COM	SUB
El/he Ella/she	ó		ió	ió
Nos./we	amos		imos	imos
Ustedes/you	aron		ieron	ieron
Ellos(as)/they	aron		ieron	ieron

Example: Yo tomé mucha agua ayer/I drank a lot of water yesterday

Pretérito imperfecto	TOM	COM	SUB
Yo/I	aba	ía	ía
Tú/you	abas	ías	ías
El/he Ella/she	aba	ía	ía
Nos./we	ábamos	íamos	íamos
Ustedes/you	aban	ían	ían
Ellos(as)/they	aban	ían	ían

Example: Yo tomaba agua cuando ella llegó/I was drinking water when she arrived

(Continued)

Table 1.5 (Continued)

		Conjugational class				
		-ar		-er		-ir
		Tomar (to drink)		Comer (to eat)		Subir (to move up)
Condicional	Yo/I	TOM	aría	COM	ería	SUB	iría
	Tú/you		arías		erías		irías
	El/he Ella/she		aría		ería		iría
	Nos./we		aríamos		eríamos		iríamos
	Ustedes/you		arían		erían		irían
	Ellos(as)/they		arían		erían		irían
Example:	Yo tomaría agua si estuviera fría/I would drink water if it were cold						
Compound tenses							
Pretérito perfecto compuesto	Yo/I	he	tomado	comido	subido		
	Tú/you	has	"	"	"		

(Continued)

Table 1.5 (*Continued*)

		tomado	comido	subido
El/he Ella/she	ha	"	"	"
Nos./we	hemos	"	"	"
Ustedes/you	han	"	"	"
Ellos(as)/they	han	"	"	"
Example:	Yo he tomado mucha agua hoy/I have drunk a lot of water today			
Pretérito pluscuamperfecto	Yo/I	había	tomado	comido	subido
	Tú/you	habías	"	"	"
	El/he Ella/she	había	"	"	"
	Nos./we	habíamos	"	"	"
	Ustedes/you	habían	"	"	"
	Ellos(as)/they	habían	"	"	"
Example:	Yo había tomado agua antes que ella llegara/I had drunk water before she arrived			

[a]Tenses have been labeled using the terminology of the Real Academia Española (1985)

tense-mood-aspect (TMA) notions, or, more often, as tense-aspect when referring to the temporal characteristics of a particular verb in a sentence.

Spanish verbs also encode agreement information relating the verb form to the executor of the action and its number (Morpheme II above) to a greater degree than do English verbs. Spanish verbs can express first, second, or third person for each singular (*yo* 'I', *tú* 'you', *él* 'he', *ella* 'she') or plural (*nosotros* [masculine]/*nosotras* [feminine] 'we', *ustedes* 'you', *ellos* [masculine]/*ellas* [feminine] 'they').

Other features of the Spanish verb phrase include auxiliaries and copulas. Like English, Spanish has an auxiliary system. Three main verbs occur as auxiliaries in Spanish. They are *haber* 'to have', *estar* 'to be', and *andar* 'to walk' (Anderson, 1995). Unlike Standard English, which uses one verb as copula, 'to be', Spanish employs two: *ser* and *estar*. Although both Spanish verbs are attributive, they have different semantic and syntactic functions. In general, *ser* refers to a constant condition (*ella es alta* 'she is tall'). *Estar* conveys attributes that are not permanent or fixed (*el perro está dormido* 'the dog is asleep') and can precede the present participle to form present progressive structures (*ella está hablando* 'she is speaking') (see Anderson, 1995; Marcos-Marín, 1975, for further discussion).

A final point concerns the classification of Spanish verbs. Spanish verb forms can be divided in two ways: by theme (thematic vowel) and by the extent to which their inflectional affixes can be predicted by general rules (Stockwell *et al.*, 1965). Classification in terms of thematic vowel inflectional endings was discussed above. Regarding inflectional predictability, verbs can be grouped as regular and irregular verbs, as in English. Regular verbs conform to most of the general rules of stem formation and affixation. Irregular verbs fall into two categories: stem irregularities and stem-affix irregularities. Stem-changing verbs, the largest group of irregular verbs in Spanish, have more than one stem form (*contar* [infinitive] 'to count': stem 1 *cuent-*, *cuento* 'I count', stem 2 *cont-*, *contamos* 'we counted'). Stem-affix irregular verbs are much smaller in number but much more frequently used in Spanish than their regular counterparts (e.g. *ser* 'to be', *estar* 'to be', *haber* 'to have', *ir* 'to go', etc.). In addition to variant stems, these verbs also have irregularities in their inflectional patterns involving changes in the theme vowel as well as aspect-tense and person-aspect markers (e.g. *ser- soy* 'I am', *eres* 'you are', *es* 'he is', etc.) (Stockwell *et al.*, 1965).

Pronoun case marking

The Spanish pronominal system is considerably more inflected than that of English. In general, Spanish pronouns can be grouped into two major categories: stressed and unstressed (Bedore, 1999). The stressed group includes subject, possessive, and prepositional pronouns. The unstressed group encompasses object (reflexive and nonreflexive) pronouns. Table 1.6 summarizes the Spanish pronominal system.

Subject pronouns often are dropped from utterances because both sentential context and the highly inflected Spanish verb forms provide sufficient information to retrieve the subject of the sentence. For this reason, Spanish is called a *pro-drop language* (see Harley, 2001, for a discussion). Yet, subject pronouns can be used to convey emphasis about who the subject of the sentence is (e.g. *ella me dió el regalo* 'she [nobody else] gave me the present') (Anderson, 1995).

Possessive pronouns and prepositional pronouns are among the possessive structures used in Spanish. Possessive pronouns are post-verbal and agree with the item that is possessed in gender and number (e.g. *el carro es mío* 'the car is mine', *las pelotas son tuyas* 'the balls are yours'). Prepositional pronouns agree with the possessor in gender and number (e.g. *los juguetes de ellos(as)* 'The toys of theirs'). Other constructions, involving possessive adjectives (e.g. *mi casa* 'my house'), are also employed in Spanish to express possession.

Unstressed pronouns, that is, object reflexive and nonreflexive groups, are considered *clitics* because they always occur next to the verb (Anderson, 1995; Bedore, 1999). They are preclitic when they are used before the verb in finite or negative imperative verbal forms (e.g. *lo corté* 'I cut it', *me corté* 'I cut myself', *¡no lo cortes!* 'don't cut it!'). They are enclitic if they are used after infinitives, present participle, or imperatives (e.g. *tenemos que ponerlo* 'we have to put it', *estamos poniéndolo* 'we are putting it', *¡pónlo!* 'put it!', respectively) (refer to Anderson, 1995; Bedore, 1999; Solé & Solé, 1977, for further discussion).

Syntax

In this section, several characteristics of Spanish syntax will be described, particularly word order structure and its variability, and structural aspects of wh- questions, negative formation, and use of complex sentences. Those features that are deemed most salient and pertinent for the purposes of this book will be presented.

Use of subject forms

A salient characteristic of Spanish is that sentences can be realized without an overt subject. Because Spanish is uniformly inflected, that is, all verb forms must be inflected, it permits omission of the subject (Lakshmanan, 1995). Indeed, as mentioned above, as a pro-drop language, the subject in a Spanish sentence can be inferred from the discourse context as well as from verbal inflection. In contrast, in English, the use of subjects is obligatory; sentences without overt subjects are considered ungrammatical. English, unlike Spanish, is not uniformly

Table 1.6 The Spanish pronominal system (adapted from Anderson, 1995; Bedore, 1999)

Person		Stressed			Unstressed	
	Subject	Possessive	Prepositional	Object nonreflexive	Object reflexive
Singular 1	yo	mío(a)	mí	me	me
2	tú usted	tuyo(a) suyo(a)	tí sí	te se/le/lo/la	te se
3	él/ella	suyo(a)	él/ella	le/lo/la	se
Plural 1	nosotros (as)	nuestro(a)	nuestros(as)	nos	nos
2	ustedes	suyo(a)	ustedes	les/los/las	se
3	ellos(as)	suyo(a)	ellos(as)	les/los/las	se

inflected; that is, verb forms occur with as well as without inflection (e.g. runs versus run). The following examples (ex. 1–4) illustrate sentences with and without overt subjects:

(1) *Los niños tienen hambre.*
The children are hungry.
(2) *Tienen hambre.*
[They] are hungry.
(3) *Yo no quiero cantar.*
I don't want to sing.
(4) *No quiero cantar.*
[I] don't want to sing.

Noun phrase word order

The default word order in Spanish for NPs is DET + NOUN + ADJECTIVE (e.g. *la casa bonita* [the house pretty] 'the pretty house') (Anderson, 1995). Most adjectives are thus placed after the noun. There are some instances where the modifier must precede the noun in Spanish. These include the use of a numeral (e.g. *tres gatos* 'three cats'), the use of attributive terms (e.g. *un gran violinista* 'a great violinist'; *un buen lector* 'a good reader'), and the use of ordinal numbers or adjectives (e.g. *el último pedazo* 'the last piece'; *la primera mujer* 'the first woman').

Sentence word order

Like English, Spanish is described as a subject-verb-object (SVO) language. Unlike English, Spanish word order is more flexible; the subject, object and verb constituents can occur in different positions within the sentence (Mackenzie, 2001). Usually, a constituent order that differs from the default SVO is used within discourse for pragmatic purposes, as, for example, to focus on a particular part of the sentence (Bedore, 1999; Qüilis & Hernández Alonso, 1990). Some examples (ex. 5–8) are shown below using the target SVO sentence *La niña tiene una trenza* 'The girl has a braid':

(5) *Tiene la niña una trenza.* (VSO)
Has the girl a braid.
(6) *Tiene una trenza la niña.* (VOS)
Has a braid the girl.
(7) *Una trenza tiene la niña.* (OVS)
A braid has the girl.
(8) *La niña una trenza tiene.* (SOV)
The girl a braid has.

In English the distinctions made in these sentences would more likely be made by adding additional stress to the focus-word without changing word order.

Question formation/movement

In most Spanish dialects, subject–verb inversion in wh- questions is obligatory. This is specifically the case where the wh- word is not part of a constituent that plays the role of adverb (Mackenzie, 2001). For example, in the interrogative sentence *¿Cuántos años tiene Elena?* [How many years has Elena?] 'How old is Elena?', subject–verb inversion is obligatory. On the other hand, in an interrogative sentence such as *¿Cómo pudo entrar el niño?* 'How was the boy able to enter?', it is acceptable to not invert the subject and verb, realizing that sentence as *¿Cómo el niño pudo entrar?*. In terms of subject placement when there is an auxiliary verb, the subject can follow either the finite verb form or auxiliary, or it can follow the verb phrase. The only exception occurs with the auxiliary verb *haber* 'to have', where the subject must always follow the verb phrase. Some examples (ex. 9–12) are provided next:

(9) *¿Dónde está comiendo la niña?*
Where is eating the girl?/Where is the girl eating?
(10) *¿Dónde está la niña comiendo?*
Where is the girl eating?
(11) *¿Qué ha hecho Juan?*
What has done Juan?/What has Juan done?
(12) **¿Qué ha Juan hecho?*
What has Juan done?

In some Spanish dialects, in particular those spoken in the Caribbean, there are instances where subject–verb inversion in wh- questions is not obligatory (Pérez-Leroux, 1990). In fact, it is usually the case that speakers typically do not invert the subject and verb, especially in sentences with second person reference. Specifically, if the subject is realized as a pronoun, the interrogative sentence does not require that the subject and verb be inverted. Some examples (ex. 13–15) follow:

(13) *¿Qué tú haces?*
What you do?/What do you do?
(14) *¿Dónde él está?*
Where he is?/Where is he?
(15) *¿Cómo ellos lo hacen?*
How they it do?/How do they do it?

Yes–no interrogative sentences are more flexible with respect to the order of the sentence constituents (Mackenzie, 2001). Subject–verb inversion is not required in these sentences, as intonational cues indicate their interrogative nature. Thus, yes–no interrogative sentences can be produced in the following ways: by raising intonation (e.g. *¿Juan está durmiendo?* 'Juan is sleeping?'), by using subject–verb inversion (e.g. *¿Está durmiendo Juan?* 'Is sleeping Juan?'), and by placing the subject after the auxiliary (e.g. *¿Está Juan durmiendo?* 'Is Juan sleeping?'). As with wh-questions, with compound verb forms that contain the auxiliary verb *haber*, the subject cannot be inserted after the auxiliary. For example, the sentence *¿Ha Juan terminado la tarea?* 'Has Juan finished the task?' is ungrammatical.

Negative sentences

Compared to English, Spanish negative sentence construction is structurally simple (Anderson, 1995). It does not require the use of an auxiliary form like 'do' in English. The negative adverb is placed before the inflected verb, as shown below (ex. 16, 17):

(16) *No sabe qué hacer.*
[S/he] not know what to do/[S/he] does not know what to do
(17) *Nunca se sabrá la verdad.*
Never will know the truth/The truth will never be known.

Spanish, like many vernacular dialects of English, permits the use of double negatives. In fact, in certain contexts, these are obligatory. Specifically, when a negative word follows the inflected verb, the negative form *no* must precede the verb. For example, the sentence 'I have done nothing' would be produced in Spanish as *yo no he hecho nada* 'I have [not] done nothing.'

In summary, this chapter has discussed features of Spanish phonology, morphology, and syntax that can be useful for cross-linguistic analysis and interpretation of communication profiles in monolingual and bilingual Spanish speakers, particularly of Latin American origin, in the USA. Specifically, interlanguage analysis would highlight both linguistic similarities and differences with an impact on language processing and, in turn, on preferential errors or differences in vulnerability to dissolution across syntactic constructions produced by the speakers. Further, as mentioned earlier, cross-linguistic data would facilitate the assessment of English-based theoretical accounts as suitable explanations of communication performance in typical and disordered speakers of other languages (Leonard, 1996; Paradis, 2001; see Anderson, Ch. 6, this volume).

For example, understanding Spanish phonological features is crucial in bilingual Spanish–English contexts. Spanish–English bilinguals may treat [d] and [ð] like allophones as in Spanish, thus pronouncing *day* and *they* in the same manner. Likewise, they may use Spanish syllabic structure in English, for example, saying [ˌɛsˈkul] and [ˌɛsˈlip] (Yavaş, 1998). Such episodes of interlanguage phonology, rather than being a disorder, represent transfer speech patterns reflecting the bilingual Spanish–English person's late acquisition of English (see Bell-Berti, ch. 20, and Centeno, ch. 3, this volume). Similarly, regarding morphosyntactic patterns, bilingual Spanish–English speakers may use Spanish structures in English, as in *the house green* 'the green house' or *she no sing* 'she doesn't sing.' In monolingual disordered situations, cross-linguistic comparisons of morphosyntactic limitations in Spanish- or English-speaking Broca's aphasic individuals have provided interesting clinical profiles with theoretical implications. Although the typically restricted verb use of Broca's aphasia is present in both language groups, error profiles are more morphologically complex in Spanish than in English, a reflection of the richer verb inflectional system in the former language. These observations have additionally been useful to make theoretical distinctions between Spanish and English speakers with Broca's aphasia (e.g. Centeno & Obler, 2001).

It is hoped that the descriptive overview presented here enhances the understanding of the Spanish language by both speech-language investigators and practitioners and stimulates their theoretical and clinical application of the presented information. Such efforts would contribute to the continuation and refinement of research on Spanish speakers and, in turn, the enhancement of clinical practice with this population.

References

Alarcos Llorach, E. (1999) *Gramática de la Lengua Española*. Madrid: Espasa.
Anderson, R.T. (1995) Spanish morphological and syntactic development. In H. Kayser (ed.) *Bilingual Speech-language Pathology: An Hispanic Focus* (pp. 41–74). San Diego, CA: Singular.
Bedore, L.M. (1999) The acquisition of Spanish. In O.L. Taylor and L.B. Leonard (eds) *Language Acquisition Across North America* (pp. 157–208). San Diego, CA: Singular.
Canfield, D.L. (1981) *Spanish Pronunciation in the Americas*. Chicago, IL: University of Chicago Press.
Centeno, J.G. (1996) Use of verb inflections in the oral expression of agrammatic Spanish-speaking aphasics. Unpublished doctoral dissertation, City University of New York.
Centeno, J.G. and Obler, L.K. (2001) Agrammatic verb errors in Spanish speakers and their normal discourse correlates. *Journal of Neurolinguistics* 14, 349–363.
Comrie, B. (1976) *Aspect*. Cambridge: University of Cambridge Press.
Gili-Gaya, S. (1981) *Resúmen Práctico de Gramática Española*. Barcelona: Biblograf.
Harley, T. (2001) *The Psychology of Language: From Data to Theory* (2nd edn). East Sussex, UK: Psychology Press.
Lakshmanan, U. (1995) Child second language acquisition of syntax. *Studies in Second Language Acquisition* 17, 301–329.
Leonard, L.B. (1996) Assessing morphosyntax in clinical settings. In D. McDaniel, C. McKee and H.S. Cairns (eds) *Methods for Assessing Children's Syntax* (pp. 287–302). London: MIT Press.
Mackenzie, I. (2001) *A Linguistic Introduction to Spanish*. Muenchen, Germany: Lincom Europa.

Marcos-Marín, F. (1975) *Aproximación a la Gramática Española*. Madrid: Cincel.

Navarro Tomás, T. (1974) *El Español en Puerto Rico*. Río Piedras, PR: Editorial Universitaria.

Ortega-Llebaria, M. (2004) Interplay between phonetic and inventory constraints in the degree of spirantization of voiced stops: Comparing intervocalic /b/ and intervocalic /g/ in Spanish and English. In T.L. Face (ed.) *Laboratory Approaches to Spanish Phonology* (pp. 237–254). New York: Mouton de Gruyter.

Paradis, M. (2001) By way of a preface: The need for awareness of aphasia symptoms in different languages. In M. Paradis (ed.) *Manifestations of Aphasia Symptoms in Different Languages* (pp. 1–7). Amsterdam: Elsevier

Parker, F. and Riley, K. (2000) *Linguistics for Non-linguists: A Primer with Exercises* (3rd edn). Boston: Allyn and Bacon.

Pérez-Leroux, A.T. (1990) The acquisition of wh- movement in Caribbean Spanish. In T.L. Mahfield and B. Plunkett (eds) *Papers in the Acquisition of Wh-questions: Proceedings of the University of Massachusetts Roundtable* (pp. 79–99). Amherst, MA: GLSA Publications.

Qüilis, A. and Fernández, J.A. (1985) *Curso de Fonética y Fonología Españolas para Estudiantes Angloamericanos*. Madrid: Consejo Superior de Investigaciones Científicas.

Qüilis, A. and Hernández Alonso, C. (1990) *Lingüística Española Aplicada a la Terapia del Lenguaje*. Madrid: Gredos.

Real Academia Española (1985) *Esbozo de una Nueva Gramática de la Lengua Española*. Madrid: Espasa-Calpe.

Schnitzer. M.L. (1989) *The Pragmatic Basis of Aphasia*. Hillsdale, NJ: Lawrence Erlbaum.

Schnitzer, M.L. (1993) Steady as a rock: Does the steady state represent cognitive fossilization? *Journal of Psycholinguistic Research* 22, 1–20.

Silva-Corvalán, C. (1983) Tense and aspect in oral Spanish narrative. *Language* 59, 760–780.

Solé, Y. and Solé, C. (1977) *Modern Spanish Syntax: A Study in Contrasts*. Lexington, MA: Heath.

Stockwell, R.P., Bowen, J.D. and Martin, J.W. (1965) *The Grammatical Structures of English and Spanish*. Chicago: University of Chicago.

Tserdanelis, G. and Wong, W.Y.P. (eds) (2004) *Language Files: Materials for an Introduction to Language and Linguistics* (9th edn). Columbus: Ohio University Press.

Yavaş, M. (1998) *Phonology: Development and Disorders*. San Diego, CA: Singular.

Zentella, A.C. (1997) Spanish in New York. In O. García and J. Fishman (eds) *The Multilingual Apple: Languages in New York City*. Berlin: Mouton de Gruyter.

Chapter 2

English Language Learners: Literacy and Biliteracy Considerations

HORTENCIA KAYSER and JOSÉ G. CENTENO

There are multiple variables that will influence literacy achievement in children. For example, language socialization practices, printed-language experiences, socioeconomic circumstances, and academic language uses have been identified. The home and parents' contributions to educational success similarly are critical (Cobo-Lewis *et al.*, 2002; Wallach & Butler, 1994). But it is the child who is faced with the formidable challenge of meeting school standards. For bilingual students, also described as *limited English proficient* (LEP) or *English language learners* (ELLs) to identify their considerable difficulty in all or some of the linguistic modalities in English (Centeno & Eng, 2005; García, 1999; Gonzalez *et al.*, 1997), this challenge is compounded by the process of learning literacy skills in two print systems, one for the first language (L1) and the other for the second language (L2), in a bilingual communication environment.

Addressing all of the issues and theoretical discussions reported on literacy development in bilingual contexts is beyond the scope of this chapter. The purpose of this chapter is to provide an overview of the issues related to the development of literacy in bilingual students, henceforth operationally identified as ELLs, in the US context. The focus is on ethnographic and sociolinguistic factors impacting literacy acquisition in Hispanic children. Although some cognitive, linguistic, and psycholinguistic phenomena will be addressed, the reader is referred to a more in-depth treatment of these issues in both monolingual Spanish and bilingual Spanish–English readers/writers presented elsewhere in this book (i.e. Ijalba & Obler, ch. 18; Iribarren, ch. 17; Ostrosky-Solís *et al.*, ch. 19, Weekes, ch. 7).

The chapter begins with a brief description of ELLs in the USA, focusing on Hispanic children. Next, an overview of literacy prerequisites, especially cognitive, linguistic, and sociocultural variables and their interactions, for literacy acquisition in monolingual and bilingual contexts will follow. In conclusion, clinical and educational implications will be addressed, giving particular attention to home environment, academic policies and approaches, and family engagement in literacy programs with ELLs.

English Language Learners in the USA: Educational and Ethnographic Realities

There were over 3.4 million children with limited English proficiency in elementary and secondary schools in the USA in 1997–2000 (US Census, 2000). Throughout the country, school systems have been attempting to meet the educational needs of these children in instructional environments that often involve limited resources and unrealistic expectations. Frequently, educational programs lack the materials, personnel, and administrative support for realistic implementation. Notably, more than one-fourth of newly hired teachers are put in a classroom without having completed their state's licensing requirements and only 5% of all teachers have more than 1 course in reading instruction. More than 2.2 million new teachers are needed. States across the country are responding by lowering standards for teachers (Children's Defense Fund, 2000). Administrators, educators, and clinical personnel may also have attitudinal responses to minority students that limit their fair management of the educational and clinical needs of these students (Kayser, 1998; Zentella, 2005). In addition, limited understanding of these students' sociocultural and linguistic realities compounds logistical challenges and biased attitudes from the educational staff. In fact, many teachers have no or minimal training in bilingualism or teaching bilingual students developing in minority contexts (García & Menken, 2006; Zentella, 2005).

Addressing the educational needs of ELLs in the USA, like other minority children in other countries, requires a broad, multidimensional analysis of their learning histories. Critical in this analysis is the home literacy and language environments. Without the realistic understanding of the foundational strengths already present in the student from home literacy experiences, some teachers may have unreceptive attitudes to parents' contributions to the education of their children. Teachers may believe that the absence of parent–child storybook reading is evidence that a child has been reared in a low-literate home and is, thus, at risk for reading difficulty (Dickinson & Tabors, 2002; Paratore et al., 2003). Teachers may think that parents who have low literacy and low English proficiency are uninterested in supporting their children's school success or that parents who are uneducated or have low English literacy lack effective parenting skills (Paratore et al., 2003; also see Zentella, 2005).

Families vary in their literacy/language backgrounds and their expectations. Parents may have been educated in their native language but do not have the same sociocultural practices of book reading that is assumed for mainstream American families (also see Restrepo & Castilla, ch. 10, for related discussion on discourse socialization and research implications). Children may possibly enter public schools with diverse language backgrounds, ages, and experiences with schooling in their native country. The roles and expectations for children in their own cultures, whether raised in their native lands or in the USA, determine the extent of their language development and literacy experiences that they bring to American clinical and educational settings (Centeno & Eng, 2005; Damico *et al.*, 2005; Harris, 2003). For example, in Mexico, children are expected to complete the 6th year of school, but may not be expected to go further unless the parents have financial resources for the children to continue a high school education. In the bilingual environment of the USA, some homes may have written materials in the native or first language through newspapers, magazines, Bibles, and information materials (i.e. brochures, pamphlets, and so forth). Family members more capable in L2 also participate in literacy socialization practices by exposing less-fluent L2 speakers to reading materials by helping them decode problem spelling patterns and words (see Zentella, 2005).

Another important aspect is that ELLs in the USA are a highly heterogeneous group. As exemplified by Latino students, there is considerable linguistic, social, cultural, and socioeconomic diversity in Hispanic students, a reflection of the unique experiences of each of their families (see Introduction of this volume for further discussion on demographic characteristics in US Hispanics). Such varying experiential trajectories have direct impact on how each Latino student handles academic language requirements (see García & Menken, 2006). Very importantly, bilingual and dialectal differences, due to contrasting degrees of Spanish–English bilingualism and the use of different Spanish dialects in their living environments, are manifested in these students' written and spoken language (Zentella, 1997). This inequality between the language students know and the language used in high-stake testing has dramatic repercussions on the students' lives, particularly because a low score in these tests would translate into inappropriate program placement, delayed grade promotion, and later graduation (García & Menken, 2006).

Socioeconomic environments similarly warrant attention as they critically shape learning opportunities in which ELLs develop. Poverty exists in many homes and communities where these children live. Their learning and educational opportunities tend to be different from those in children from a mainstream culture (Centeno & Eng, 2005). As mentioned earlier, there is a lack of school resources for many children who live in impoverished regions, that is, schools may not have the necessary materials for teaching and learning (Paratore *et al.*, 2003; Pew Hispanic Center, 2002; US Census Bureau, 2000).

Hence, the complexities involved in educating ELLs warrant innovative, ecologically sound approaches grounded in the comprehensive knowledge of students' life experiences. Without these understandings, as it happens in many of the present academic settings, the foundation of education, literacy, is often presented to these children in poorly equipped instructional settings in English, a language that many of them do not know, have minimal skills in, or have not developed well, by a teaching staff that may have unfair expectations and/or limited training to educate bilingual students from minority environments. The result and reality for many Hispanic children is that there is a high dropout rate (e.g. Cubans have the lowest while Mexican students have the highest) (see García & Menken, 2006).

Literacy

Although children are expected to effectively learn to read and write without difficulty when provided with the necessary experiential and academic opportunities to meet literacy expectations of their cultural group, a large number of them experience difficulties. Lyon (1998) states that 5% of children learn to read effortlessly. He further states that research literature suggests that another 20–30% of children learn to read relatively easily once exposed to formal instruction, with any instructional emphasis. Unfortunately, he reports that about 60% of children have much more formidable challenges and, from this group, 20–30% will consider reading to be the most difficult task in their schooling.

Successful literacy development may not occur without appropriate social and academic support and intact personal linguistic/cognitive abilities in the literacy learners. How children manage to negotiate and develop cognitive and linguistic prerequisites for (bi)literacy has been examined from different perspectives. While psychology and linguistics have provided important descriptions on the linguistic–cognitive interactions in literacy development (e.g. Bialystok, 2001; Durgunoğlu, 1997), applied linguistics, sociolinguistics, and education have contributed with linguistic and contextual aspects, such as the role of cultural experiences, settings, and language functions in literacy skills (e.g. Damico *et al.*, 2005; Zentella, 2005). Next, a survey of some of these aspects will be briefly discussed as they apply to monolingual and bilingual literacy skills.

Literacy prerequisites: Cognitive, linguistic, and cultural considerations

Understanding literacy development requires the analysis of print experiences, their concomitant linguistic and cognitive operations, and the sociocultural environment shaping those experiences and operations (Bialystok, 2001; Damico *et al.*, 2005; Durgunoğlu, 1997; Kamhi & Catts,

2005; Wallach & Butler, 1994). Literacy home environments provide children with their initial encounters with print and prepare them for later literacy experiences in school. Print socialization routines vary from home to home. Broadly speaking, while in low-print contexts children minimally experience early graphic (letters/graphemes)–auditory (sounds/phonemes) associations preliminary to literacy, in high-print situations, children are socialized to learn about sound–letter associations and the functions of print through multiple activities and literate artifacts, such as crayons for 'writing letters', rhyming games, and joint book reading with their caregivers (Wallach & Butler, 1994; also see Neuman & Dickinson, 2002). In fact, an area of literacy development that has received considerable attention is the relationship of phonological awareness to literacy development. That is, early experiences recognizing and manipulating sounds before learning to read provide an initial foundation for later literacy learning (Bialystok, 2001; Durgunoğlu *et al.*, 1993; Tabors & Snow, 2002). There is compelling evidence that a child's ability to discriminate, segment, and blend phonemes may be an important psycholinguistic prerequisite for instruction and acquisition of reading (see Meschyan & Hernández, 2004, for a review). Yet, the relationships between phonology and literacy in the processing of an alphabetic script seem to be complex and reciprocal, rather than unidirectional (see Swank & Larrivee, 1998, for a review).

Because differences in high–low print stimulation are culturally determined, home literacy scenarios require individual attention. Each home exposes a child to literacy in unique ways that ultimately are reflected in each child's literacy gains. The cultural ways that students use language and literacy at home and in their communities (i.e. child–caregiver dyadic collaborations as in joint book reading, functions of literacy [e.g. informational, instructive, leisure, etc.]) are represented in the extent of print awareness and related linguistic–cognitive interactions individually brought by each student to school (see Damico *et al.*, 2005; Wallach & Butler, 1994; Zentella, 2005). Further, as oral-literate language domains are in continuous reciprocity throughout an individual's life (Wallach & Butler, 1994), understanding the overall language performance in each individual student must involve a broad and comprehensive analysis of his/her linguistic history and the cultural scenarios that shaped it (see Harris, 2003). With bilingual students, as will be discussed later, that analysis would require the examination of contexts, modalities, and functions for L1 and L2 use since birth (Centeno & Eng, 2005).

Formal instruction should continue the developmental progression in the growth of literacy skills started in the home. Effective literacy experiences in school should be designed to promote a child's acquisition of both lower- and higher-level linguistic and cognitive processes required for successful print management (see Durgunoğlu, 1997; Kamhi & Catts, 2005). Lower-level processes involve letter recognition, grapheme–phoneme associations, word recognition, and lexical access; and higher-level components relate to concept activation (word meaning), syntactic analysis, sentence comprehension, and intersentential text integration (Durgunoğlu, 1997; Kamhi & Catts, 2005). Further, beyond the cognitive skills (e.g. attention, discrimination, and integration) called upon to process language at such low and high levels of literacy demands, cognition additionally participates in literacy tasks in the form of the socioculturally mediated representational knowledge that each individual develops through experiential learning in his/her life environments and applies to reading and writing activities. Prior cognitive schemata (mental representations) and their storage strength in memory, as well as accompanying language (i.e. topics, vocabulary, discourse routines, and so forth), are important aspects in reading comprehension, story development in writing, and overall language use (Blachowicz, 1994; Wallach & Butler, 1994). Thus, meaning-making demands and language requirements in literacy tasks are tightly linked to their developmental culturally contextualized experiences (Bialystok, 2001; Damico *et al.*, 2005; Harris, 2003).

Biliteracy: Negotiating the acquisition of two print systems

The preceding linguistic, cognitive, and sociocultural factors in monolingual literacy learning similarly apply to bilingual speakers. Yet, bilingual learners face two major challenges as they acquire literacy skills. First, they have to face two print systems, one for L1 and the other for L2, and second, they do not generally use both systems to the same extent, in the same contexts, or for the same purposes in their daily bilingual routines.

Regarding the first challenge, although Spanish and English employ alphabetic scripts in written language (i.e. single letters and letter combinations [graphemes] correspond to sounds [phonemes]), Spanish involves a regular (transparent) orthography whereas that of English is irregular (opaque) (see Ijalba & Obler, 18; Iribarren, ch. 17; Weekes, ch. 7, this volume for pertinent discussion). In terms of the second difficulty faced by bilingual readers/writers, it is well recognized that bilingual speakers generally tend to use their two languages in contrasting ways, involving different contexts, modalities, and linguistic skills, which, in turn, impose different cognitive demands. Bialystok (2001) suggests bilingual speakers' language use could be viewed as a continuum of three domains, namely, oral, literate, and metalinguistic, involving increasing levels of cognitive complexity unique to the communication scenarios of each language (see Centeno, ch. 3, this volume for further discussion).

Durgunoğlu's (1997) discussion on the development of bilingual reading provides a useful approach to summarize the above challenges faced by bilingual learners when they have considerable linguistic competence in L1. To Durgunoğlu, the development of reading skills in L2 is closely tied to the extent of linguistic knowledge in L1. Acquisition of L2 literacy, according to Durgunoğlu, depends on cross-language transfer involving prior linguistic, literate, and conceptual knowledge the learner has in L1 that can enhance analysis and acquisition in L2. In broad terms, linguistic knowledge refers to the learner's skills and strategies to process syntactic, morphological, lexical, and metalinguistic tasks in L1 that can be applied to similar linguistic areas in L2. Literacy variables basically involve meaning-making strategies employed to understand decontextualized L1 uses (i.e. language free of cues, such as facial expressions, pictures, or any other physical aspect that would enhance meaning) as in written texts that prepare the bilingual learner for reading comprehension in L2.

Finally, prior conceptual knowledge pertains to topic awareness in order to understand a reading. Durgunoğlu suggests that this area may impose difficulties on the bilingual person due to a cultural mismatch because, when reading in L2, the bilingual person may not have the background cultural knowledge and assumptions taken for granted by the writer of the text. Indeed, constructing text meaning, whether to develop a story in writing or to understand a story in spoken or written texts, calls upon an individual's world knowledge (i.e. specific content domains – history, mathematics, procedural information [how to milk a cow, fix a car, etc.] – and interpersonal norms-relationships, values, etc.) (Kamhi & Catts, 2005).

There is considerable evidence suggesting that linguistic and literate abilities in the native language transfer to and enhance L2 learning. In particular, phonological awareness, as mentioned earlier, an important predictor of literacy skills in monolingual learners, similarly facilitates bilingual literacy acquisition. For example, Meschyan and Hernández (2004) found that good phonological–orthographic ability in L1 enhanced linguistic gains in L2 (i.e. vocabulary and test results in L2). Similarly, Durgunoğlu *et al.* (1993) suggested that building children's phonological awareness in the first language would transfer and help improve the child's reading ability in English. The best predictors of literacy development in both Spanish and English for native Spanish-speaking children were their phonological awareness and word-recognition skills in Spanish. However, as mentioned earlier, there is evidence that phonology–literacy interactions may be very complex and reciprocal rather than unidirectional, as shown by monolingual data (see Swank & Larrivee, 1998).

Despite the evidence supporting cross-linguistic transfer, some studies have highlighted certain areas hindering this process. For example, MacWhinney (1997) points out that, in the initial stages of L2 development, syntactic interpretation strategies in L1 bias the bilingual learner's processing of L2 syntactic patterns (i.e. word order). This phenomenon, however, gradually changes over time when the learner gains competence in L2 and changes interpretive settings in the direction of the native L2 users' settings. Other factors, such as phonological differences between the two languages, may impose problems on the acquisition of biliteracy skills (e.g. see Gonzales & García, 1995; Gorman & Gillam, 2004; Ijalba & Obler, ch. 18, this volume, for phonological issues in Spanish–English biliteracy). All in all, the preceding evidence suggests that understanding the development of bilingual reading must acknowledge the role of facilitating and nonfacilitating cross-linguistic phenomena, the complex inter-relationships between phonology and literacy operations, and the effect of proficiency in each language.

The process of biliteracy acquisition similarly needs to be interpreted within the sociocultural and ethnographic scenarios in which ELLs live, described earlier. Cognitive and linguistic phenomena in literacy acquisition are embedded in the social, political, educational, and personal factors that define the student's environment in which learning takes place (Bialystok, 2001; Kaufman, 1998). The interplay of external conditions, such as the quantity and quality of the teaching approaches used in school and L1 support in the curriculum and school at large, and more internal and personal phenomena, such as learning opportunities provided at home and the student's attitude to each language, has direct consequences on the development and maintenance of literacy skills in both languages.

Clinical and Educational Implications

The multiple factors and complexities involved in literacy development in bilingual children impose challenges on clinical interventionists and educators, as predicated earlier in this chapter. The demands imposed by developmental processes additionally interact with the management confines brought upon practitioners by official guidelines. For example, in the USA, the No Child Left Behind (NCLB) legislation, a reauthorization of the *Elementary and Secondary Education Act* (ESEA) of 1965, makes schools accountable for student performance and teacher quality. It also enhances fairness and inclusiveness in American education (US Department of Education, 2006). Despite its potential benefits, the NCLB has made literacy development and academic achievement a challenge for school administrators, teachers, parents, and children who are ELLs in the USA. Broadly speaking, the NCLB requires extensive coordination and availability of teaching resources (e.g. availability of qualified staff, appropriate teaching materials, close student monitoring) for schools to provide the most effective quality instruction that facilitate student performance and meet official expectations.

Snow *et al.* (1998) propose a plausible framework for literacy instruction that may be useful as a clinical and educational basis to address the literacy needs of ELLs. This approach predicts successful reading in young children by focusing on three important areas impacting literacy acquisition: child-based, school-based, and family-based factors. These factors include: value placed on literacy; emphasis on achievement; availability and use of reading materials; and parent–child book reading. Specifically, within the classroom and clinical setting, literacy may be stimulated through the use of varied materials that will develop from lower-level skills, such as word recognition and lexical access, to higher-level demands, such as syntactic analysis and narrative interpretation. Using a wide variety of reading materials from magazines, books, to pamphlets that children review, collect, write, and read about would provide important literacy experiences.

Snow *et al.*'s (1998) approach may be combined with principles of two-way immersion, or dual-language, teaching programs for enhanced learning in both languages. In fact, dual-language pedagogical approaches, in which both languages are valued as part of the curriculum and daily interactions, have been successful in facilitating comparable language and academic achievement in both languages in bilingual students (Oller & Eilers, 2002; Zecker, 2004). Similarly, some schools have developed innovative approaches to improve academic success in ELLs. For instance, based on the importance of supporting the student's culture and findings suggesting facilitating cross-linguistic transfer in language and literacy, several New York City schools have greatly improved performance in academic testing in Latino ELLs by increasing these students' opportunities to formally study Spanish (García & Menken, 2006).

Literacy instruction must similarly acknowledge the facilitating role of the home language environment (Brisk & Harrington, 2000). Family engagement, however, requires sensitive and realistic approaches. We cannot assume that all children who are ELLs come from homes that do not value literacy, have parents who do not want their children to achieve academically, do not have reading materials, and do not share book reading in the home. We can assume that families will be different, children will have different experiences with literacy, and that their experiences can be used to foster strengths to learning in school (see Zentella, 2005).

Finally, despite the use of systematic and well intended bilingual instructional philosophies, linguistic outcomes in bilingual students additionally depend on the linguistic influences from the community and the students' own personal attitudes to each of their languages. Oller and Eilers (2002) showed that, even though bilingual Spanish–English students in the Miami area exhibited gains in both languages after long-term two-way instruction, their performance in English tended to be better than in Spanish on all tested areas (i.e. oral language and academic performance). These students, by far, preferred to use English for communication socially. Indeed, linguistic assimilation to English, with resulting increases in English proficiency and loss in the first language, is a reality in younger generations of bilingual groups in the USA (e.g. Kaufman, 1998; Oller & Eilers, 2002). Intergenerational differences in acculturation can similarly be manifested in language proficiencies among members of the same bilingual group (see Brozgold & Centeno, ch. 5, this volume). This phenomenon is likely to occur in bilingual students throughout the world, as sociolinguistic forces shaping language use outside the school play a critical role in language maintenance and loss. Ultimately, L2, the language of the majority, which is the language used with peers, read and watched in the media, and perceived to have higher prestige than L1, becomes the dominant language (Kaufman, 1998).

Hence, academic efforts combined with personal and societal variables impact the final oral and literate language gains in bilingual students. Because oral and literate language practices in both languages continuously interact, facilitating contexts of bilingual/biliterate development requires great effort involving administrators, educators, clinicians, families, and students themselves. Within this process, however, acknowledging the instructional potential of the learning resources available in the home, accepting the student's sociocultural background respectfully, and minimizing the mismatch between personal language/literacy experiences and academic language demands should be critical requirements. This approach, in turn, would support the student's culture, enhance student and parental engagement, and prevent inappropriate educational and remedial decisions on the bilingual student's behalf (Gonzalez *et al.*, 1997; Verhoeven, 1997; Zentella, 2005).

References

Bialystok, E. (2001) *Bilingualism in Development: Language, Literacy, and Cognition.* New York: Cambridge University Press.

Blachowicz, C.L.Z. (1994) Problem-solving strategies for academic success. In G.P. Wallach and K.G. Butler (eds) *Language Learning Disabilities in School-Age Children and Adolescents: Some Principles and Applications* (pp. 304–322). Boston: Allyn and Bacon.

Brisk, M.E. and Harrington, M.M. (2000) *Literacy and Bilingualism: A Handbook for All Teachers.* Mahwah, NJ: Lawrence Erlbaum.

Centeno, J.G. and Eng, N. (2005) Bilingual speech-language pathology consultants in culturally diverse schools: Considerations on theoretically-based consultee engagement. *Journal of Educational and Psychological Consultation* 16, 333-347.

Children's Defense Fund (2000) *State of America's Children Yearbook*. Washington, DC: Beacon Press.

Cobo-Lewis, A.B., Pearson, B.Z., Eilers, R.E. and Umbel, V. (2002) Effects of bilingualism and bilingual education on oral and written Spanish skills: A multifactor study of standardized test outcomes. In D.K. Oller and R.E. Eilers (eds) *Language and Literacy in Bilingual Children* (pp. 98–117). Clevedon, UK: Multilingual Matters.

Damico, J.S., Nelson, R.L. and Bryan, L. (2005) Literacy as a sociolinguistic process for clinical purposes. In M. Ball (ed.) *Clinical Sociolinguistics* (pp. 242–249). Malden, MA: Blackwell.

Dickinson, D.K. and Tabors, P.O. (2002) Fostering language and literacy in classrooms and homes. *Young Children* 57, 10–18.

Durgunoğlu, A.Y. (1997) Bilingual reading: Its components, development, and other issues. In A.M.B. de Groot and J.F. Kroll (eds) *Tutorials in Bilingualism: Psycholinguistic Perspectives* (pp. 255–276). Mahwah, NJ: Lawrence Erlbaum.

Durgunoğlu, A.Y., Nagy, W.E. and Hancin-Bhatt, B.J. (1993) Cross-language transfer of phonological awareness. *Journal of Educational Psychology* 85, 453–465.

García, E. (1999) *Student Cultural Diversity: Understanding and Meeting the Challenge* (2nd edn). Boston: Houghton Mifflin.

García, O. and Menken, K. (2006) The English of Latinos from a plurilingual and transcultural angle: Implications for assessment and schools. In S.J. Nero (ed.) *Dialects, Englishes, Creoles, and Education* (pp. 167–183). Mahwah, NJ: Lawrence Erlbaum.

Gonzales, J.E. and García, C.R.H. (1995) Effects of word linguistic properties on phonological awareness in Spanish children. *Journal of Educational Psychology* 87, 193–201.

Gonzalez, V., Brusca-Vega, R. and Yawkey, T. (1997) *Assessment and Instruction of Culturally and Linguistically Diverse Students with or At-risk of Learning*. Boston: Allyn and Bacon.

Gorman, B.K. and Gillam, R.B. (2004) Phonological awareness in Spanish: A tutorial for speech-language pathologists. *Communication Disorders Quarterly* 25, 13–22.

Harris, J.L. (2003) Toward an understanding of literacy issues in multicultural school-age populations. *Language, Speech, and Hearing Services in Schools* 34, 17–19.

Kamhi, A.G. and Catts, H.W. (2005) Language and reading: Convergences and divergences. In H.W. Catts and A.G. Kamhi (eds) *Language and Reading Disabilities* (2nd edn, pp. 1–25). Boston, MA: Pearson.

Kaufman, D. (1998) Children's assimilatory patterns and L1 attrition. *Proceedings of the Annual Boston University Conference on Language Development* 22, 409–420.

Kayser, H. (1998) *Assessment and Intervention Resource for Hispanic Children*. San Diego: Singular.

Lyon, G.R. (1998) *Overview of Reading and Literacy Initiatives*. On WWW at www.nichd.nih.gov/about/crmc/edb/r_overview.htm. Accessed 23.11.05.

MacWhinney, B. (1997) Second language acquisition and the competition model. In A.M.B. de Groot and J.F. Kroll (eds) *Tutorials in Bilingualism: Psycholinguistic Perspectives* (pp. 113–142). Mahwah, NJ: Lawrence Erlbaum.

Meschyan, G. and Hernández, A.E. (2004) Cognitive factors in second-language acquisition and literacy learning. In C.A. Stone, E.R. Silliman, B.J. Ehren and K. Apel (eds) *Handbook of Language and Literacy* (pp. 73–81). New York: The Guilford Press.

Neuman, S.B. and Dickinson, D.K. (2002) *Handbook of Early Literacy Research*. New York: Guilford Press.

Oller, D.K. and Eilers, R. (2002) Balancing interpretations regarding the effects of bilingualism: Empirical outcomes and theoretical possibilities. In D.K. Oller and R.E. Eilers (eds) *Language and Literacy in Bilingual Children* (pp. 281–292). Clevedon, UK: Multilingual Matters.

Paratore, J.R., Melzi, G. and Krol-Sinclair, B. (2003) Learning about the literate lives of Latino families. In D.M. Barone and L.M. Morrow (eds) *Literacy and Young Children* (pp. 101–120). New York: Guilford Press.

Pew Hispanic Center (2002) *2002 National Survey of Latinos*. Washington, DC: Pew Hispanic Center.

Snow, E.E., Burns, M.S. and Griffin, P. (1998) *Preventing Reading Difficulties in Young Children*. Washington, DC: National Academy Press.

Swank, L.K. and Larrivee, L.S. (1998) Phonology, metaphonology, and the development of literacy. In R. Paul (ed.) *Exploring the Speech–Language Connection* (pp. 253–297). Baltimore: Paul H. Brookes.

Tabors, P.O. and Snow, C.E. (2002) Young bilingual children and early literacy development. In S.B. Neuman and D.K. Dickinson (eds) *Handbook of Early Literacy Research* (pp. 159–178). New York: Gilford Press.

US Census Bureau (2000) *Census, 2000*. On WWW at http://www.census.gov. Accessed 10.10.05.

US Department of Education (2006) *A Guide to Education and No Child Left Behind*. On WWW at http://www.ed.gov/nclb/overview/intro/guide/guide.pdf. Accessed 24.04.06.

Verhoeven, L. (1997) Sociolinguistics and education. In F. Coulmas (ed.) *Handbook of Sociolinguistics* (pp. 389–404). Oxford, UK: Blackwell Publishers.

Wallach, G. and Butler, K. (1994) Creating communication, literacy, and academic success. In G.P. Wallach and K.G. Butler (eds) *Language Learning Disabilities in School-Age Children and Adolescents: Some Principles and Applications* (pp. 2–26). Boston: Allyn and Bacon.

Zecker, L.B. (2004) Learning to read and write in two languages: The development of early biliteracy abilities. In C.A. Stone, E.R. Silliman, B.J. Ehren and K. Apel (eds) *Handbook of Language and Literacy: Development and Disorders* (pp. 248–265). New York: Guilford Press.

Zentella, A.C. (1997) *Growing up Bilingual*. Malden, MA: Blackwell.

Zentella, A.C. (2005) Perspectives on language and literacy in Latino families and communities. In A.C. Zentella (ed.) *Building on Strength: Language and Literacy in Latino Families and Communities* (pp. 1–12). New York: Teachers College Press.

Chapter 3
Bilingual Development and Communication: Implications for Clinical Language Studies

JOSÉ G. CENTENO

Bilingual speakers' linguistic performance is a complex phenomenon. Bilingual development depends on each learner's individual communicative experiences in the first (L1) and second language (L2), including contexts, modalities, and language-use practices, throughout life (Grosjean, 2004). In addition, bilingual speakers' discourse generally shows special expressive features reflecting individual acquisition history in each language and conversational routines typical of language-contact situations. While there is a sizeable body of literature on development, sociolinguistic contexts, and typical language practices in both child and adult bilinguals, there is little research yet that explores the interaction among these phenomena and their clinical applications (Gutiérrez-Clellen et al., 2000; Roberts, 1998).

The purpose of this chapter is to address this set of links, discussing the theoretical basis of bilingual speakers' language performance as they apply to clinical communication research and practice. Particularly, this chapter discusses bilingual children and adults' acquisition phenomena and expressive features to highlight relationships between developmental background, sociolinguistic variables of language use, language practice patterns, and proficiency. The chapter starts with an overview of bilingual development in young and late learners, continues with a summary of special bilingual expressive behaviors, and concludes with a discussion of the implications of both acquisition and communication features in the methodology and data interpretation in clinical language studies with bilingual speakers. Although many of the phenomena addressed here have been extensively described in the literature, in view of the tutorial nature of this chapter, discussions survey crucial issues and make reference to important studies for further reading.

The Acquisition of Bilingual Skills in Children and Adults: An Overview

Bilingual development has broadly been classified into *simultaneous* or *sequential bilingualism*. Generally, simultaneous bilingual acquisition occurs when children are regularly exposed to two languages from a very early age whereas sequential acquisition involves an introduction to L2 from late childhood onwards (McLaughlin, 1978; Romaine, 1995). In both acquisitional contexts, linguistic gains depend on the learner's personal and environmental circumstances regulating exposure and practice in L1 and L2. In the next two sections, variables specific to simultaneous acquisition in children and successive bilingualism in older children and adults are summarized.

Bilingual children

Simultaneous bilingualism has been described in several ways. For instance, *bilingualism as a first language* or *bilingual first language acquisition* identifies a regular dual-language exposure from birth (De Houwer, 1998; Meisel, 1990). By contrast, *preschool successive* and *incipient bilingualism* specify an onset of daily L2 exposure or minimal L2 skills at the time of preschool enrollment, respectively (Kayser, 2002). Yet, despite the terminology, what seems to be crucial in these young learners' linguistic gains is their sociolinguistically regulated input experiences at home and school (De Houwer, 1990; Romaine, 1995). Specifically, simultaneous bilinguals' skills in L1 and L2 are correlatable solely to the linguistic input in their daily sociolinguistic experiences, including communication environments and discourse practices (De Houwer, 1990; 1998).

The impact of input factors, such as presentation contexts and parental discourse strategies, in young bilinguals' language development has been well documented. For example, different L1 and L2 contexts may result in bilingual children's overall 'distributed' lexical knowledge with some vocabulary elements known in L1 and others in L2 (Oller & Pearson, 2002: 10). Also, some input experiences seem to have a greater impact than others on the quantity of learning. Patterson (2002) reports bilingual toddlers' vocabulary size in each language showed a stronger positive correlation to the amount (input) of reading than to the minimal effect of hours of TV-watching in either language. Similarly, parental discourse patterns provide important input that is reflected in bilingual children's utterances. Almgren and Idiazabal (2001) showed that language-specific verb-tense use in bilingual Basque–Spanish children's conversation reflected the distributional frequency of their parents' verb-tense use in monolingual discourse in Basque or Spanish. Further, Lanza (2001) supports that interactional discourse strategies used by each parent during conversation may indeed compel the bilingual child's clear separation of languages or mixed use of both languages in the same utterance.

Regarding school settings, Romaine (1995) describes shifts in bilingual children's language dominance after their daily input environments changed upon school enrollment. Coming into school with a predominant L1 exposure at home and incipient L2 skills, many immigrant children in England tend to change from an L1-dominance pattern to monolingual performance levels in both L1 and L2 after regular attendance to an English-speaking school and continued L1 exposure at home. In fact, dominance shifts may occur whenever input in one of a bilingual child's two languages ceases for prolonged periods of time resulting in *language loss* or *attrition* (Kessler, 1984). In sum, daily input routines to young simultaneous bilinguals constitute a key determinant of development, maintenance, or loss of skills in L1 or L2. Understanding such communication patterns and their changes over time is crucial to interpret individual L1–L2 proficiency differences in each bilingual child.

Bilingual adults

Sequential (successive or consecutive) bilingualism generally refers to older children and adults acquiring L2 skills in naturalistic contexts, as *second language acquisition* (SLA), or in classroom environments, as *foreign language* (FL) *learning* (Ritchie & Bhatia, 1996). In contrast to young learners, later learners' bilingual development involves multiple variables beyond the sociolinguistic dynamics at home and school. Several developmental phenomena have been highlighted to account for older bilinguals' linguistic gains, namely, the age of L2 learning, the distinction between rate and extent of language attainments, motivation, contextually regulated demands of linguistic presentation, and learning opportunities.

Maturational age-related constraints in bilingual development initially referred to a time-restricted *critical period* for language development from birth to puberty reflecting progressive lateralization of cerebral language sites (Lenneberg, 1967; Penfield & Roberts, 1959). However, the evidence for childhood versus adult L2 abilities is more complex, as Hyltenstam and Abrahamsson (2003) argue in their excellent recent review. While most evidence suggests that younger learners have better results than older learners, it also shows more flexible time-windows for L2 acquisition, which may extend beyond puberty. It is true that early L2 exposure and continuous use, measured in terms of length of residence (LOR) or age of arrival (AOA), may facilitate L2 performance in several tasks, such as sentence repetition and grammaticality judgment (Flege *et al.*, 2002; Johnson & Newport, 1989). Yet, some postpubertal L2 learners have shown L2 native-like performance in several linguistic areas, such as grammaticality judgment and pronunciation (Johnson & Newport, 1989; Yavaş, 1996). Hence, age-related restrictions may be viewed as a gradual decrease in cerebral plasticity resulting in separate *sensitive periods* or *multiple critical periods* for different linguistic skills (Johnson & Newport, 1989; Seliger, 1978).

Understanding the role of age in SLA is complex and requires the examination of confounding factors, particularly rate versus final outcome measurements and the learner's personality variables. Based on their review of the research, Krashen *et al.* (1979) argued that older learners may acquire L2 skills faster but, in the long run, younger learners become more proficient. While adult L2 learners may bring more mature and experienced linguistic and cognitive skills and strategies to the experimental paradigms, evidence irrefutably confirms that child L2 learners' final achievement in L2 tends to be better.

Nevertheless, special personal traits in exceptional late L2 learners remind us not to consider older bilinguals a uniform group. For instance, Novoa *et al.* (1988) present evidence of a talented late multilingual speaker with special cognitive, motivational, and educational strengths. Birdsong (1992) and White and Genesee (1996) report on outlying cases in their bilingual subject pool showing some exceptional L2 performance among late L2 learners in L2 grammatical intuition tasks. Based on the greater cognitive flexibility found in talented monolingual language learners (Schneiderman & Desmarais, 1988) and attitudinal requirements for L2 learning (Novoa *et al.*, 1988), it may very well be that talented late L2 learners represent a neuropsychologically distinctive cohort of motivated individuals fortunately afforded the social and educational opportunities for L2 learning.

Complex linguistic demands in late L2 learners' acquisitional environments need to be considered, particularly because differences in the manner and context of acquisition are concomitant with different modes of language practices and processing strategies (Seliger, 1996). Several important arguments capture the formal–informal communication challenges in late bilingual development. Krashen (1982) proposes an account targeting SLA learning in formal or informal contexts. Krashen argues that a formal language development context (i.e. foreign-language classrooms), or *language learning*, emphasizes the understanding of linguistic rules whereas an informal language development context (i.e. routine discourse), or *language acquisition*, directs the speaker's attention to linguistic content in a naturalistic, conversational setting. Thus, manner of linguistic input in these learning situations determines the salience of, and attention to, target L2 form for the learner, be it adjustments by a native speaker or a more competent interlocutor during conversation in SLA contexts or actual explanations of L2 errors by an instructor in formal FL scenarios (Gass, 1997; Long, 1996). Yet, of these two environments, classroom instruction seems to work more effectively than naturalistic exposure in promoting L2 grammatical development in SLA. When combined with sufficient opportunity to practice, classroom instruction can maximize consciousness, learning, and proficiency (Long, 1983). Lastly, in more cognitive terms, Bialystok (2001) suggests bilingual speakers' language use could be viewed as a continuum of three domains, namely, oral, literate, and metalinguistic, involving increasing levels of cognitive complexity as defined by demands in control, attention, and analysis. As bilingual speakers process tasks at each of the above linguistic levels, they must control their attention resources to analyze specific mental representations involved in performing the target tasks.

Finally, the social context of bilingual development deserves attention in sequential bilinguals as it does for simultaneous learners. Because social environments with limited learning opportunities may present several challenges (e.g. language and literacy experiences that are not commensurate with standard mainstream language practices; Roseberry-McKibbin, 2001), it is critical to understand how such phenomena may have an impact on bilingual speakers' linguistic development. In fact, in culturally and linguistically diverse (CLD) populations, an individual's limited formal language skills may reflect different language-learning experiences and educational opportunities, not necessarily language deficits (Gutiérrez-Clellen & Peña, 2001). Indeed, Snow *et al.* (1991) argue that academic language experiences result in better ability to perform academic tasks, such as defining words. Their evidence was that the older bilingual students they tested provided better definitions in the language in which they had been educated than in their L1.

All in all, older children and adults in dual-language learning contexts are exposed to a constellation of variables that go beyond the input-based development in young simultaneous bilinguals. Understanding linguistic gains in late bilingualism requires the examination of interacting factors, including age, rate versus complete attainments, motivation, informal-formal contextual demands, and access to learning opportunities, for each bilingual speaker throughout life.

Expressive Features of Bilingual Discourse

Conversational features in bilingual communication warrant particular attention in clinical communication. Bilingual speakers' expressive routines represent cross-linguistic interactions that need to be understood to avoid the inaccurate labeling of typical expressive behaviors as clinical deficits. Most crucially, transfer, borrowing, language mixing, attrition, and, in some circumstances, dialectal influences, deserve particular examination.

First-language effects in situations of language contact, often described as 'transfer', 'interference', or 'cross-linguistic influence' (Romaine, 1995: 52), may occur at different linguistic levels. While phonological L1 influence in L2 speech production is commonly recognized as *accent* (see Bell-Berti, ch. 20, this volume), transfer effects from L1 to L2 can be seen at grammatical, morphological, lexical, and orthographic levels, as well (e.g. Hoffman, 1991). For example, in grammatical transfer, a bilingual speaker would use L1 word order, pronouns, determiners, prepositions, and verb features when communicating in L2. Utterances produced by a Spanish–English bilingual such as *The house red* 'The red house', *She no go yesterday* 'She didn't go yesterday' show the use of Spanish noun–adjective word order and the absence of auxiliaries (does) in Spanish negation. Similarly, regarding vocabulary, an L1–L2 influence would be seen in *Robert makes his homework* for 'Robert does his homework'. Here the Spanish–English speaker does not differentiate between 'making' and 'doing', as one must in Standard English, as Spanish only requires one lexical entry *hacer* for actions that use either *make* or *do* in English (Centeno, 2006; also see Anderson & Centeno, ch. 1, this volume for additional areas of possible cross-linguistic Spanish–English influences).

Lexical items in bilingual discourse may also manifest as permanent or temporary cross-linguistic *lexical borrowings*. Unlike the semantic nature of L1–L2 lexical transfers above, borrowed or loan words occur cross-linguistically to fill a lexical gap (Bhatia & Ritchie, 1996). They may be permanently assimilated into the language after phonological and morphological adaptation of the original word (e.g. *pizza* from Italian to English, *estrés* 'stress' and *cliquear* 'to click' from English to Spanish; Romaine, 1995). In other cases, such *loan words* include a specific word partially assimilated in the language of discourse when the bilingual speaker feels stressed or fatigued, or does not have a word expressing the same meaning in the language of discourse (e.g. *piñata* – object used originally in some Spanish-speaking countries at children's parties) (Centeno, 2006; Hoffman, 1991).

Bilinguals may also mix their two languages in conversation. Poplack (1980) describes three types of *language switches*: tag switching, and intersentential and intrasentential switching. In tag switches, a tag phrase in one language is inserted in an utterance produced in the other language (e.g. by the way, imagine that!). In contrast, intersentential switches occur at clause or sentence boundaries (Sometimes I start a sentence in English *y termino en Español* /Sometimes I start a sentence in English and finish it in Spanish) whereas intrasentential switches take place within clause or sentence boundaries (El estaba caminando raro *like a zombie* /He was walking strangely like a zombie). Language mixing is not restricted to adult bilinguals' speech. It starts early in bilingual development when children regularly exposed to two languages are socialized into parental discourse strategies in bilingual homes (Lanza, 2001). In addition, young bilingual children may produce mixed utterances when they don't have sufficient morphosyntactic resources in either language to generate an entire structural string in one language (Nicoladis & Genesee, 1997). There is much debate about the theoretical underpinnings of language-mixing in children and in adults, however, it is clear that language mixes do not happen at random and require the understanding of grammatical, social, and psychological factors (Bhatia & Ritchie, 1996; MacSwan, 2004).

Bilinguals' L1 skills may also change due to a lack or a reduction of domains for L1 use. Primary *language attrition* occurs in many bilinguals receptively and expressively in those circumstances lacking the regular multimodal L1 stimulation of monolingual scenarios (Seliger, 1996). Some L1 difficulties include the marked reduction or loss of verb tenses, simplification of sentence structure, difficulty with making grammaticality judgments, dysfluency, and lexical retrieval problems (e.g. Seliger, 1996; Silva-Corvalán, 1991; Zentella, 1997).

Finally, bilingual groups sharing neighborhoods with other bilingual or dialectal groups may show the effects of cross-linguistic influence, particularly in the structure and vocabulary. For instance, Spanish–English teenagers living in the same area and attending the same schools as African–Americans may take aspects of African–American Vernacular English (AAVE) dialect (e.g. '... she Jewish ... she going to have the baby' (copula deletion), 'when she have the baby...' (lack of 3rd person -s suffix) (Zentella, 1997: 158, 172). In sum, both young and older bilingual speakers exhibit particular expressive features at different linguistic levels (e.g. lexical, syntactic, morphological, etc.) resulting from cross-linguistic influences (transfer, borrowings, mixing, and dialectal effects) or language practices (attrition).

Implications for Clinical Communication Research with Bilingual Speakers

The preceding discussion underscores the complexity in bilingual speakers' language performance as a reflection of both acquisitional heterogeneity among bilinguals and typical communication features in dual-language oral expression. Linguistic gains in both young and older bilinguals represent an interaction of sociolinguistically regulated input and, more strongly in older learners, the participation of individual factors, such as age, motivation, informal–formal contextual demands, and access to learning opportunities. Because such variables may change over time for each speaker, language proficiency emerges as an individual multidimensional phenomenon responding to dynamic fluctuations in contexts, modalities, and skills of language use. In this scenario, the interaction of language acquisition, proficiency, and expressive patterns of language use imposes challenges on the clinical communication investigator.

First, defining who is bilingual and determining proficiency levels in each language present researchers with difficult challenges. Rather than being a monolingual in each language, bilingual speakers' L1 and L2 skills are likely to be anywhere between minimal to near-native or native mastery as linguistic abilities are differentially shaped by the degree of experiential practice in each language (Centeno & Obler, 2001). Second, because both languages are not uniformly used across all experiences, bilingual speakers' overall linguistic knowledge is summative in nature with both languages complementing each other as a result of their context-specific use (Grosjean, 2004). Lastly, in view of bilingual speakers' communication representing a continuous cross-linguistic interaction, typical expressive features in bilingual contexts need to be understood to distinguish nonpathological language differences from genuine pathological communicative deviations in both young and older bilinguals (Kayser, 2002; Obler *et al.*, 1995).

Clearly, realistic understanding of language use and proficiency in both young simultaneous and older sequential bilinguals requires knowledge of their language history, social contexts of language learning, and background communication routines (De Houwer, 1998; Grosjean, 1989; Paradis, 1987). What crucially stands out in this process is the domain-specific nature of the linguistic gains exhibited by the bilingual learner/ user. Because differences in the manner and context of acquisition imply different modes of language practices and processing strategies (Seliger, 1996), the careful assessment of bilingual subjects' proficiency levels relative to their specific acquisitional backgrounds is warranted in both typical and disordered speakers. Specifically, systematic efforts to correlate bilingualism history and self-assessment with proficiency measures would enhance the appropriate selection and classification of research participants, stimuli and task development, language mode during task administration, and linguistic interpretation (see Kohnert *et al.*, 1998; Vaid & Menon, 2000). In addition, for clinicians relying on the research for evidence-based practices, careful assessment and classification of bilingual research participants would facilitate the understanding of the specific bilingual clients to whom findings can be generalized (Roberts, 1998; also see De Houwer, 1998; Grosjean, 2004; Obler *et al.*, 1982). Further, concerning expressive routines, knowledge of the speakers' typical expressive patterns, such as mixing, borrowing, attrition behaviors, or dialectal influences, would allow the use of suitable measures and interpretive approaches for utterance analysis in studies of typical and disordered bilingual speakers (Bhatia & Ritchie, 1996; Grosjean, 1989; 2004; Gutiérrez-Clellen *at al.*, 2000). Indeed, systematic comparisons between typical expressive routines and disordered communication in bilingual children and adults may yield valuable clinically relevant data (Muñoz *et al.*, 1999; Nicoladis & Genesee, 1997).

In sum, developing a composite of bilingual research participants' background linguistic information, based on developmental and typical expressive patterns, seems critical to understand language usage and proficiency as well as implement appropriate procedures in clinical communication research. Although understanding bilinguals' communication abilities goes beyond linguistic features, as predicated throughout this volume (e.g. Ansaldo & Marcotte, ch. 16; Brozgold & Centeno, ch. 5; Goldstein, ch. 13), failure to acknowledge the preceding experiential bases would compromise both methodological and interpretive approaches used to explicate bilinguals' language performance and, in turn, the development and improvement of evidenced-based clinical methods to be used with this population.

References

Almgren, M. and Idiazabal, I. (2001) Past tense verb forms, discourse context, and input features in bilingual and monolingual acquisition of Basque and Spanish. In F. Genesee and J. Cenoz (eds) *Trends in Bilingual Acquisition* (pp. 107–130). Amsterdam: John Benjamins.

Bhatia, T.K. and Ritchie, W.C. (1996) Bilingual language mixing, universal grammar, and second language acquisition. In W.C. Ritchie and T.K. Bhatia (eds) *Handbook of Second Language Acquisition* (pp. 627–688). San Diego, CA: Academic Press.

Bialystok, E. (2001) *Bilingualism in Development: Language, Literacy, and Cognition.* Cambridge: Cambridge University Press.

Birdsong, D. (1992) Ultimate attainment in second language acquisition. *Language* 68, 706–765.

Centeno, J.G. (2006) *Tutorials in Bilingualism for Speech-language Pathologists.* Unpublished manuscript.

Centeno, J.G. and Obler, L.K. (2001) Principles of bilingualism. In M. Pontón and J.L. Carrión (eds) *Neuropsychology and the Hispanic Patient: A Clinical Handbook* (pp. 75–86). Mahwah, NJ: Lawrence Erlbaum.

De Houwer, A. (1990) *The Acquisition of Two Languages: A Case Study.* Cambridge: Cambridge University Press.

De Houwer, A. (1998) By way of introduction: Methods in studies of bilingual first language acquisition. *International Journal of Bilingualism* 2, 249–263.

Flege, J.E., MacKay, I.R.A. and Piske, T. (2002) Assessing bilingual dominance. *Applied Psycholinguistics* 23, 567–598.

Gass, S.M. (1997) *Input, Interaction, and the Second Language Learner.* Mahwah, NJ: Lawrence Erlbaum.

Grosjean, F. (1989) Neurolinguists, beware! The bilingual is not two monolinguals in one person. *Brain and Language* 36, 3–15.

Grosjean, F. (2004) Studying bilinguals: Methodological and conceptual issues. In T.K. Bhatia and W.C. Ritchie (eds) *The Handbook of Bilingualism* (pp. 32–63). Malden, MA: Blackwell.

Gutiérrez-Clellen, V.F. and Peña, E. (2001) Dynamic assessment of diverse children: A tutorial. *Language, Speech, and Hearing Services in Schools* 32, 212–224.

Gutiérrez-Clellen, V.F., Restrepo, M.A., Bedore, L.M., Peña, E. and Anderson, R.T. (2000) Language sample analysis in Spanish-speaking children: Methodological considerations. *Language, Speech, and Hearing Services in Schools* 31, 88–98.

Hoffmann, C. (1991) *An Introduction to Bilingualism*. London: Longman.

Hyltenstam, K. and Abrahamsson, N. (2003) Maturational constraints in SLA. In C. Doughty and M. Long (eds) *Handbook of Second Language Acquisition* (pp. 539–588). Malden, MA: Blackwell.

Johnson, J.S. and Newport, E.L. (1989) Critical periods effects in second language learning: The influence of maturational state on the acquisition of English as a second language. *Cognitive Psychology* 21, 60–99.

Kayser, H.R. (2002) Bilingual language development and language disorders. In D.E. Battle (ed.) *Communication Disorders in Multicultural Populations* (3rd edn) (pp. 205–232). Boston: Butterworth-Heinemann.

Kessler, C. (1984) Language acquisition in bilingual children. In N. Miller (ed.) *Bilingualism and Language Disability: Assessment and Remediation* (pp. 26–54). London: Croom Helm.

Kohnert, K.J., Hernández, A.E. and Bates, E. (1998). Bilingual performance on the Boston Naming Test: Preliminary norms in Spanish and English. *Brain and Language* 65, 422–440.

Krashen, S. (1982) *Principles and Practice in Second Language Acquisition*. London: Pergamon Press.

Krashen, S., Long, M. and Scarcella, R. (1979) Age, rate, and eventual attainment in second language acquisition. *TESOL Quarterly* 13, 573–582.

Lanza, E. (2001) Bilingual first language acquisition: A discourse perspective on language contact in parent–child interaction. In F. Genesee and J. Cenoz (eds) *Trends in Bilingual Acquisition* (pp. 107–130). Amsterdam: John Benjamins.

Lenneberg, E.H. (1967) *Biological Foundations of Language*. New York: Wiley.

Long, M. (1983) Does second language instruction make a difference? A review of research. *TESOL Quarterly* 17, 359–382.

Long, M. (1996) The role of the linguistic environment in second language acquisition. In W.C. Ritchie and T.K. Bhatia (eds) *Handbook of Second Language Acquisition* (pp. 413–454). San Diego, CA: Academic Press.

MacSwan, J. (2004) Code-switching and grammatical theory. In T.K. Bhatia and W.C. Ritchie (eds) *The Handbook of Bilingualism* (pp. 283–311). Malden, MA: Blackwell.

McLaughlin, B. (1978) *Second-language Acquisition in Childhood*. Hillsdale, NJ: Lawrence Erlbaum.

Meisel, J. (1990) *Two First Languages: Early Grammatical Development in Bilingual Children*. Dordrecht: Foris.

Muñoz, M.L., Marquardt, T.P. and Copeland, G. (1999) A comparison of codeswitching patterns of aphasic and neurologically normal bilingual speakers of English and Spanish. *Brain and Language* 66, 249–274.

Nicoladis, E. and Genesee, F. (1997) Language development in preschool bilingual children. *Journal of Speech-Language Pathology* 21, 258–270.

Novoa, L., Fein, D. and Obler, L.K. (1988) Talent in foreign languages: A case study. In L.K. Obler and D. Fein (eds) *The Exceptional Brain: Neuropsychology of Talent and Special Abilities* (pp. 294–303). New York: Guilford.

Obler, L.K., Centeno, J.G. and Eng, N. (1995) Bilingual and polyglot aphasia. In L. Menn, M. O'Connor, L.K. Obler and A. Holland (eds) *Non-fluent Aphasia in a Multilingual World* (pp. 132–143). Amsterdam: John Benjamins.

Obler, L.K., Zattore, R.J., Galloway, L. and Vaid, J. (1982) Cerebral lateralization in bilinguals: Methodological issues. *Brain and Language* 15, 40–54.

Oller, D.K. and Pearson, B.Z. (2002) Assessing the effects of bilingualism: A background. In D.K. Oller and R.E. Eilers (eds) *Language and Literacy in Bilingual Children* (pp. 3–21). Clevedon, UK: Multilingual Matters.

Paradis, M. (1987) *The Assessment of Bilingual Aphasia*. Hillsdale, NJ: Lawrence Erlbaum.

Patterson, J.L. (2002) Relationships of expressive vocabulary to frequency of reading and television experience among bilingual toddlers. *Applied Psycholinguistics* 23, 493–508.

Penfield, W. and Roberts, L. (1959) *Speech and Brain Mechanisms*. New York: Atheneum.

Poplack, S. (1980) Sometimes I start a sentence in English y termino en español: Toward a typology of code-switching. *Linguistics* 18, 581–618.

Ritchie, W.C. and Bhatia, T.K. (1996) Introduction. In W.C. Ritchie and T.K. Bhatia (eds) *Handbook of Second Language Acquisition* (pp. 1–46). San Diego, CA: Academic Press.

Roberts, P.M. (1998) Clinical research needs and issues in bilingual aphasia. *Aphasiology* 12, 119–130.

Romaine, S. (1995) *Bilingualism* (2nd edn). Oxford: Blackwell.

Roseberry-McKibbin, C. (2001) Serving children from the culture of poverty: Practical strategies for speech-language pathologists. *ASHA Leader* 6, 4–16.

Schneiderman, E.I. and Desmarais, C. (1988) A neuropsychological substrate for talent in second language acquisition. In L.K. Obler and D. Fein (eds) *The Exceptional Brain: Neuropsychology of Talent and Special Abilities* (pp. 103–126). New York: Guilford.

Seliger, H. (1978) Implications of a multiple critical period hypothesis for second language learning. In W.C. Ritchie (ed.) *Second Language Acquisition Research: Issues and Implications* (pp. 11–19). San Diego: Academic Press.

Seliger, H. (1996) Primary language attrition in the context of bilingualism. In W.C. Ritchie and T.K. Bhatia (eds) *Handbook of Second Language Acquisition* (pp. 605–626). San Diego, CA: Academic Press.

Silva-Corvalán, C. (1991) Spanish language attrition in a contact situation with English. In H.W. Seliger and R.M. Vago (eds) *First Language Attrition* (pp. 151–171). Cambridge: Cambridge University Press.

Snow, C.E., Cancino, H., De Temple, J. and Schley, S. (1991) Giving formal definitions: A linguistic or metalinguistic skill? In H. Bialystok (ed.) *Language Processing in Bilingual Children* (pp. 90–112). Cambridge: Cambridge University Press.

Vaid, J. and Menon, R. (2000) Correlates of bilinguals' preferred language for mental computations. *Spanish Applied Linguistics* 4, 325–342.

White, L. and Genesee, F. (1996) How native is near-native? The issue of ultimate attainment in adult second language acquisition. *Second Language Research* 12, 233–265.

Yavaş, M. (1996) Differences in voice onset time in early and late Spanish–English bilinguals. In J. Jensen and A. Roca (eds) *Spanish in Contact: Issues in Bilingualism* (pp. 131–141). Sommerville, MA: Cascadilla Press.

Zentella, A.C. (1997) *Growing Up Bilingual*. Malden, MA: Blackwell.

Chapter 4

Neurolinguistic Aspects of Bilingualism

MARTIN R. GITTERMAN and HIA DATTA

The study of language and the brain (i.e. neurolinguistics) has fascinated scholars for many years. Research on the neurolinguistics of bilingualism, given our multilingual society, takes on added significance. The overview presented in this chapter will focus largely on the bilingual aphasia literature and the related topic of language organization in the brain. Included will be reference to the assessment and treatment of bilinguals with aphasia, an issue of particular concern to the many speech-language pathologists (SLPs) working with bilingual clients. Mention of advances in neuroimaging as contributing to an understanding of the bilingual brain will be incorporated. Other topics covered are the critical period hypothesis, the related topic of the highly talented language learner, and translation, including pathological performance in translation. Space constraints have made it necessary to cover only a portion of the topics that could have been included and to limit the degree of detail for each of the topics selected. Nevertheless, the reader is presented with a substantive overview of the field. The term *bilingual* is used throughout the chapter to refer to two or more languages, thus avoiding the need to make distinctions between *bilingual* and *multilingual*. The terms L1 and L2 are used interchangeably with *first language* and *second language*, respectively.

While the notion of *bilingual*, as used in this chapter, may refer to any two (or more) languages, a framework is established which is applicable to the study of Spanish–English bilinguals. As mentioned in the introduction of this volume, an understanding of this population is critical for both researchers and practitioners in clinical communication, given the extremely large worldwide Hispanic population. Of particular concern to the issues discussed in this chapter, Goldstein (2000) reports, in reference to Arámbula (1992), the occurrence of about 32,000 to 35,000 strokes annually in Hispanics in the USA alone, thus highlighting the need to understand the dynamics of aphasia in this population.

Bilingual Aphasia

Researchers have been publishing case studies of bilinguals with aphasia for many years (see Albert & Obler, 1978, Paradis, 1977, 2004, for comprehensive overviews). Paradis (1977: 65) outlines a number of distinct patterns of recovery, of which parallel recovery ('when the languages are similarly impaired and restored at the same rate') is the most prevalent (found in 56 of the 138 cases he reviewed). Paradis notes that the percentage of cases of parallel recovery in his sample is undoubtedly lower than would be found in a more representative sampling, as researchers tend to report the more exceptional cases. In nonparallel recovery patterns, a cover term for a number of distinct patterns, clear differences in either rate of restitution or measure of impairment are found in the languages in question. The existence of nonparallel patterns of recovery in bilingual patients with aphasia is consistent with a model of language organization in the brain in which bilingualism influences patterns of localization. Of note, the occurrence of nonparallel patterns of recovery does not constitute proof of mono-lingual/bilingual differences in localization, nor do such patterns of recovery constitute the sole basis for speculating about such differences.

Albert and Obler (1978) suggest a greater right hemisphere role in bilinguals. This suggestion, focusing on a laterality-based difference in the brain of bilinguals, has sparked extensive debate. Paradis (1998), for example, argues that any greater use of the right hemisphere in bilinguals may result from a greater reliance on pragmatic factors (associated with the right hemisphere) in the second (and presumably weaker) language. He argues that monolingual and bilingual brains do not differ either 'neurofunctionally' or 'neuroanatomically' (see also, Mendelsohn, 1988). The suggestion that bilingualism might influence the cerebral representation of language can be viewed historically as part of a broader neurolinguistic framework focusing on the possible influence of nonbiological factors on language organization in the brain, bilingualism being one of these factors (Gitterman, 2005; Gitterman & Sies, 1990).

Researchers, for example, have hypothesized that tone languages might involve greater participation of the right hemisphere, as non-linguistic tone is subserved by the right hemisphere. Similarly, as nonlinguistic visuospatial activities are linked to the right hemisphere, it is natural to question whether processing sign language, because it is visuospatial, might be a more right hemisphere activity than spoken language. The evidence, however, suggests that the left hemisphere is primarily responsible for processing both tone and sign languages (April & Han, 1980; Poizner *et al.*, 1987). In addition to hypothesized laterality differences in monolinguals and bilinguals, research has addressed within-hemisphere differences. Ojemann and Whitaker (1978), for example, using electrical stimulation, report on differential within-hemisphere impairment in the languages of the bilinguals they studied, including one Spanish–English bilingual. Other researchers have focused on comparing subcortical to cortical areas regarding the representation of language.

Fabbro and Paradis (1995), studying bilingual patients with aphasia, relate their subcortical lesions to particular types of language impairment. It is suggested that localization of language, cortical versus subcortical, might be dependent on the strategies used in acquiring a language.

Researchers will continue to study bilingual aphasia and the related issue of language representation in the brain (see Goral *et al.*, 2002 for additional discussion, including an outline of areas where additional research is needed). Such research will be of interest to a broad range of professionals, including SLPs. The increased focus on work in bilingualism in recent years has, for example, resulted in the production of the *Bilingual Aphasia Test* (BAT) (Paradis, 1987), an assessment instrument available to SLPs in a wide variety of languages. This comprehensive test, containing numerous language tasks, is aimed at facilitating valid assessment of post-stroke fluency across language pairs in various bilingual groups, using linguistically and culturally equivalent content. Versions of the test are available in a broad range of languages (including both English and Spanish), thus providing a valuable resource to speech-language clinicians. One part of the test enables clinicians to assess in great detail a client's abilities in each of a number of languages. This testing involves numerous tasks (e.g. spontaneous speech, sentence repetition, derivational morphology, spontaneous writing). Another part of the BAT requires patients, among other things, to engage in translation tasks. Spanish is included in combination with a number of other languages (e.g. English, Italian, Portuguese, Basque) in this part of the test (see, also, Fabbro, 1999).

Researchers are addressing the needs of bilingual clients in other ways as well. For example, some authors have stressed the importance of understanding pre-morbid linguistic routines, such as within-language dialect differences and bilingual communication features (e.g. language mixing, attrition, and so forth), in assessing bilingual clients (Centeno, 2005; Obler *et al.*, 1995). In addition, researchers are trying to gain a greater understanding of the impact of treatment in only one of the languages spoken by a bilingual aphasic speaker and possible generalization to the untreated language (Fabbro, 1999; Paradis, 2004). In one study, involving Catalan–Spanish bilinguals with aphasia, Junqué *et al.* (1989) report that treatment provided in only Catalan resulted in improvement in both Catalan and Spanish, with improvement in Catalan surpassing that observed in Spanish. All would agree that more remains to be learned about the dynamics of treatment in only language in bilinguals (in particular, both the extent and characteristics of this carryover phenomenon), but studies such as Junqué *et al.* (1989) are bringing us closer to an understanding of this process (see Fabbro, 1999, Gitterman, 2005, for additional discussion of both assessment and treatment).

Recent advances in neuroimaging techniques have enabled researchers to study neurolinguistic processes of healthy bilinguals as well. These tools have been critical in helping researchers gain a greater understanding of the neural basis of language localization in the brain and the neurophysiology of the underlying linguistic mechanisms. Currently, *positron emission tomography* (pet), *functional magnetic resonance imaging* (fMRI), and *event-related potentials* (ERPs) are the most popular imaging tools in such research. PET is a process that creates images of the brain from measures of radioactively labeled chemicals that have been injected into the bloodstream. In fMRI, magnetic fields and radio waves are used to produce high-quality two- or three-dimensional images of the brain while the participant is doing a particular task. ERP methods involve placement of electrodes on the scalp to detect and measure patterns of electrical activity emanating from the brain.

Although neuroimaging has been an indispensable research tool, current literature still makes apparent the many unanswered questions that await additional investigation. For example, with respect to language localization, some researchers suggest overlapping areas for the two languages of a bilingual (Dehaene *et al.*, 1997; Klein *et al.*, 1999; Perani *et al.*, 1998). Others (see, for example, Kim *et al.*, 1997) suggest that late bilinguals activate different cortical areas for their two languages. The findings of Kim *et al.* (1997) are supported by Wattendorf *et al.* (2001) in their study of German-French-English speakers. Horowitz *et al.* (2001), however, in a study using narration tasks with American Sign Language and English, report on an overlapping representation of languages, with evidence of extended activation for L2 (see Urbanik *et al.*, 2001, for similar findings). Hernández *et al.* (2000), in a comprehensive study of early Spanish–English bilinguals, report that similar areas of the brain are activated in a picture naming task in both languages (Spanish and English) of their participants. Although these findings are consistent with those found in a number of previous studies, they suggest that the results of their fMRI study must be interpreted with caution. They indicate that fMRI alone might be insufficient to provide the answers being sought in areas such as language localization. Future research, it is argued, should combine various neuroimaging methods. Research on language processing, nevertheless, does show general consensus on how L2 acquisition-age influences L2 syntax and semantics, i.e. earlier bilinguals are more native-like than later ones (Weber-Fox & Neville, 1996).

Fortunately, the factors accounting for the seemingly contradictory findings in many of the studies are becoming better understood. It appears that the task employed (i.e. comprehension versus production), level of linguistic probe (e.g. phonological, lexical, syntactic, or some combination), age of second language acquisition, length and frequency of second language use, proficiency in second language, method of second language learning, and linguistic proximity of the languages being investigated, to name a few, influence cerebral localization of language. Current findings suggest that language areas overlap more in early proficient bilinguals for lexical-semantic comprehension tasks, while the brain is likely to recruit different areas in late, nonproficient bilinguals for language production tasks (Kim *et al.*, 1997; Perani *et al.*, 1998).

The Critical Period

It is generally agreed that children tend to outperform adults in language learning (see Centeno, ch. 3, for pertinent discussion). Lenneberg (1967) links this performance dichotomy to a neurologically based critical period. Language lateralization (claimed by Lenneberg to occur at puberty), resulting in a loss of plasticity in the brain, is argued to be the basis for the age-related differences in language learning. The critical period hypothesis, as proposed by Lenneberg, has been the subject of much controversy. Krashen (1973), for example, argues that lateralization takes place much earlier than puberty (suggesting age five as a possibility). Relatedly, Dulay *et al.* (1982) assert that an explanation for child–adult differences must not be limited to the neurological domain. To provide one example, they suggest that 'affective factors' (with adults generally being more self-conscious than children) might help to explain the poorer performance of adults (who approach the task of language acquisition with a mindset less conducive to acquisition than one finds in children). Similarly, Butler and Hakuta (2004) caution against making overly broad claims regarding biologically based factors to explain child–adult differences in language performance.

Some research has suggested that there is a neurological explanation only for performance in phonology, but not in other aspects of language, such as syntax. Scovel (1988: 65), for example, in advocating such a position, speaks of a 'Joseph Conrad phenomenon' to describe the 'mismatch between the potential for perfect lexical and syntactic performance and the impossibility of perfect phonological learning in a second language, if acquired after puberty'. Supporting evidence is provided by studies such as Scovel (1981) in which native speakers of American English were able to identify highly proficient non-native adult learners (representing a wide range of languages, e.g. Spanish, Arabic, Chinese, Swedish) from native speech samples with great accuracy, but had difficulty distinguishing between the two groups in their written samples. This viewpoint is, to say the least, not universally accepted (see, for example, Patkowski, 1980, who argues in support of a critical period for the acquisition of syntax). In fact, most issues about the critical period remain subject to debate, including even linking a particular age or ages to language performance (see Hyltenstam & Abrahamsson, 2003, for a substantive overview).

Suffice it to say, however, that a neurologically based critical period will continue to be explored in future research attempting to explain age-related differences in language learning. As such, the concept of a critical period is integral to the study of the neurolinguistics of bilingualism. Future research will continue to shed light on the nature and causes of child–adult differences in language learning and its confounding variables (see Centeno, ch. 3, this volume for further discussion). Nonetheless, because both educators and clinicians will, undoubtedly, continue to apply this knowledge in their respective professions, it must be noted that researchers recognize that there are exceptions among both children and adults to the critical period hypothesis. Some adults, in fact, are categorized as truly talented, as we discuss next.

Talent

Talented adult second language learners develop proficiency in a second language with greater ease, less effort, and faster than most adult second language learners. Schneiderman and Desmaris (1988) propose a neuropsychological theory to explain this phenomenon. They suggest that the L1 interference evident in most adult L2 learners results from the tendency of these learners to employ their L1 parameters or, in neurolinguistic terms, their L1 neural patterns in learning their L2. The basis for success in talented L2 learners is argued to be their cognitive flexibility, a flexibility resulting in the use of a new set of parameters or neural networks in learning a second language. This flexibility is employed both in learning the syntax and in establishing native-like articulation in the target language.

Neurologically, the right hemisphere is thought to be more flexible in creating new neural pathways to accommodate the acquisition of novel stimuli, while the left hemisphere is associated more with efficiency and automaticity of processing and, hence, incapable of much neurocognitive flexibility. There is some evidence of greater right hemisphere participation in learning new stimuli (Goldberg & Costa, 1981; Reynolds & Jeyes, 1978). Consistent with this claim, Papcun et al. (1974) report a stronger right ear advantage (indicating greater left hemisphere participation) in expert Morse-code operators compared to naive participants. Interestingly, as stated earlier, some researchers have suggested greater right hemisphere participation in the second language than in the first language (see, also, Obler et al., 1975).

Schneiderman and Desmaris (1988) propose that the right hemisphere initially plays a significant role in language acquisition while the left hemisphere organizes language into descriptive and automatic processing systems over time. Critically, it is suggested that typical adults make greater use of their existing more automatic and set left-hemisphere L1 processing strategies for the L2 acquisition process, as well. In so doing, these adults fail to derive the benefit of flexibility linked with alternative strategies or neural mechanisms in processing their L2, leading to somewhat less native-like second language output. Talented adults, on the other hand, maximize use of the right hemisphere in learning L2, thus attaining more native-like L2 output, without the degree of L1 interference experienced by the more typical adult. Of course, future research will have to provide additional evidence on what all would, undoubtedly, agree are these very tentative suggestions about the talented second language learner.

Translation

Translation is a task in which, to some extent, all language learners engage. Whether translation at the word level occurs directly between word forms in the two languages, or involves accessing word meanings (concepts) prior to producing the target forms, has been greatly debated. Models examining word processing have been employed to represent the process of word translation within a theoretical framework. In one such model, the *Concept Mediation Model* (CMM), it is proposed that bilinguals, irrespective of their proficiency in L2, translate from L2 to L1 via concepts, that is, not by accessing L1 words directly (Potter *et al.*, 1984). In another model, the *Revised Hierarchical Model* (RHM), it is suggested that in the earlier stages of bilingualism, the second language learner accesses L2 words via L1, whereas in the later stages (more balanced bilingualism), L2 words can be mediated through concepts, relying less on L1 (Kroll & Stewart, 1994). Thus, in the early stages of bilingualism, associations from L2 to L1 are stronger than associations from L1 to L2. In an L2 to L1 translation task, the less balanced bilingual is, therefore, expected to be faster than the more balanced bilingual, as the former group would translate directly from L2 to L1 without accessing the associated concepts. Translation from L1 to L2, on the other hand, would involve concept mediation before entering the L2 lexicon, thus increasing translation time.

In studies examining translation, where bilinguals carry out lexical translations from their L1 to L2 and vice versa, results reveal that participants are faster from L2 to L1 than from L1 to L2 (Alvarez *et al.*, 2003; Kroll & Stewart, 1994). The direct lexical links present in L2 to L1 translation are seemingly not available when translating from L1 to L2, thus accounting for the longer translation time taken in L1 to L2 translation. These data are consistent with the RHM.

The neurolinguistics of bilingualism literature also incorporates the study of breakdown in translation in some individuals with aphasia. Fabbro (1999), for example, outlines different types of deficits in translation found in bilinguals with aphasia (e.g. the inability to translate, the compulsion to translate [*spontaneous translation*], translating better into one's less proficient language than into one's more proficient language [*paradoxical translation*]). A greater understanding of these deficits will undoubtedly follow additional research. Researchers have attempted to provide further insight into the neurolinguistic dynamics of translation. Price *et al.* (1999), for example, suggest a particular location of the translation mechanism in the brain, as suggested by their fMRI research (see, also, Paradis, 1982).

Conclusion

Remarkable progress has been made in advancing our understanding of the bilingual brain. Future research will, in part due to the availability of neuroimaging, provide answers to the many questions still waiting to be answered. While these answers will be of interest on their own, they will also provide a framework within which more informed judgments can be made about second language teaching by educators and about assessment and treatment by SLPs.

References

Albert, M.L. and Obler, L.K. (1978) *The Bilingual Brain: Neuropsychological and Neurolinguistic Aspects of Bilingualism.* New York: Academic Press.

Alvarez, R.P., Holcomb, P.J. and Grainger, J. (2003) Accessing word meaning in two languages: An event-related brain potential study of beginning bilinguals. *Brain and Language* 87, 290–304.

April, R.S. and Han, M. (1980) Crossed aphasia in a right-handed bilingual Chinese man. *Archives of Neurology* 37, 342–346.

Arámbula, G. (1992) Acquired neurological disabilities in Hispanic adults. In H. Langdon (ed.) *Hispanic Children and Adults with Communication Disorders: Assessment and Intervention* (pp. 373–407). Gaithersburg, MD: Aspen.

Butler, Y.G. and Hakuta, K. (2004) Bilingualism and second language acquisition. In T.K. Bhatia and W.C. Ritchie (eds) *The Handbook of Bilingualism* (pp. 114–144). Malden, MA: Blackwell.

Centeno, J.G. (2005) Working with bilingual individuals with aphasia: The case of a Spanish–English bilingual client. *American Speech-Language-Hearing Association Division 14: Perspectives on Communication Disorders and Sciences in Culturally and Linguistically Diverse Populations* 12, 2–7.

Dehaene, S., Dupoux, E., Mehler, J., Cohen, L., Paulesu, E., van de Moortele, P.-F., Lehericy, S. and Le Bihan, D. (1997) Anatomical variability in the cortical representation of the first and second language. *Neuroreport* 8, 3809–3815.

Dulay, H., Burt, M. and Krashen, S. (1982) *Language Two.* New York: Oxford University Press.

Fabbro, F. (1999) *The Neurolinguistics of Bilingualism: An Introduction.* East Sussex, UK: Psychology Press.

Fabbro, F. and Paradis, M. (1995) Differential impairments in four multilingual patients with subcortical lesions. In M. Paradis (ed.) *Aspects of Bilingual Aphasia* (pp. 139–176). Oxford, UK: Pergamon.

Gitterman, M.R. (2005) Aphasia in multilingual populations. In M.J. Ball (ed.) *Clinical Sociolinguistics* (pp. 219–229). Malden, MA: Blackwell.

Gitterman, M.R. and Sies, L.F. (1990) Aphasia in bilinguals and ASL signers: Implications for a theoretical model of neurolinguistic processing based on a review and synthesis of the literature. *Aphasiology* 4, 233–239.

Goldberg, E. and Costa, L.D. (1981) Hemisphere differences in the acquisition and use of descriptive systems. *Brain and Language* 14, 144–173.

Goldstein, B. (2000) *Cultural and Linguistic Diversity Resource Guide for Speech-Language Pathologists.* San Diego, CA: Singular.

Goral, M., Levy, E.S. and Obler, L.K. (2002) Neurolinguistic aspects of bilingualism. *The International Journal of Bilingualism* 6, 411–440.

Hernández, A.E., Martinez, A. and Kohnert, K. (2000) In search of the language switch: An fMRI study of picture naming in Spanish–English bilinguals. *Brain and Language* 73, 421–431.

Horowitz, B., Amunts, K., Bhattacharya, R., Patkin, D. and Braun, A. (2001) Activation of Broca's area during language production by speech and American Sign Language: Cytoarchitectural mapping and PET. Poster presented at the Annual Meeting of Society for Cognitive Neuroscience, San Francisco.

Hyltenstam, K. and Abrahamsson, N. (2003) Maturational constraints in SLA. In C.J. Doughty and M.H. Long (eds) *The Handbook of Second Language Acquisition* (pp. 539–588). Malden, MA: Blackwell.

Junqué, C., Vendrell, P., Vendrell-Brucet, J.M. and Tobena, A. (1989) Differential recovery in naming in bilingual aphasics. *Brain and Language* 36, 16–22.

Kim, K.H.S., Relkin, N.R., Lee, K. and Hirsch, J. (1997) Distinct cortical areas associated with native and second languages. *Nature* 338, 171–174.

Klein, D., Milner, B., Zatorre, R., Zhao, V. and Nikelski, J. (1999) Cerebral organization in bilinguals: A PET study of Chinese–English verb generation. *Neuroreport* 10, 2841–2846.

Krashen, S.D. (1973) Lateralization, language learning, and the critical period: Some new evidence. *Language Learning* 23, 63–74.

Kroll, J.F. and Stewart, E. (1994) Category interference in translation and picture naming: Evidence of asymmetric connections between bilingual memory representations. *Journal of Memory and Language* 33, 149–174.

Lenneberg, E.H. (1967) *Biological Foundations of Language.* New York: John Wiley and Sons.

Mendelsohn, S. (1988) Language lateralization in bilinguals: Facts and fantasy. *Journal of Neurolinguistics* 3, 261–291.

Obler, L.K., Centeno, J.G. and Eng, N. (1995) Bilingual and polyglot aphasia. In L. Menn, M. O'Connor, L.K. Obler and A. Holland (eds) *Non-Fluent Aphasia in a Multilingual World* (pp. 132–143). Amsterdam: John Benjamins.

Obler, L.K., Albert, M.L. and Gordon, H. (1975) Asymmetry of language dominance in Hebrew–English bilinguals. Paper presented at the thirteenth meeting of the Academy of Aphasia, Victoria, Canada.

Ojemann, G.A. and Whitaker, H.A. (1978) The bilingual brain. *Archives of Neurology* 35, 409–412.

Papcun, G., Krashen, S., Terbeek, D., Remington, R. and Harshman, R. (1974) Is the left hemisphere specialized for speech, language and/or something else? *Journal of the Acoustical Society of America* 55, 319–327.

Paradis, M. (1977) Bilingualism and aphasia. In H. Whitaker and H.A. Whitaker (eds) *Studies in Neurolinguistics* (Vol. 3, pp. 65–121). New York: Academic Press.

Paradis, M. (1982) Alternate antagonism with paradoxical translation behavior in two bilingual aphasia patients. *Brain and Language* 15, 55–69.

Paradis, M. (1987) *The Assessment of Bilingual Aphasia*. Hillsdale, NJ: Lawrence Erlbaum.

Paradis, M. (1998) Aphasia in bilinguals: How atypical is it? In P. Coppens, Y. Lebrun and A. Basso (eds) *Aphasia in Atypical Populations* (pp. 35–66). Mahwah, NJ: Lawrence Erlbaum.

Paradis, M. (2004) *A Neurolinguistic Theory of Bilingualism*. Amsterdam: John Benjamins.

Patkowski, M.S. (1980) The sensitive period for the acquisition of syntax in a second language. *Language Learning* 30, 449–472.

Perani, D., Paulesu, E., Galles, N.S., Dupoux, E., Dehaene, S., Bettinardi, V., Cappa, S.F., Fazio F. and Mehler, J. (1998) The bilingual brain: Proficiency and age of acquisition of the second language. *Brain* 21, 1841–1852.

Poizner, H., Klima, E.S. and Bellugi, U. (1987) *What the Hands Reveal about the Brain*. Cambridge, MA: MIT Press.

Potter, M.C., So, K.F., Von Eckardt, B. and Feldman, L.B. (1984) Lexical and conceptual representation in beginning and proficient bilinguals. *Journal of Verbal Learning and Verbal Behavior* 23, 23–38.

Price, C.J., Green, D.W. and von Studnitz, R. (1999) A functional imaging study of translation and language switching. *Brain* 122, 2221–2235.

Reynolds, D.M. and Jeyes, M.A. (1978) A developmental study of hemisphere specialization for recognition of faces in normal subjects. *Cortex* 14, 511–520.

Schneiderman, E.I. and Desmaris, C. (1988) In L.K. Obler and D. Fein (eds) *The Exceptional Brain: Neuropsychology of Talent and Special Abilities* (pp. 103–126). New York: The Guilford Press.

Scovel, T. (1981) The recognition of foreign accents in English and its implications for psycholinguistic theories of language acquisition. *Proceedings of the 5th International Association of Applied Linguistics* (pp. 389–401). Montreal: Laval University Press.

Scovel, T. (1988) *A Time to Speak: A Psycholinguistic Inquiry into the Critical Period for Human Speech*. New York: Newbury House.

Urbanik, A., Binder, M., Sobiecka, B. and Kozub, J. (2001) fMRI study of sentence generation by bilinguals differing in proficiency levels. *Revista di Neuroradiologia* 14, 11–16.

Wattendorf, E., Westerman, B., Zappatore, D., Franceschini, R., Ludi, G., Radu, E.W. and Nitsch, C. (2001) Different languages activate different fields in Broca's area. *Neuroimage* 13, S624.

Weber-Fox, C. and Neville, H.J. (1996) Maturational constraints on functional specializations for language processing: ERP and behavioral evidence in bilingual speakers. *Journal of Cognitive Neuroscience* 8, 231–256.

Chapter 5

Sociocultural, Societal, and Psychological Aspects of Bilingualism: Variables, Interactions, and Therapeutic Implications in Speech-Language Pathology

ALIZAH Z. BROZGOLD and JOSÉ G. CENTENO

Understanding bilingual speakers extends beyond the examination of their linguistic and cognitive processes. Bilingualism is a phenomenon in which the interpretation of language usage practices and proficiency also requires the analysis of the relationships between sociocultural phenomena and psychological variables, and the pertinent individual and societal factors. Besides its formal structural elements (e.g. syntax, morphology, and so forth), language can also be characterized in psychological terms as a tool to internalize culture and its concomitant affective connections (Hamers & Blanc, 2001; Pérez-Foster, 1998). Linguistic experiences in interactional routines provide the basis for the acquisition of linguistic elements that also convey both sociocultural information and emotions associated with the acquisition contexts (Ochs, 1986; Pavlenko, 2004). Bilingual speakers may experience their first (L1) and second (L2) languages[1] in different cultural environments with contrasting language usage patterns and different emotional connections (Pavlenko, 1998; Torres, 1997). Further, because bilingual development often occurs in minority contexts, emotional and affective associations to each language may stem not only from microsocial individual factors in the bilingual person's sociocultural reality but also from the larger macrosocial societal scenario operating on the bilingual speaker's ethnic group (Centeno, 2007b; Duncan, 1989).

There is clinical value in exploring the psychoemotional consequences of the interconnection among sociocultural dimensions, societal dynamics, and language use/identity in bilingual contexts. Indeed, while language choice in intervention with bilingual speakers must acknowledge a multitude of factors including the speaker's stage of bilingual development and the language usage of the family (Gutiérrez-Clellen, 1999), some scholars argue that bilingualism is a continuum in which individual language usage and proficiency may vary as a function of each bilingual speaker's ethnic identity and experienced cultural domains (Hamers & Blanc, 2001; Romaine, 1995). For example, in a study by Fishman *et al.* (1971), use of Spanish in a Puerto Rican community in New York City depended on the specific life domain, with the family being the most likely place for Spanish use, followed by friendship, religion, work, and education. A more recent study of a Puerto Rican community in a New York suburb found that most residents (61% of adults and 81% of teenagers) reported using both Spanish and English rather than either language exclusively, and that both languages coexist across cultural domains (Torres, 1997). However, while Spanish was the language preferred for speaking to parents and spouses, the younger cohort did not identify Spanish 'as the language or even a language of the United States' (Torres, 1997: 29). In addition, to these young bilinguals, English was important for educational reasons whereas Spanish was not. These examples speak to the psychological valence associated with each language as a reflection of both internal group dynamics and societal pressures on minority groups. Many bilinguals might know one language better because the educational system has schooled them in it, yet feel a stronger affective attachment to another language which was learned and used in the home (Romaine, 1995).

The purpose of this chapter is to discuss the possible interconnections among sociocultural realities, societal contexts, psychological variables, and language use/allegiance in bilingual speakers, and bring forth their possible implications in clinical communication services with bilingual speakers, particularly language choice for intervention. We draw from a broad multidisciplinary base of research and theoretical accounts, particularly sociolinguistic and ethnopsychological in nature, for our clinical arguments. Assessment issues will not be discussed here, as they have been discussed extensively in earlier works (e.g. Anderson, 2002; Centeno & Obler, 2001; Kayser, 1995; Reyes, 1995; Roberts, 2001). We focus on language decisions for intervention keeping in mind that, prior to treatment, bilingual clients have been assessed using culturally and linguistically valid testing protocols in both languages, consistent with the clients' background experiences.

The chapter is structured in three sections that will examine how language learning and usage intersect with psychological elements in bilingual speakers. For the sake of our argument, information has been divided into three sections addressing language usage in bilinguals within the context of acculturation, the bilingual speaker's psyche, and minority–majority societal relations. Some of the issues in these sections are not easily separable because they actually represent multiple interconnections of both individual and societal factors. In the first section, we discuss how language, embedded as an element in the process of acculturation, may represent ethnic identity. Next, we describe language as a processor of psychological and emotional phenomena, followed by an overview of language as a societal experience in intergroup relations. The chapter will conclude with clinical implications of the preceding phenomena for the selection of language for clinical intervention with bilingual speakers.

Language and Acculturation

The interaction between language and ethnic identity needs to be examined within the complex and larger context of acculturation. The classic definition of acculturation by Redfield *et al.* (1936: 149) was as follows: 'Acculturation comprehends those phenomena which result when groups of individuals having different cultures come into continuous first-hand contact with subsequent changes in the original cultural patterns of either or both groups.' This definition emphasized acculturation as a collective or group phenomenon. Contemporary thinking has focused more on how contact between distinct cultures results in changes in the psychology of the individual (Berry, 2002; Berry & Sam, 1996). Unlike acculturation models focusing on the psychological and social processes supporting L2 acquisition (e.g. Schumann, 1978), acculturation is currently conceptualized as a *multidimensional process* involving a gradual change in the individual along many directions in addition to language, including ethnic identity, cognitive styles, attitudes, and acculturative stress.

The range of acculturation strategies may include not only assimilation of the dominant cultural practices and integration, but also extinction of native cultural customs, separation, and marginality (Berry & Sam, 1996; Domino, 1992). Acculturation is often assessed according to the mode of identification with the majority group on a continuum from marginality to traditionality, assimilation, and, ultimately, biculturality. This range accounts for the experience of immigrants who, as a minority in a majority society, may choose to maintain their cultural heritage and language in a separate community within the new country. There is evidence that individuals explore various strategies before eventually settling on one that is more useful and/or satisfying than another. While the strategy of integration within the dominant or majority culture may be preferred by many, others opt for separation.

The factors that determine an individual's acculturation strategies are complex. They include not only personal predispositions (e.g. level of social skills and general adaptability or hardiness), but also level of proficiency in the language of the new culture, as well as the extent to which the new culture may permit an individual's or group's acculturation strategy. For instance, Hispanic immigrants who wish to integrate themselves into Anglo society experience a stronger pull to immerse themselves in Anglo cultural media, including English language television, music, and magazines, in addition to socializing with English, as opposed to Spanish, speakers. These efforts generally result in increased proficiency levels in English. Yet, while such individuals may eventually feel better integrated into Anglo society, many challenges and losses may accompany that process of acculturation.

As immigrants traverse that continuum of acculturation, they may experience a range of psychological conflicts and even crises. The new immigrant needs to acquire a new set of cultural scripts that include not only verbal language but also nonverbal communication, such as proxemics, eye contact, and facial expressions of emotion. Smart and Smart (1995) described the difficult stages of psychological adjustment among Hispanic immigrant communities. Although their subjects may have felt some 'initial joy and relief' upon coming to the USA, later ambivalence (i.e. 'post-decisional regret') was common, as well as symptomatic manifestations of stress (Smart & Smart, 1995: 392). The adjustment process took time, with a gradual reorganization of cultural identity.

Hence, embedded within acculturative changes and adaptations, *cultural or ethnic identity* formation occurs. The process, like acculturation itself, happens gradually, 'subject to change along various dimensions: over time or across generations in a new culture, in different contexts, and with age and development' (Phinney, 2003: 63). Ethnic identity is one aspect of acculturation in which the individual develops subjective feelings about his/her ethnicity and a sense of belonging in an ethnic group. Although acculturation has been measured in terms of social affiliation, cultural practices, and self-identification, the most frequent index of acculturative adaptations is language, including assessment of primary language spoken or written, language preference, language proficiency, or language use (Marín *et al.*, 2003).

Because language links individual and collective group identities and is a tool to internalize culture (Hamers & Blanc, 2001; Tabouret-Keller, 1997), it is not surprising that language may predict ethnic identity. However, the relationship between cultural affiliation and language is not uniform among bilingual speakers. Fishman (1997: 330) points out that, while for some people, 'language is the prime indicator and expression of their own and another's ethnicity; for others, language is both merely marginal and optional (i.e., detachable) vis-a-vis their ethnicity'. Nevertheless, though the link between language and ethnicity is conditioned by social, contextual, and historical circumstances, a 'detached' perspective on language and ethnicity does not prevent the language–cultural affiliation link from being experienced as a vital and basic element in social organization.

Indeed, identification with the language of an ethnocultural group depends on many factors, such as age, social context, length of residence in the country where the language is spoken, and so forth, which vary among bilingual speakers. There is considerable diversity in terms of the extent of acculturation, including language allegiance, within the members of an ethnic group (Hidalgo, 1993). As mentioned earlier, Torres (1997) found that, within a Puerto Rican bilingual community, there were different attitudes to English and Spanish, depending on the speaker's age. Particularly, for all members of the group, the use of Spanish was supported for affective reasons towards the family and culture. Interestingly, for the younger generation in the group, Spanish did not seem to have another role. They judged English as their best language and the language of education. Similarly, Matute-Bianchi (1991) carefully studied adaptations and ethnic identifications in high school students of Mexican descent in a rural California community. One central finding was that the students were quite culturally heterogeneous and had a range of strategies and accommodations to the American schooling process. They differed in terms of social identification and language use as well as dress codes. Specifically, regarding cultural affiliation and language abilities, recent immigrants still referred to Mexico as home and were mostly unilingual in Spanish. They also had varying levels of proficiency in English, and dressed differently from the other Mexican students, often being stigmatized by other students for their manner of dress. Other immigrant students that had been living in the USA longer were bilingual and still maintained strong connections with Mexico. Students considered Mexican–American were US-born and were English speakers with minimal skills in Spanish. They exhibited prominent acculturation to the US lifestyles.

There is also marked variability in the language identities of bilinguals as a group. Nero (2005) observed a large heterogeneity in the linguistic identities reported by bilingual college students upon administration of a language questionnaire. Despite being English-dominant, a large number of these bilingual students reported having more than one native language and that English, their dominant language, was not their native language. According to Nero, these observations are reflective of the students' simultaneous access to, and affiliation with, more than one language and culture. Such differential access has consequences for the level of proficiency in the students' languages, their attitudes towards the languages and affiliated groups, and the cultural knowledge that comes from participating in the various groups. Nero (2005: 201) adds that, in some cases, students' attitudes may change over time as those that consider themselves 'recent immigrants' in the first year of college (and identify with their native language more strongly than with English) might feel less like 'outsiders' later in their college years. Taken together, the foregoing studies consistently support arguments against the use of monolithic views of bilingual speakers, which do not realistically capture the full range of linguistic repertory and acculturative identities of bilingual speakers (see Nero, 2005).

In general, understanding the relationships, challenges, and outcomes in the interaction between ethnic identity formation and acculturation is complex. Research has shown that both personal and societal factors need to be assessed as each individual experiences his/her culture in the context of a larger majority society (see Centeno, 2007b, for a review). Research has also shown that cultural acceptance/rejection may vary according to gender, generation, urban versus rural locations, socio-economic circumstances, and length of residence in the USA (Hidalgo, 1993; Torres, 1997; Zentella, 1997).

The Interaction between Language and Psyche in Bilingual Speakers

Psychologists and psychoanalysts have focused on how the bilingual individual integrates and expresses the dual nature of the self when first and second languages and cultures combine. For instance, Pérez-Foster (1998: 61) coined the term 'bilingual self' to capture this sense of duality in the bilingual individual. As a psychoanalyst treating bilinguals in psychotherapy, she has eloquently described how the bilingual's internal self-representations can be differentially subsumed by two different languages. For example, the first language, with its associations to early mother/infant interactions, contains echoes of unconscious experience, while the second language may evoke the more objective experience of formal learning. Similarly, Altarriba and Morier (2004) argue that internal psychological conflict and acculturative stress will be expressed in the complex interplay of the two languages. In treatment, for example, the bilingual's choice of conducting therapy in English may be a way of fending off exploration of psychological conflicts that would more easily come to the fore in the language in which those earlier emotional connections were first established.

Research and anecdotal evidence suggests that specific emotions have different nuances in individual languages; a phenomenon that may involve adaptive challenges during the acculturation process. The indivisibility of language and culture is a key assumption here, as acquiring a second language requires learning a different reference frame for behavior and attitudes and even different ways of viewing and understanding individual emotions. For example, according to Dewaele and Pavlenko (2002), some words in English imply that emotions are conceptualized as passive states that are externally imposed or caused. This is reflected in adjectives and pseudoparticiples, such as 'worried'. In a sense, as individuals acquire a second language, they learn a new way of expressing their emotional/internal life. It is possible to think that acculturation may bring an adapted repertory of emotional scripts and vocabulary, at times leading to transformation of personal emotional scripts. Consequently, the initial phases of linguistic/cultural learning often entail a sense of emotional dislocation.

Autobiographical narratives written by bilingual authors have also been rich sources of information on the affective tones that permeate bilinguals' experiences in their two languages (Pavlenko, 1998). Kaplan (1994: 59) refers to these narratives as 'language memoirs' that chronicle the process of the writers' dislocation from their native language and culture and gradual translation into a new subjective self that incorporates elements of both the first and second languages and cultures. Similarly, the feelings of loss that accompany the process of assimilation into Anglo culture have been described by many Latino authors (e.g. Anzaldua, 1987; Rodriguez, 1982; Stavans, 2001).

In his autobiography, Rodriguez (1982: 198) describes how his parents' eagerness to assimilate and consequent relinquishment of Spanish in their household resulted in a 'falling away' of connection with his parents and a subsequent loss of emotional intimacy. As he gained English as a 'public language', he lost Spanish as his 'private language' with all its affective ties to childhood. While Rodriguez ultimately came to view his initial loss and subsequent assimilation as a gain, Anzaldua (1987: 79) asserted her ethnic identity as a Chicana with the following rallying cry: 'Ethnic identity is twin to linguistic identity. Until I can take pride in my language, I cannot take pride in myself ... Until I am free to write bilingually and to switch codes without having to translate ... my tongue will be illegitimate.'

Finally, Stavans (2001: 15) suggests that the 'losses' accompanying the metamorphosis of Latino immigrants from 'alien citizens to full-status citizens' may also turn into 'assets': 'The vanishing of a collective identity – Hispanics as eternally oppressed – necessarily implies the creation of a refreshingly different self. Confusion, once recycled, becomes effusion and revision.' Or, as Salman Rushdie said about the process of acquiring a new linguistic and cultural self (quoted in Pavlenko, 1998: 18): ' ... It is not normally supposed that something always gets lost in translation. I cling, obstinately, to the notion that something can also be gained.'

An approach that may be employed by psychologists to explore the psychological functions and nuances of L1 and L2 involves the collection of a 'psycholinguistic history' (Pérez-Foster, 1998: 103). Using an interview format, the practitioner presents the client with questions looking at psychodevelopmental factors, as well as current usage of both languages, to clarify emotional associations and situational contexts pertinent to each language. For example, some questions to probe into those areas would be: does the bilingual consider Spanish the language of his/her early feelings of disempowerment and/or abuse? Is English the language of affective disengagement because it was learned at the time of separation and individuation from primary caregivers?, and so forth. In communication disorders, similar information on affective disposition to each language may be obtained using questions on language use practices, language preferences, and personal feelings about each language, similar to those questions in acculturation scales (see Marín *et al.*, 2003, for a discussion). This information can give potent clues on the respective psychoaffective valences of the languages. When analyzing this information, however, it is important to bear in mind there is considerable variability in bilingual speakers in terms of their language-culture identities, as mentioned earlier regarding acculturation. Because language is deeply connected to cultural experiences and bilinguals experience and feel each culture differently, their language identities and emotions will reflect their individual language-culture realities.

Language Use and Motivation in a Societal Context

In addition to the motivational and affective factors accompanying acculturation and language experiences in bilingual speakers, researchers have also examined the interactions between individual social behaviors and societal attitudes. Hamers and Blanc (2001), for example, cite studies about L2 learning that emphasize the social factors. One finding is that differences in rate of L2 learning seem to vary depending on individual differences in social skills. After linguistic aptitude, motivation for learning L2 is the second most important factor in predicting achievement in acquiring L2. This motivation will be influenced by both practical and integrative reasons – the latter being reflected in the desire to resemble the speakers in the L2 community. Linking attitudes and motivations to language learning and practice situations in bilingual contexts might not be an implausible notion as 'highly motivated individuals are likely to seek out a greater amount of input than those less motivated' and, in turn, avail themselves of more practice scenarios (Cummins, 1991: 85; also see Centeno, ch. 3, this volume).

However, L2 learners' willingness to seek rich and meaningful L2 experiences may be tempered by attitudes of L2 native speakers to minority individuals. Interactional possibilities between L2 learners and native L2 speakers may be limited when native L2 individuals refuse to interact with minority individuals who may be perceived as incompetent or illegitimate L2 users (Pavlenko, 2000). Also, some L2 native speakers may find such interactions unrewarding and avoid contact (Wong Fillmore, 1991). In optimal learning scenarios, certain facilitating attributes are necessary in both learner and speaker. Personality, social style, social competence, motivation, and attitudes in both learners and speakers of L2 can affect language learning (Wong Fillmore, 1991).

Individual affective disposition in minority L2 learners requires the examination of the social–psychological processes participating in intergroup relations in a multiethnic society. Schumann (1978) posited that acculturation and bilingual attainment depends on the interaction of both *social distance* and *psychological distance* between the L2 learner and L2 speaker. In broad terms, the more politically, socially, economically, and culturally distant two groups feel, the farther the social and psychological distances between the two. In defiance, the subordinate minority may resist learning the language of the dominant majority. Similarly, Ogbu (2002) provides a useful taxonomy to explain attitudinal differences in minorities. Ogbu distinguishes between immigrant or voluntary minorities from nonimmigrant or nonvoluntary minorities. Although these two groups live in the same majority society and may experience similar prejudices, they react to it differently. Briefly, voluntary minorities chose to move to a new country and, while facing prejudice, perceive themselves doing better than in their country of origin and seek the tools to overcome barriers in the new country. They see emigration to the homeland as an option. In contrast, involuntary minorities, incorporated through colonization, conquest, birth, or slavery, live in a country against their will. Their limited motivational disposition reflects a history of mistreatment.

Lack of support and pressure from the majority group has an impact on the self-perceptions of members of a minority group and their adherence to their own culture and language (Centeno, 2007b). In the face of prejudice and discrimination, members of a minority group may assert their group identity, including their language, as a way to deal with the threats to their sense of self (Phinney, 2003). Some members of the minority group will unwillingly tend to shift to the majority language, as the minority language is seen as lacking prestige and not associated with academic achievement and economic progress (Appel & Muysken, 1987; Grosjean, 1982). They may also encourage their young to emphasize learning the majority language to protect them from the negative experiences they had as immigrants and to prevent them from being stigmatized later in life (Grosjean, 1982). Also, children of a stigmatized minority may decide not to use their native language so as not to be differentiated from the children of the majority group (Grosjean, 1982).

Hence, the sociopolitical scenario in which minority individuals live cannot be separated from their motivational and affective disposition to the two cultures they experience daily (Centeno, 2007b; also see Zentella, 2003). Acculturative adaptations are diverse because they reflect individual life histories. However, they represent important personality processes resulting from individual expectations and goals as well as societal pressures. It is of paramount importance for speech-language clinicians to bear in mind that cultural identification and its effect on L2 learning involve the interaction of both individual and societal factors.

Clinical Implications in Speech-Language Intervention

This chapter has outlined some of the critical and complex social, cultural, and psychological issues to be considered when pursuing intervention with bilingual speakers in speech-language pathology. Central to our discussion was the tenet that language usage in bilinguals needs to be interpreted within the context of acculturation, the bilingual speaker's psyche, and minority–majority societal relations. Although all three areas may not always be easily separable, our discussion underscores that language decisions for therapy would benefit from the understanding of bilingual speakers' individual language experiences and their culture–emotion associations within their home and in relation to the majority society at large. Because bilinguals represent considerable heterogeneity in terms of their extent of acculturation, language identities, and levels of bilingualism (Centeno, 2007b; Nero, 2005; Rodriguez & Olswang, 2002; Torres, 1997; Zentella, 1997, 2003), the interaction between sociocultural history and psychological phenomena requires individual attention. Further, it is important to be mindful that, very often in minority situations, both microsocial individual elements, involving conflict and stigma, cannot be divorced from the macrosocial societal circumstances differentiating languages along sociopolitical lines. Societal attitudes to minority groups have repercussions in the life of minority individuals, the perception of their culture (including their language), and the education of their children (Centeno, 2007b; Duncan, 1989; Hamers & Blanc, 2001; Mahon *et al.*, 2003).

Hence, like in contexts of psychological and educational services (e.g. Altarriba & Bauer, 1998; Altarriba & Morier, 2004; Nero, 2005), speech-language clinicians' awareness of the interplay between language, culture, motivational disposition, and societal attitudes is not just a matter of theoretical interest but is a critical factor in the successful provision of clinical services to the bilingual client (see Centeno, 2007a). For example, encouraging the bilingual client to 'choose' English as the language of treatment may, for one family, be a valued step toward acculturation and assimilation but, for another family, symbolize a demeaning loss of cultural identity and ethnic pride. In addition to these powerful psychosocial factors, despite the paucity in the literature on speech-language intervention with bilingual speakers, there is interdisciplinary theoretical and clinical ground suggesting the importance of sociocultural factors and emotional valence in therapeutic contexts with bilingual clients.

The ethnopsychology literature gives us preliminary evidence suggesting that memories seem to be encoded in a language-specific manner (Schrauf & Rubin, 2000). It also tells us that emotional content may be a facilitating factor linked to information retrieval in bilingual individuals; memories of information experienced in the native language are typically more intense and richer in terms of emotional valence when recounted in that specific language (Schrauf, 2000). Although some concerns have been raised on this research (e.g. lack of theory) (see Altarriba & Morier, 2004; Heredia & Brown, 2004, for a discussion), these preliminary works have several strengths. Because participants consistently reported information in the language that it was experienced, these studies suggest the possible connection between emotional experiences and the specific language of the experiences. Further, these studies give an applied interpretation to bilingual memory beyond theoretical constructs that has clinical value for the social and naturalistic enhancement of language retrieval/use in clinical settings. This latter strength is particularly important, based on reports that culture-specific linguistic elements may be useful to create or eliminate emotional distance, and recreate events more accurately during therapy (Altarriba & Morier, 2004).

The speech-language pathology, sociolinguistics, and neurolinguistics literature similarly provides support to the importance of language usage and culture–emotion connections in therapy. First, emotions have been argued to be part of the cognitive mechanism which, in combination with perception, attention, and memory, supports learning and, in turn, therapeutic language gains in bilingual children (Kohnert & Derr, 2004). Second, language(s) used in treatment must reflect daily communication routines and contexts, and proficiency levels (Centeno, 2003, 2005; Gutiérrez-Clellen, 1999; Roberts, 2001). Third, while emotions experienced in each language during acquisitional stages seem to have a powerful role regulating 'affective strengths' for each language in bilingual children (Pearson *et al.*, 1997: 54), such emotional associations may enhance or discourage language choice for expression after a stroke (see Paradis, 1989, for a review). Also, as claimed regarding unilingual speakers, therapy activities involving language and concepts meaningfully related to the clients' past seem to have a positive role in enhancing participation and language recall during therapy (Harris, 1997).

In summary, the combination of theoretical principles and empirical evidence from various disciplines, including ethnopsychology, speech-language pathology, sociolinguistics, and neurolinguistics, may be useful for language selection when treating the communicatively impaired bilingual person. In addition to language proficiency results from testing, language choice in intervention with bilingual speakers would benefit from acknowledging the individual affective interconnections among sociocultural dimensions, societal dynamics, and language use/identity. Prior to selecting the language of intervention, a thorough sociolinguistic interview, examining language use practices, language preferences, and feelings towards each language, would be extremely valuable. This interview would provide important information to assess contextual variables of language use as well as motivational and psychological factors that will influence language selection for treatment (also see Centeno, 2007a). Also, language choice must be respectful of the preferences of the family and/or client, and, obviously, whether therapy is conducted monolingually or bilingually, the intervention program must be based on the client's available resources in his/her language(s). As culturally competent clinicians, our language treatment of bilingual individuals must be based on the realistic understanding of the complex interaction among language use, ethnic/linguistic identity, and psychoemotional processes. The overall goal is to enhance communication in the most optimal contexts, keeping in mind the cultural and linguistic rights of the individual.

Notes

1. It is understood that, for many bilinguals, there is no first or second language because both languages are learned simultaneously from birth. Some authors identify this bilingual environment as *bilingualism as a first language or bilingual first language acquisition* (De Houwer, 1995; Meisel, 1990). However, in this chapter, we use L1 and L2 to identify languages used by two different ethnocultural groups regardless of the bilingual context.

References

Anderson, R.T. (2002) Practical assessment strategies with Hispanic students. In A.E. Brice (ed.) *The Hispanic Child: Speech, Language, Culture, and Education* (pp. 143–184). Boston: Allyn and Bacon.

Altarriba, J. and Bauer, L.M. (1998) Counseling the Hispanic client: Cuban Americans, Mexican Americans, and Puerto Ricans. *Journal of Counseling and Development* 76, 389–395.

Altarriba, J. and Morier, R. (2004) Bilingualism: Language, emotions, and mental health. In T.J. Bhatia and W.C. Richie (eds) *The Handbook of Bilingualism* (pp. 250–280). Malden, MA: Blackwell.

Anzaldua, G. (1987) *Borderland/La Frontera: The New Mestiza*. San Francisco, CA: Aunt Lute Books.

Appel, R. and Muysken, P. (1987) *Language Contact and Bilingualism*. London: Edward Arnold.

Berry, J.W. (2002) Conceptual approaches to acculturation. In K.M. Chun, P.B. Organista and G. Marín (eds) *Acculturation: Advances in Theory, Measurement, and Applied Research* (pp. 17–38). Washington, DC: American Psychological Corporation.

Berry, J.W. and Sam, D.L. (1996) Acculturation and adaptation. In J.W. Berry, M.H. Segall and I. Kagitcibasi (eds) *Handbook of Cross-cultural Psychology* (Vol. 3, pp. 291–326). Boston: Allyn and Bacon.

Centeno, J.G. (2003) Evaluating communication skills in bilingual students: Important considerations on the role of the speech-language pathologist. In E. Watkins (ed.) *ELL Companion to Reducing Bias in Special Education Evaluation* (pp. 171–178). Minneapolis: Department of Education.

Centeno, J.G. (2005) Working with bilingual individuals with aphasia: The case of a Spanish–English bilingual client. *American Speech-Language-Hearing Association Division 14: Perspectives on Communication Disorders and Sciences in Culturally and Linguistically Diverse Populations* 12, 2–7.

Centeno, J.G. (2007a) Considerations for an ethnopsycholinguistic framework for aphasia intervention with bilingual speakers. In A. Ardila and E. Ramos (eds) *Speech and Language Disorders in Bilinguals.* New York: Nova Science.

Centeno, J.G. (2007b) From theory to realistic praxis: Service-learning as a teaching method to enhance speech-language pathology services with minority populations. In A.J. Wurr and J. Hellebrandt (eds) *Learning the Language of Global Citizenship: Service-learning in Applied Linguistics.* Bolton, MA: Anker.

Centeno, J.G. and Obler, L.K. (2001) Principles of bilingualism. In M. Pontón and J.L. Carrión (eds) *Neuropsychology and the Hispanic Patient: A Clinical Handbook* (pp. 75–86). Mahwah, NJ: Lawrence Erlbaum.

Cummins, J. (1991) Interdependence of first- and second-language proficiency in bilingual children. In E. Bialystok (ed.) *Language Processing in Bilingual Children* (pp. 70–89). Cambridge: Cambridge University Press.

De Houwer, A. (1995) Bilingual language acquisition. In P. Fletcher and B. MacWinney (eds) *The Handbook of Child Language.* London: Basil Blackwell.

Dewaele, J.M. and Pavlenko, A. (2002) Emotion vocabulary in interlanguage. *Language Learning* 52, 263–322.

Domino, G. (1992) Acculturation of Hispanics. In S.B. Knouse, P. Rosenfeld and A.L. Culbertson (eds) *Hispanics in the Workplace.* Newbury Park, CA: Sage.

Duncan, D.M. (1989) Issues in bilingualism research. In D.M. Duncan (ed.) *Working with Bilingual Language Disability* (pp. 18–35). London: Chapman and Hall.

Fishman, J.A. (1997) Language and ethnicity: The view from within. In F. Coulmas (ed.) *The Handbook of Sociolinguistics* (pp. 327–343). Oxford: Blackwell.

Fishman, J.A., Cooper, R.L. and Ma, R. (eds) (1971) *Bilingualism in the Barrio.* Bloomington: Indiana University Press.

Grosjean, F. (1982) *Life with Two Languages: An Introduction to Bilingualism.* Cambridge: Harvard University.

Gutiérrez-Clellen, V.F. (1999) Language choice in intervention with bilingual children. *American Journal of Speech-Language Pathology* 8, 291–302.

Hamers, J.F. and Blanc, M.H.A. (2001) *Bilinguality and Bilingualism* (2nd edn). Cambridge: Cambridge University.

Harris, J.L. (1997). Reminiscence: A culturally and developmentally appropriate language intervention for older adults. *American Journal of Speech-Language Pathology* 6, 19–25.

Heredia, R.R. and Brown, J.M. (2004) Bilingual memory. In T.J. Bhatia and W.C. Richie (eds) *The Handbook of Bilingualism* (pp. 225–249). Malden, MA: Blackwell.

Hidalgo, M. (1993) The dialectics of Spanish language loyalty and maintenance on the U.S.–Mexico border: A two–generation study. In A. Roca and J.M. Lipsky (eds) *Spanish in The United States: Linguistic Contact and Diversity* (pp.47–74). Berlin: Mouton de Gruyter.
Kaplan, A. (1994) On language memoir. In A. Bammer (ed.) *Displacements: Cultural Identities in Question* (pp. 59–70). Bloomington: Indiana University Press.
Kayser, H. (1995) Assessment of speech and language impairments in bilingual children. In H. Kayser (ed.) *Bilingual Speech-Language Pathology: An Hispanic Focus* (pp. 243–264). San Diego: Singular.
Kohnert, K. and Derr, A. (2004) Language intervention with bilingual children. In B.A. Goldstein (ed.) *Bilingual Language Development and Disorders in Spanish–English Speakers* (pp. 311–338). Baltimore: Paul H. Brookes.
Mahon, M., Crutchley, A. and Quinn, T. (2003) New directions in the assessment of bilingual children. *Child Language Teaching and Therapy* 19, 237–244.
Marín, G., Organista, P.B. and Chun, R.M. (2003) Acculturation research: current issues and findings. In G. Bernal, J.E. Trimble, A.K. Burlew and F.T.L. Leong (eds) *Handbook of Racial and Ethnic Minority Psychology* (pp. 208–219). Thousand Oaks, CA: Sage Publications
Matute-Bianchi, M. (1991) Situational ethnicity and patterns of school performance among immigrant Mexican-descent students. In M. Gibson and J. Ogbu (eds) *Minority Status and Schooling* (pp. 205–247). New York: Garland.
Meisel, J. (1990) *Two First Languages: Early Grammatical Development in Bilingual Children*. Dordrecht: Foris.
Nero, S. (2005) Language, identities, and ESL pedagogy. *Language and Education* 19, 194–211.
Ochs, E. (1986) Introduction. In B.B. Schieffelin and E. Ochs (eds) *Language Socialization across Cultures* (pp. 1–13). Cambridge: Cambridge University Press.
Ogbu, J.U. (2002) Cultural amplifiers of intelligence: IQ and minority status in cross-cultural perspective. In J. Fish (ed.) *Race and Intelligence: Separating Science from Myth* (pp. 241–280). Mahwah, NJ: Erlbaum.
Paradis, M. (1989) Bilingual and polyglot aphasia. In F. Boller and J. Grafman (eds) *Handbook of Neuropsychology* (Vol. 2, pp. 117–140). New York: Elsevier.
Pavlenko, A. (1998) Second language learning by adults: testimonies of bilingual writers. *Issues in Applied Linguistics* 9, 3–19.
Pavlenko, A. (2000) Access to linguistic resources: key variables in second language learning. *Estudios de Sociolingüística* 1, 85–106.
Pavlenko, A. (2004) 'Stop doing that, *la Komu Skazala!*': Language choice and emotions in parent–child communication. *Journal of Multilingual and Multicultural Development* 25, 179–203.
Pearson, B., Fernández, M., Lewedeg, V. and Oller, K. (1997) The relation of input factors to lexical learning by bilingual infants. *Applied Psycholinguistics* 18, 41–58.
Pérez-Foster, R. (1998) *The Power of Language in the Clinical Process: Assessing and Treating the Bilingual Person*. Northvale, NJ: Jason Aronson.
Phinney, J.S. (2003) Ethnic identity and acculturation. In K.M. Chun, P.B. Organista and G. Marín (eds) *Acculturation: Advances in Theory, Measurement, and Applied Research* (pp. 63–82). Washington, DC: American Psychological Association.
Redfield, R., Linton, R. and Herskovits, M. (1936) Memorandum for the study of acculturation. *American Anthropologist* 38, 149–152.

Reyes, B.A. (1995) Considerations in the assessment and treatment of neurogenic communication disorders in bilingual adults. In H. Kayser (ed.) *Bilingual Speech-language Pathology: An Hispanic Focus* (pp. 153–182). San Diego: Singular.

Roberts, P.M. (2001) Aphasia assessment and treatment for bilingual and culturally diverse clients. In R. Chapey (ed.) *Language Intervention Strategies in Adult Aphasia* (4th edn, pp. 208–234). Baltimore, MD: Williams and Wilkins.

Rodriguez, B. and Olswang, L.B. (2002) Cultural diversity is more than group differences: An example from the Mexican American community. *Contemporary Issues in Communication Science and Disorders* 29, 154–164.

Rodriguez, R. (1982) *Hunger of Memory: The Education of Richard Rodriguez: An Autobiography.* New York: Bantam Books.

Romaine, S. (1995) *Bilingualism* (2nd edn). London, UK: Blackwell Publishers.

Schrauf, R.W. (2000) Bilingual autobiographical memory: Experimental studies and clinical cases. *Culture and Psychology* 6, 387–417.

Schrauf, R.W. and Rubin, D.C. (2000) Internal languages of retrieval: The bilingual encoding of memories for the personal past. *Memory and Cognition* 28, 616–623.

Schumann, J. (1978) The acculturation model for second language acquisition. In R.C. Gingras (ed.) *Second Language Acquisition and Foreign Language Teaching* (pp. 27–50). Arlington: Center for Applied Linguistics.

Smart, J.F. and Smart, D. (1995) Acculturative stress of Hispanics: Loss and challenges. *Journal of Counseling and Development* 73, 390–396.

Stavans, I. (2001) *The Hispanic Condition: The Power of a People.* New York: Harper Collins.

Tabouret-Keller, A. (1997) Language and identity. In F. Coulmas (ed.) *The Handbook of Sociolinguistics* (pp. 315–326). Oxford, UK: Blackwell Publishers.

Torres, L. (1997) *Puerto Rican Discourse: A Sociolinguistic Study of a New York suburb.* Mahwah, NJ: Lawrence Erlbaum.

Wong Fillmore, L. (1991) Second-language learning in children: A model of language learning in social context. In E. Bialystok (ed.) *Language Processing in Bilingual Children* (pp. 49–69). Cambridge: Cambridge University Press.

Zentella, A.C. (1997) Spanish in New York. In O. Garcia and J. Fishman (eds) *The Multilingual Apple: Languages in New York City* (pp. 167–202). Berlin: Mouton de Gruyter.

Zentella, A.C. (2003) José, can you see? Latin responses to racist discourse. In D. Sommer (ed.) *Bilingual Games: Some Literary Investigation* (pp. 51–66). New York: Palgrave MacMillan.

Chapter 6
Cross-linguistic Research: The Convergence of Monolingual and Bilingual Data

RAQUEL T. ANDERSON

During the last three decades, there has been an increase of published research on language acquisition and use across a variety of languages (e.g. Berman & Slobin, 1994; Slobin, 1985). This increase has resulted in great gains in our understanding of how language 'works', that is, how language is structured and what factors impact its development and different manifestations. For researchers and clinicians who work with linguistically diverse populations, access to such research has certainly improved how the study of language acquisition and disorders is approached and how services are provided to individuals with language disorders. This increase is clearly visible for Spanish. Studies have described developmental patterns in children who are acquiring Spanish as a first language from varied theoretical perspectives (e.g. Anderson, 1998; Johnson, 1995; López-Ornat, 1997; Torrens & Wexler, 1996). In addition, studies on atypical acquisition (e.g. Anderson, 2001; Restrepo & Gutiérrez-Clellen, 2001) and on acquired disorders (e.g. Centeno & Obler, 2001, 2003; Cuetos et al., 2002), although not extensive, are readily available to both researchers and clinicians.

While the increase in data from Spanish speakers provides those working with this language group necessary and relevant information, it is important to note that most of the research has been conducted with monolingual speakers of the language. For those working with Spanish speakers in a language contact situation such as the bilingual context in the USA, the usefulness of such data has been questioned (Kayser, 1995), especially for clinical populations where decisions concerning the presence of disability and intervention goals have to be established. As Centeno notes (ch. 3, this volume), because the target population's language skill and developmental path may differ due to sociolinguistic variables present in language contact situations, monolingual data have often not been considered relevant for individuals in a bilingual context.

The purpose of the present chapter is to discuss how cross-linguistic data, both monolingual and bilingual and from a variety of languages, can aid both researchers and clinicians in speech-language pathology who work with Spanish-speaking populations from different *socio-linguistic contexts*. The value of cross-linguistic data in the study of how language is organized will be presented. In addition, particular ways in which such data can inform both research and clinical work with Spanish speakers will be described. The focus will be on their application to child populations, both typical and atypical, although cross-linguistic data can certainly guide research and practice with adult populations, as well (e.g. Bates *et al.*, 1991; Menn & Obler, 1990). The discussion will center mainly on grammatical development, as this area has been studied extensively in language acquisition in both monolingual and bilingual populations.

The General Value of Cross-linguistic Data

Cross-linguistic investigations provide both researchers and practitioners in clinical communication with descriptions of developmental patterns that aid in understanding how the process of acquisition in typical and atypical populations occurs. These descriptive data thus provide a framework for identifying developmental disorders and how different language functions/forms emerge in the process of both normal and atypical acquisition. Most of the initial studies were descriptive in nature (e.g. Bowerman, 1973, in Jakubowicz, 1996). These, in turn, focused mainly on describing how different languages follow similar, as well as dissimilar, developmental paths. The data were then used to test theoretical explanations for the mechanisms underlying language development and disorders.

More recent studies have approached cross-linguistic study from an alternative perspective. Although this perspective also describes and compares patterns across languages, it develops its research paradigm, and, thus, methodology, based on particular theoretical approaches to language acquisition and use (Jakubowicz, 1996). The data are collected or re-evaluated to test particular predictions concerning language development from the theoretical perspective under scrutiny. Hence, the research is not merely descriptive in nature, but *theory-driven*. Such research serves to evaluate the strength of various theoretical constructs concerning how language develops and what may account for the patterns noted in a variety of disordered populations, such as those with specific language impairment (e.g. Ravid *et al.*, 2003; Wexler, 2003). Cross-linguistic data are, thus, essential for testing theories of acquisition, as any theory must explain both similarities and differences noted across language groups.

The Cross-linguistic Data: Monolingual Versus Bilingual Populations

A careful look at the cross-linguistic data available suggests that there are four main types of research endeavors: (1) monolingual speaker data on one language group for comparison with previous research on other languages or for description of the patterns observed in the target language (e.g. Pizzuto & Caselli, 1994; Restrepo & Gutiérrez-Clellen, 2001); (2) monolingual speaker data on two different languages following similar methodological procedures (e.g. Gathercole & Min, 1997; Pérez-Leroux & Schulz, 1999); (3) comparison of language skills across two (or more) languages spoken by a bilingual/multilingual individual (e.g. Paradis & Genesee, 1996; Sinka & Schelleter, 1998); and (4) description of language patterns in one language spoken by a bilingual/multilingual person (e.g. Bayley *et al.*, 1998). Thus, cross-linguistic data can be of two main types: (1) cross-language comparisons across individuals, and (2) cross-language comparisons within individuals. In the former type, both bilingual and monolingual individuals are studied. In the latter type, languages are contrasted as they are used by one individual, either bilingual or multilingual.

One of the issues that arises from a monolingual-versus-bilingual participant dichotomy is that researchers/clinicians who work with one or the other population question the usefulness of the data obtained from studies with individuals that do not share the same language experiences. Furthermore, for those working with bilingual individuals, issues pertaining to the sociolinguistic environment and experience may also impact the applicability of the research with individuals in language contact situations. Examples of these aspects include when the two languages were acquired and the particular social context in which they are learned.

Studies of early acquisition of two languages suggest that both similarities and differences in developmental patterns between monolingual and bilingual children exist. For example, a study on the grammatical development of French–English learning toddlers by Paradis and Genesee (1996) reported that grammatical skill, at least for the structures targeted in each language, paralleled what had been reported in the English and French monolingual developmental research. On the other hand, other researchers suggest that, although certain aspects of development parallel what is observed in monolingual children, differences in the patterns of use of certain grammatical forms may emerge. Data from the analysis of samples obtained from Dutch–French and German–Italian children acquiring the two languages simultaneously report that for grammatical forms where pragmatics and syntax interact, and where these languages are similar at the surface level, *cross-linguistic influence* occurs (Hulk & Müller, 2000). Thus, depending on the target languages being acquired, there may be cross-linguistic influence and thus development may differ from what has been reported in monolingual data.

Furthermore, data from children who are learning a second language sequentially (i.e. generally after 3 years of age, McLaughlin, 1978) suggest both similar and distinct patterns of development from those of monolingual learners. For example, in a study of the acquisition of English auxiliary forms by two Hebrew-speaking children who were learning English as a new language, Armon Lotem (1998) noted that particular errors produced by the children did not follow the expected forms observed in monolingual learners of the target language. These nontarget responses could not be solely explained by first language transference, that is, Hebrew structure impacting acquisition. This suggests that both general language-learning principles, as well as information available from the first language to second language learners, influence development. Similar findings have been reported for second language learners of other language pairs (e.g. Gass & Selinker, 2001; Lakshmanan, 1995).

Applying Cross-linguistic Data to Research and Clinical Practice with Spanish-speakers

Because of the differences and similarities that have been reported, researchers and clinicians may find it difficult to discern how cross-linguistic data, both monolingual and bilingual, may aid them as they unravel the processes underlying Spanish acquisition and use. Data from a variety of sources, languages, and populations can assist both clinicians and researchers working with the Spanish-speaking population across the world. What is essential is that the data be understood within the context in which it was gathered, and used to the extent that it can help us to understand how language works and how it may be impacted by a variety of factors.

Cross-linguistic data and research applications

Individuals studying language abilities/disabilities with Spanish-speaking populations can use cross-linguistic data for two main purposes: (1) comparison, and (2) development of methodology to evaluate the explanatory power of various theoretical approaches to the study of language. Contrasting what has been reported across a variety of languages and language learners, including Spanish, gives researchers relevant information concerning the regularities of language, including patterns of acquisition in typical and atypical populations. For example, research on Spanish-speaking children in bilingual learning contexts as well as monolingual environments demonstrates that they follow a similar developmental path with respect to the determiner system (see Anderson & Centeno, ch. 1, for relevant discussion on Spanish morphosyntax). Studies with children who were learning Basque and Spanish (Ezeizabarrena, 1997; Idiazabal, 1995), as well as children who were acquiring Spanish in a monolingual community (Baauw, 2001), show very early acquisition of this system, thus suggesting that, during the early stages of development, the determiner system in Spanish is robust, regardless of the language learning environment.

Cross-linguistic research also provides information about language aspects that may be impacted by language-specific or environmental factors. For example, a study on novel word learning by Gathercole and Min (1997) evaluated word-meaning biases in children from three language backgrounds: English, Spanish, and Korean. Preschool children were taught new words and were tested to determine to which new objects they would apply the label they had just learned. These new objects were similar to the original object in various aspects, specifically shape, substance, and/or function. Results supported the proposal that the structure of the target language impacts the children's extension of the meaning of a word to new objects. Specifically, the language groups differed with respect to the object qualities they used as cues for extending the meaning of the newly learned word. While Spanish-speaking and English-speaking children used shape as a cue, the Korean-speaking cohort demonstrated a preference for utilizing substance-based characteristics for extending word meanings. Thus, cross-language (and cross-population) comparisons can inform us on those aspects of language that are universal, or shared across linguistic varieties, and those that are influenced by the specific language environment.

Because cross-linguistic data focus on comparisons, they are important for testing the explanatory power of various theories concerning how language is acquired, and how it is affected by factors such as sociolinguistic environment and disability. Any theory that attempts to explain the mechanisms underlying language acquisition, as well as how language is structured, must draw on a variety of sources, among different languages and different language learners. This approach is necessary as language is a shared faculty. Researchers who work with Spanish speakers can thus use the cross-linguistic data to develop similar methodologies and to test the explanatory power of various theoretical constructs.

Cross-linguistic data and clinical applications

A common belief among clinicians is that only data that are specific to the target language – and even its dialectal variants – and obtained from populations that share similar sociolinguistic characteristics should be used for clinical application. This approach has stemmed, in part, from the pattern where children often were incorrectly diagnosed as presenting a language disability because their performance was contrasted to that of children who were learning the same language but in different contexts. In particular, concerns were raised about the use of monolingual data for clinical decision-making when working with children in a language contact situation (Anderson, 2003; Restrepo & Silverman, 2001). While this strategy may be problematic, data from a variety of sources can be used by clinicians to establish linguistically and culturally fair assessment and intervention strategies. The difficulty lies not in the value of the data, but in how it is used.

How can seemingly disparate data aid clinicians? First, by studying regularities and differences across languages, clinicians can identify those aspects of language that are more universal in nature, and thus less prone to be impacted by environmental factors, and those that are readily impacted by contextual idiosyncrasies. Such an approach, in turn, is beneficial for the development of assessment techniques and methodologies that can be applied across language groups. For example, the study of tense and aspect in Spanish-speakers, as well as in other language groups, suggests that different verbs have inherent biases toward a particular aspect. Verbs that are stative (e.g. *estar*, *ser* 'to be'), or refer to activities (e.g. *caminar* 'to walk'), because they do not have an explicit or definable ending, tend to receive imperfective marking more frequently (e.g. *caminaba*, *estaba*), in contrast to those verbs that have a definable end-point, such as verbs of accomplishments and achievements (e.g. *dormirse* 'to fall sleep', *correr una milla* 'to run a mile') (see Anderson & Centeno, ch. 1, for a discussion on Spanish verb morphology). These latter forms clearly indicate the completion of an activity. Spanish acquisition data suggest that children begin to use perfective aspect with verbs of accomplishment and achievement and imperfective aspect with stative and activity verbs. As they develop language, Spanish-speaking children extend the use of both aspects across all verb types. Research with Spanish-speaking children in a language contact situation and with varied levels of Spanish proficiency show that use of the feature aspect begins to be restricted to particular verb types, similar to the pattern noted in monolingual acquisition (Bayley *et al.*, 1998). Thus, this reduction in contrastive use of aspect within verb types appears to be related to general language skill. Clinicians who may be interested in evaluating verb morphology in children who are in a language contact situation can actually use these data to develop testing probes that consider the patterns of acquisition, and still provide information concerning how proficient children are in their language, in this case Spanish.

Having both monolingual and bilingual data at their disposal, clinicians can also identify factors that impact language performance and, therefore, adjust their clinical interventions accordingly. In this way, they are cognizant of the client and background information they need to interpret their client's performance. Without such data, it would be difficult to identify these important factors that can assist clinicians in the interpretation of an individual's language skills.

In summary, it is important for clinicians to recognize the value of cross-linguistic research, both monolingual and bilingual, and across a variety of languages. Such research provides a more comprehensive picture of what language is rather than simply relying on within-language comparisons. Further, it can particularly show how language is impacted by environmental factors and what aspects of language are significant for study, thus enhancing linguistic assessment in our clients. What is essential to understand is how cross-linguistic comparison is to be used. For speech-language professionals who treat language-disordered individuals, it is of paramount importance to have as much knowledge as possible of the construct being studied: language. The confluence of data from a variety of languages and language groups will increase such knowledge. Although this chapter focused on child language issues, a similar cross-language approach may actually be informative in both research and practice with clinical adult populations (e.g. Bates *et al.*, 1991; Menn & Obler, 1990), as well.

References

Anderson, R.T. (1998) The development of grammatical case distinctions in the use of personal pronouns in Spanish-speaking preschoolers. *Journal of Speech, Language and Hearing Research* 41, 394–406.

Anderson, R.T. (2001) Learning an inflectional morpheme in Spanish by children with typical language skills and children with specific language impairment (SLI). *International Journal of Language and Communication Disorders* 36, 1–19.

Anderson, R.T. (2003) Practical assessment strategies with Hispanic students. In A.E. Brice (ed.) *The Hispanic Child: Speech, Language, Culture and Education* (pp. 143–184). Boston, MA: Allyn and Bacon.

Armon Lotem, S. (1998) What to do with *have* and *be*: Auxiliary verbs in child second language acquisition. *University of Maryland Working Papers in Linguistics* 6, 1–11.

Baauw, S. (2001) Expletive determiners in child Dutch and Spanish. *BUCLD 25 Proceedings*, 82–93.

Bates, E., Wulfeck, B. and MacWhinney, B. (1991) Cross-linguistic research in aphasia: An overview. *Brain and Language* 41, 123–148.

Bayley, R., Alvarez-Calderón, A. and Schecter, S.R. (1998) Tense and aspect in Mexican-origin children's Spanish narratives. In E.V. Clark (ed.) *The Proceedings of the Twenty-ninth Annual Child Language Research Forum* (pp. 221–230). Stanford, CA: Center for the Study of Language and Information.

Berman, R.A. and Slobin, D.I. (1994) *Relating Events in Narrative: a Crosslinguistic Developmental Study*. Hillside, NJ: Lawrence Erlbaum.

Centeno, J.G. and Obler, L.K. (2001) Agrammatic verb errors in Spanish speakers and their normal discourse correlates. *Journal of Neurolinguistics* 14, 349–363.

Centeno, J.G. and Obler, J. (2003) Agramatismo expresivo en español. In E. Matute and F. Leal (eds) *Introducción al Estudio del Español desde una Perspectiva Multidisciplinaria* (pp. 469–486). Guadalajara, México: Universidad de Guadalajara.

Cuetos, F., Aguado, G., Izura, C. and Ellis, A.W. (2002) Aphasic naming in Spanish: Predictors and errors. *Brain and Language* 82, 344–365.

Ezeizabarrena, M.J. (1997) Morfemas de concordancia con el sujeto y los objetos en el castellano infantil. In A.T. Pérez-Leroux and W.R. Glass (eds) *Contemporary Perspectives on the Acquisition of Spanish. Volume 1: Developing Grammars* (pp. 21–36). Sommerville, MA: Cascadilla Press.

Gass, S.M. and Selinker, L. (2001) *Second Language Acquisition.* Mahwah, NJ: Erlbaum.

Gathercole, V.C.M. and Min, H. (1997) Word meaning biases or language-specific effects? Evidence from English, Spanish, and Korean. *First Language* 17, 31–56.

Hulk, A. and Müller, N. (2000) Bilingual first language acquisition as the interface between syntax and pragmatics. *Bilingualism: Language and Cognition* 3, 227–244.

Idiazabal, I. (1995) First stages in the acquisition of noun phrase determiners by a Basque–Spanish bilingual child. In C. Silva-Corvalán (ed) *Spanish in Four Continents: Studies in Language Contact and Bilingualism* (pp. 260–278). Washington, DC: Georgetown University Press.

Jakubowicz, C. (1996) Crosslinguistic investigation. In D. McDaniel, C. McKee and H.S. Cairns (eds) *Methods for Assessing Children's Syntax* (pp. 257–285). Cambridge, MA: MIT Press.

Johnson, C.M. (1995) Verb errors in the early acquisition of Mexican and Castilian Spanish. In E.V. Clark (ed.) *The Proceedings of the Twenty-ninth Annual Child Language Research Forum* (pp. 221–230). Standford, CA: Center for the Study of Language and Information.

Kayser, H. (ed.) (1995) *Bilingual Speech-Language Pathology: An Hispanic Focus.* San Diego, CA: Singular.

Lakshmanan, U. (1995) Child second language acquisition of syntax. *Studies in Second Language Acquisition* 17, 301–329.

López-Ornat, S. (1997) What lies between a pre-grammatical and a grammatical representation? Evidence on nominal and verbal form-function mappings in Spanish from 1;7 to 2;1. In A.T. Pérez-Leroux and W.R. Glass (eds) *Contemporary Perspectives on the Acquisition of Spanish. Volume 1: Developing Grammars* (pp. 3–20). Sommerville, MA: Cascadilla Press.

McLaughlin, B. (1978) *Second-language Acquisition in Childhood.* Hillsdale, NJ: Lawrence Earlbaum.

Menn, L. and Obler, L.K. (1990) *Agrammatic Aphasia (Vol. 1–3).* Amsterdam: John Benjamins.

Paradis, J. and Genesee, F. (1996) Syntactic acquisition in bilingual children. *Second Language Acquisition* 18, 1–25.

Pérez-Leroux, A. and Schulz, P. (1999) The role of tense and aspect in the acquisition of factivity: Children's interpretation of factive complements in English, German and Spanish. *First Language* 19, 29–54.

Pizzuto, E. and Caselli, M.C. (1994) The acquisition of Italian verb morphology in a cross-linguistic perspective. In Y. Levy (ed.) *Other Children, Other Languages* (pp. 137–187). Hillsdale, NJ: Erlbaum.

Ravid, D., Levie, R. and Ben-zvi, G.A. (2003) The role of language typology in linguistic development: Implications for the study of language disorders. In Y. Levy and J. Schaeffer (eds) *Language Competence Across Populations: Toward a Definition of Specific Language Impairment* (pp. 171–196). Mahwah, NJ: Erlbaum.

Restrepo, M.A. and Gutiérrez-Clellen, V.F. (2001) Article use in Spanish-speaking children with specific language impairment. *Journal of Child Language* 28, 433–452.

Restrepo, M.A. and Silverman, S.W. (2001) Validity of the Spanish Preschool Language Scale-3 for use with bilingual children. *American Journal of Speech-Language Pathology* 10, 382–393.

Sinka, I. and Schelleter, C. (1998) Morphosyntactic development in bilingual children. *International Journal of Bilingualism* 2, 301–326.

Slobin, D.I. (ed.) (1985) *The Crosslinguistic Study of Language Acquisition.* Hillsdale, NJ: Erlbaum.

Torrens, V. and Wexler, K. (1996) Clitic doubling in early Spanish. *BUCLD 20 Proceedings* 780–791.

Wexler, K. (2003) Lenneberg's dream: Learning, normal language development, and specific language impairment. In Y. Levy and J. Schaeffer (eds) *Language Competence Across Populations: Toward a Definition of Specific Language Impairment* (pp. 11–62). Mahwah, NJ: Erlbaum.

Chapter 7

The Cognitive Neuropsychology of Language Disorders among Spanish Speakers

BRENDAN STUART WEEKES

Speech-language pathology students and practitioners need conceptual frameworks to assess and treat communication disorders among Spanish speakers, including cognitive models to generate predictions about language problems that follow damage to the brain. Cognitive neuropsychologists use cognitive models to explain why language impairments occur (see Caramazza, 1986). This contrasts with the traditional syndrome approach in language pathology (Zurif *et al.*, 1989). Cognitive neuropsychology involves a reciprocal relationship between theories of normal language processing and clinical investigations of acquired disorders of language. Data from case studies of clinical patients are used to develop theories of language processing, and patterns of impaired and preserved language are interpreted within models of normal processing. A pattern of acquired impairment is assumed to reflect selective breakdown or *functional dissociation* in modular processing systems. The cognitive neuropsychological approach has been applied to communication problems in Spanish.

The aim of this chapter is to illustrate how a *conceptual framework* can be used to generate predictions about language impairments including naming (anomia), reading (dyslexia) and writing (dysgraphia) in Spanish. Data from single case studies of aphasic Spanish speakers will be reviewed to illustrate how a model assuming modular representations for phonology, orthography, and semantics can explain disorders in reading and spelling (i.e. in the mappings between print and sound) (see Figure 7.1). The motivation for this chapter is to encourage practitioners to apply cognitive models to clinical work. The focus of the chapter will be on patterns of acquired dyslexia and dysgraphia because these disorders are the best documented disorders of communication in Spanish.

Cognitive Models of Reading and Writing in English

Much of our understanding of normal reading and writing in English comes from cognitive modeling. Early modular views (Coltheart, 1978)

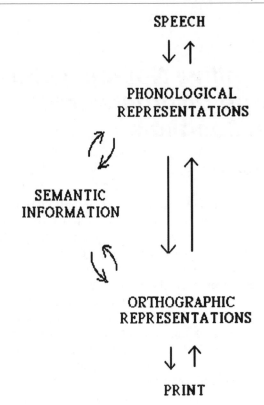

SPEECH

PHONOLOGICAL
REPRESENTATIONS

SEMANTIC
INFORMATION

ORTHOGRAPHIC
REPRESENTATIONS

PRINT

Figure 7.1 The interactive triangle framework of reading and writing

and recent computational models (Coltheart *et al.*, 2001; Plaut *et al.*, 1996) have been enhanced by case studies of aphasic patients. The dissociations between impaired and preserved reading and writing in acquired surface and phonological dyslexia/dysgraphia illustrate this point. Surface dyslexia in English refers to poor reading of irregularly spelled words and preserved reading of regular words and nonwords (e.g. *zint*). The impairment to irregular word reading is most severe for low-frequency words that have an abstract meaning (e.g. *indict*). Surface dyslexics produce regularization errors (e.g. *yacht* → [jɑtʃɪd]) reflecting mispronunciation of graphemes. A grapheme refers to single/multiletter orthographic representation of a phoneme. The patient may also misunderstand homophones (e.g. the word *stake* is defined as an edible piece of meat). Surface dysgraphic patients produce incorrect but phonologically plausible spellings for irregular words (e.g. *yacht* → *yot*) and produce homophone confusions when writing (e.g. he ordered *stake* for dinner).

Phonological dyslexia refers to poor reading of nonwords and preserved reading of words even if they are irregularly spelled. Some phonological dyslexics show an effect of imageability on oral reading where concrete nouns (e.g. *dog*) are read aloud better than abstract words (e.g. *justice*). Similarly, phonological dysgraphic patients spell nonwords poorly but write regular and irregular words without error. Deep dyslexia is an extreme form of phonological dyslexia where patients make semantic, visual, and morphological errors (e.g. *justice* is read as *peace*). Deep dysgraphic patients make errors writing words to dictation (e.g. symphony → *orchestra*).

Coltheart *et al.* (2001) proposed a *multiroute computational model* to explain normal and impaired oral reading in English. This model has a *lexical semantic* pathway available for reading known words and a *direct lexical* pathway that can read without contacting the meaning of the word. The model also contains a *nonlexical* grapheme-to-phoneme route that is mandatory for correct reading of nonwords but cannot be used to read irregular words correctly. Plaut *et al.* (1996) proposed a *connectionist model*, which assumes two bidirectional routes, a *semantic* pathway and a *phonological* pathway, are available for normal reading. Connectionist models eschew lexical whole word representations in favor of components at the level of the onset (beginning), vowel, and coda (end) of syllabic structure. Thus, the terms *lexical-semantic* and *nonlexical* grapheme to phoneme used by Coltheart are *semantic* and *phonological* pathways respectively for Plaut. The differences between modular and nonmodular models are that Plaut assumes that reading of nonwords in the phonological pathway proceeds via a process of analogy and not by rules; and Coltheart assumes independent direct lexical and lexical-semantic pathways but Plaut does not.

Can Models of Reading and Writing in English be Applied to Spanish?

Some writers have argued that because of the transparent nature of the Spanish spelling system – where orthography maps onto phonology in a regular and consistent manner – reading and writing in Spanish is always mediated by phonology and, hence, is nonlexical (Ardila, 1991). However, this is not correct. Spanish speakers develop a lexicon for known words and this is accessed for normal reading and writing. This can be seen in the effects of frequency and imageability on normal performance (also see Iribarren, ch. 17, this volume). Thus, Valle-Arroyo (1996) proposed a dual route model that assumes a lexical-semantic pathway for reading in Spanish.

Evidence from case studies in aphasia supports the view that lexical-semantic and nonlexical pathways are normally available for reading and writing in Spanish. Cuetos *et al.* (1996) reported a Spanish-speaking patient, AD, who could read words correctly (90% correct) but who had difficulty reading nonwords (36% correct). They labeled this pattern *phonological dyslexia* in Spanish. AD's word recognition and comprehension were normal as were speech production and repetition, and there were no effects of lexical variables such as word frequency, grammatical class, or imageability on reading. Cuetos *et al.* (1996) argued AD could not assemble phonemes in a nonlexical reading pathway, which they assumed was necessary to read nonwords in Spanish. Similarly, Cuetos *et al.* (2003) report examples of poor nonword reading among Spanish patients with dementia, and Iribarren *et al.* (1999) reported Spanish speakers who were able to read words but not nonwords. All of these patients support a model where nonword reading in Spanish requires a nonlexical reading pathway. This is depicted in Figure 7.1 as arrows between orthography and phonology. The nonlexical pathway is damaged for phonological dyslexics leading to reliance on the lexical-semantic pathway (see Ferreres *et al.*, 2003).

Ruíz *et al.* (1994) reported two patients who made semantic errors when reading words and who read nonwords poorly. They labeled this *deep dyslexia* (see also Cuetos & Ellis, 1999; Davies & Cuetos, 2005; Ferreres & Miravalles, 1995). Semantic errors suggest reliance on the lexical-semantic pathway as, if the nonlexical reading pathway were available, the incorrect reading of related words activated in the lexicon would be inhibited. The lexical-semantic pathway is shown in Figure 7.1 as arrows between orthography, semantics, and phonology.

Phonological and deep dyslexia suggest a nonlexical reading pathway is necessary for normal oral reading in Spanish as, without it, semantic reading errors are produced. However, the existence of a lexical-semantic pathway for oral reading in Spanish is yet to be proven. If nonword reading is more difficult than word reading and more susceptible to brain damage, then poor reading of nonwords alone would not count as evidence that words are not read via a nonlexical pathway. More convincing evidence of dissociable reading pathways will come from a case who cannot use the lexical-semantic pathway but who can read words correctly (i.e. the reverse dissociation to phonological and deep dyslexia in Spanish). If this hypothetical case were reported it could not be argued that the dissociation between poor nonword and word reading is a consequence of task difficulty.

Iribarren et al. (1996) reported *surface dyslexia* in Spanish (also see Iribarren, ch. 17, this volume). The key symptom is production of errors when reading words with highly lexicalized stress in Spanish. The regular pattern of stress assignment in Spanish requires the penultimate syllable of a word to carry stress. However, some words (e.g. *corazón* 'heart') break this rule by assigning stress at the end of the word. Surface dyslexics misapply the rule (e.g. reading *coraZON* as *coRAzon*). Other manifestations of surface dyslexia are lexical effects on reading and homophone errors (e.g. *vaso* 'glass' defined as *spleen*). According to Iribarren *et al.* (1996), surface dyslexia reflects impairment to a lexical-semantic pathway for reading in Spanish. Without this pathway, reading is overly reliant on the nonlexical pathway. As the nonlexical pathway contains no lexical representations, surface dyslexic patients cannot assign appropriate stress to irregular words. However, nonword reading in surface dyslexia remains intact. Surface dyslexia suggests that word and nonword reading are dissociable skills in Spanish.

A corresponding pattern of errors can be observed among patients with acquired dysgraphia in Spanish. Iribarren *et al.* (2001) report two patterns of dysgraphia. In the first, surface dysgraphia, one patient had impaired writing of homophones and irregular words and, in the second, phonological dysgraphia, a different patient showed impaired writing of nonwords with preserved writing of irregular words (see also Ardila *et al.*, 1996). Irregularly spelled words in Spanish contain phonemes with multiple spellings (e.g. /k/ is spelled either as *c* [when followed by <a>, <o>, <u>, or liquid consonants; e.g. contra, clase]; *qu* [when followed by <e> or <i>; e.g. que], or *k* [in some exception words; e.g. kilo]). Iribarren *et al.* (2001) argued that surface and phonological dysgraphia show that lexical and nonlexical pathways are available for writing in Spanish (see also Cuetos, 1993).

Predictions

One prediction from the framework shown in Figure 7.1 is that impairments to the mappings between print and sound should impact on reading and writing in Spanish in a graded fashion. For example, abolition of the direct pathway means access to phonology from print, or conversely from phonology to print, will be severely impaired. This would explain the relatively rare occurrence of acquired deep dyslexia/dysgraphia in Spanish whereby semantic errors are produced in reading and writing. Milder damage to the direct route produces the commonly reported pattern of phonological dyslexia/dysgraphia that is poor reading of nonwords without semantic errors due to the possibility of reading/writing via the damaged direct reading pathway.

Impaired access to the lexical-semantic pathway will result in acquired surface dyslexia and dysgraphia in Spanish. The rationale for this claim comes from connectionist models. These models assume that semantic knowledge is used to prevent regularization errors in normal reading and writing by inhibiting competing and possibly more common pronunciations of subword components (Patterson *et al.*, 1994). Inhibition allows the cognitive system to settle on the correct but atypical or less common pronunciation (or spelling) of an irregular word. According to this view, more common pronunciations or spellings of irregular words will dominate in reading and writing without support from semantic memory resulting in regularization errors.

One prediction that follows is that impairments to semantic memory will be associated with surface dyslexia and surface dysgraphia in Spanish. These phenomena could manifest in a number of ways. As noted by Iribarren *et al.* (2001), 17% of polysyllabic words have stress on the last syllable (most words ending in a consonant, e.g. favor) and some are stressed three or more syllables from the last (e.g. *rápido* 'fast') although these words are rare (3%) (Alcoba & Murillo, 1998). Other irregularities from print to sound include the silent letter < h > ; the written letter < x > , which can be pronounced as /s/ as in *xenofobia*, /gs/ as in *examen*, /ks/ as in *tórax* 'thorax', and /h/ as in México; the letter < y > which takes a vocalic value as a conjunction and a consonantal value in other contexts; and the letter < r > , which at the beginning of a word or before < n > must be read as if it were < rr > . Irregularities from print to sound include the sound /b/, spelled < b > in some words and < v > in others; the sound /g/, written as < g > (as in *gas*) or < gu > (*guerra* 'war') depending on what sound follows; the sound /x/, spelled < j > (as in *jefe* 'boss') or g (before < e > or < i > as *general* and *giro* 'turn'); the sound /s/, spelled as < z > (as in *zapato* 'shoe') or c (before < e > and < i >); the sound /j/ , written as < y > as in *ya* 'already' and < ll > as in *valle* 'valley'; the spelling of < rr > is /r/ at the beginning of words and /ʃ/ in between vowels. In addition, in American Spanish and in some dialects of Spain, the sound /s/ can be spelled < s > or < c > (again before < e > and < i >) (also see Anderson & Centeno, ch. 1, this volume).

Support from semantic memory might be required to recall the correct pronunciation and stress when reading rare words and may also be necessary to recall correct spellings of such words when writing from memory or dictation (though see Del Ser *et al.*, 1997 for a contrasting view on reading in dementia).

Conclusion

The triangle framework depicted in Figure 7.1 assumes that proficient reading and writing in Spanish depends on a division of labor between lexical-semantic and direct pathways without reference to hypothetical modules (cf. Roch-Lecours *et al.*, 1999). One direction for future research is why literacy is slow to develop in some Spanish speakers (Gimenez de la Pena, 2004). There is evidence that Spanish children learn to read and to spell using a variety of strategies and selective problems in the acquisition of literacy can resemble acquired phonological and surface dyslexia in Spanish (Defior *et al.*, 1996; Dominguez & Cuetos, 1992; Jimenez & Hernández, 2000; Valle-Arroyo, 1996). Further study of single cases – both acquired and developmental – must be motivated by predictions derived from models in the tradition of classical cognitive neuropsychology. Such studies can reveal evidence of the cognitive processes used to read and write in Spanish as well as of the modularity in the language processing system. Ultimately, this approach will lead to evidence- and theory-grounded treatment methods for reading and writing problems in Spanish speakers (Weekes & Coltheart, 1996).

References

Alcoba, S. and Murillo, J. (1998) Intonation in Spanish. In D. Hirst and R. Di Cristo (eds) *Intonation Systems*. Cambridge: Cambridge University Press.

Ardila, A. (1991) Errors resembling semantic paralexias in Spanish speaking aphasics. *Brain and Language* 41, 437–445.

Ardila, A., Rosseli, M. and Ostrosky-Solis, F. (1996) Agraphia in the Spanish language. *Aphasiology* 10, 723–729.

Caramazza, A. (1986) On drawing inferences about the structure of normal cognitive systems from the analysis of patterns of impaired performance: The case for single-patient studies. *Brain and Cognition* 5, 41–66.

Coltheart, M. (1978) Lexical access in simple reading tasks. In G. Underwood (ed.) *Strategies of Information Processing* (pp. 151–216). London: Academic Press.

Coltheart, M., Rastle, K., Perry, C., Langdon, R. and Ziegler, J. (2001) DRC: A dual route cascaded model of visual word recognition and reading aloud. *Psychological Review* 108, 204–256.

Cuetos, F. (1993) Writing processes in a shallow orthography. *Reading and Writing: An Interdisciplinary Journal* 5, 17–28.

Cuetos, F. and Ellis, A.W. (1999) Visual paralexias in a Spanish-speaking patient with acquired dyslexia: A consequence of visual and semantic impairments? *Cortex* 35, 661–674.

Cuetos, F. and Labos, E. (2001) The autonomy of the orthographic pathway in a shallow language: Data from an aphasic patient. *Aphasiology* 15, 333–342.

Cuetos, F., Martinez, T., Martinez, C., Izura, C. and Ellis, A.W. (2003) Lexical processing in Spanish patients with probable Alzheimer's disease. *Cognitive Brain Research* 17, 549–561.

Cuetos, F., Valle-Arroyo, F. and Suarez, M.P. (1996) A case of phonological dyslexia in Spanish. *Cognitive Neuropsychology* 13, 1–24.

Davies, R. and Cuetos, F. (2005) Acquired dyslexia in Spanish: A review and some observations on a new case of deep dyslexia. *Behavioural Neurology* 16, 85–101.

Defior, S., Justicia, F. and Martos, F. (1996) The influence of lexical and sublexical variables in normal and poor Spanish readers. *Reading and Writing* 8, 487–497.

Del Ser, T., Gonzalez-Montalvo, J.-I., Martinez-Espinosa, S., Delgado-Villapalos, C. and Bermejo, F. (1997) Estimation of pre-morbid intelligence in Spanish people with the word accentuation test and its application to the diagnosis of dementia. *Brain and Cognition* 33, 343–356.

Dominguez, A. and Cuetos, F. (1992) Desarrollo de las habilidades de reconocimiento de palabras en niños con distinta competencia lectora. *Cognitiva* 42, 193–208.

Ferreres, A.R., Lopez, C. and China, N. (2003) Phonological alexia with consonant-vowel dissociation in non word reading. *Brain and Language* 84, 399–413.

Ferreres, A.R., Martinex Cuitino, M. and Olmedo, A. (2005). Acquired surface alexia in Spanish: A case report. *Behavioural Neurology* 16, 71–84.

Ferreres, A.R. and Miravalles, G. (1995) The production of semantic paralexias in a Spanish-speaking aphasic. *Brain and Language* 49, 153–172.

Gimenez de la Pena, A. (2004) Dyslexia in Spanish. In I. Smythe, J. Everatt and R. Salter (eds) *International Book of Dyslexia* (pp. 184–197). Chichester, UK: John Wiley and Sons.

Iribarren, I.C., Jarema, G. and Lecours, A.R. (1996) The assessment of surface dyslexia in a regular orthography, Spanish: A case study. *Brain and Cognition* 32, 196–198.

Iribarren, I.C., Jarema, G. and Lecours, A.R. (1999) Lexical reading in Spanish: Two cases of phonological dyslexia. *Applied Psycholinguistics* 20, 407–428.

Iribarren, I.C., Jarema, G. and Lecours, A.R. (2001) Two different dysgraphic syndromes in a regular orthography, Spanish. *Brain and Language* 77, 166–175.

Jimenez, J.E. and Hernández, I. (2000) Word identification and reading disorders in the Spanish language. *Journal of Learning Disabilities* 33, 44–60.

Patterson, K., Graham N. and Hodges, J. (1994) Reading in Alzheimer's type dementia: A preserved ability? *Neuropsychology* 8, 395–407.

Plaut, D.C., McClelland, J.D., Seidenberg, M.S. and Patterson, K. (1996) Understanding normal and impaired word reading: Computational principles in quasi-regular domains. *Psychological Review* 103, 56–115.

Roch-Lecours, A., Dieguez-Vide, F., Bohm, P., Tainturier, M.J., Gold, D. and Peña-Casanova, J. (1999) Acquired dyslexias and dysgraphias (I): A cognitive model for the analysis of disturbances of reading and writing in Spanish. *Journal of Neurolinguistics* 12, 95–114.

Ruíz, A., Ansaldo, A.I. and Lecours, A.R. (1994) Two cases of deep dyslexia in unilingual Hispanophone aphasics. *Brain and Language* 46, 245–256.

Valle-Arroyo, F. (1989) Errores en lectura y escritura: Un modelo dual. *Cognitiva* 2, 35–63.

Valle-Arroyo, F. (1996) Dual route models in Spanish: developmental and neuropsychological data. In M. Carreiras, J.E. Garcia-Albea and N. Sebastian (eds) *Language Processing in Spanish* (pp. 89–118). Hillsdale, NJ: Lawrence Erlbaum.

Weekes, B. and Coltheart, M. (1996) Surface dyslexia and surface dysgraphia: Treatment studies and their theoretical implications. *Cognitive Neuropsychology* 13, 277–315.

Zurif, E.B., Gardner, H. and Brownell, H.H. (1989) The case against the case against group studies. *Brain and Cognition* 10, 237–255.

Chapter 8

Ethical and Methodological Considerations in Clinical Communication Research with Hispanic Populations

JOSÉ G. CENTENO and WILLARD GINGERICH

Conducting clinical communication studies with culturally and linguistically diverse (CLD) groups imposes challenges on the investigator. Particularly, research must be guided by sensitivity and respect to the population being studied, especially considering the realistic understanding of the different normative phenomena of the group (Kayser, 1995; Silverman, 1997). A crucial concern is ensuring that the development and implementation of the different steps of the research protocol reflect the typical social, cultural, socioeconomic, educational, and linguistic factors of the target group (Hammer, 2000; Kayser, 1995; Marín & Marín, 1991; Mertens, 1998). The investigators' lack of sensitivity to, and understanding of, the group's typical dynamics would seriously compromise even initial steps in the study, such as access to the community, as well as the ethical and methodological integrity of the research effort.

The purpose of this chapter is to provide an overview of the most important principles on clinical communication research with CLD populations with an emphasis on issues relevant to Hispanic groups in the USA. As ethics in research is integral to the planning and implementation of the research protocol, we will start with a discussion on the legal and ethical guidelines in clinical communication investigations. We will continue with descriptions of demographic and cultural aspects of the Hispanic community in the USA and consider the ramifications of these variables for the research process. Next, we will address methodological considerations in clinical communication investigations on Hispanic individuals in the USA. Finally, we will conclude with implications of the above discussions for future research in clinical communication in CLD groups, particularly in Hispanic communities.

Ethical Considerations in Research

The Code of Ethics of the American Speech-Language-Hearing Association (ASHA) considers the rights and welfare of research participants of paramount importance (ASHA, 2002). ASHA's professional guidelines are consistent with the federal mandate on protection of individuals recruited to participate in research. In its *Belmont Report*, the National Commission for the Protection of Human Subjects in Biomedical and Behavioral Research (1979) identifies three ethical principles and six norms to guide research. The three ethical principles, namely, beneficence, respect, and justice, respectively describe the positive outcomes to humanity that research should have, the courteous and respectful treatment that research participants should receive, and ensures that procedures are nonexploitative and fairly administered. The six norms of scientific research emphasize the use of valid designs, the participation of competent researchers, the explanation of both compensation and possible consequences of the research methods to the participants, and the appropriate selection and voluntary participation of participants in the study.

Regarding minorities, the National Institutes of Health (NIH) and Alcohol, Drug Abuse, and Mental Health Administration (ADMHA) specifically enacted policies requiring the inclusion of women and minorities in study populations (NIH, 1990; 1994). These policies are consistent with findings on the *under-representation of ethnic minorities* documented in the literature (Burlew, 2003).

Such official policies provide legal grounds to enforce fair research procedures. Yet, despite those governmental regulations, there are additional considerations necessary to implement sensitive research steps and make accurate methodological and analytical decisions. We next provide an overview of such considerations.

Demographic Overview of the Hispanic Population in the USA

Individuals with a Spanish origin or descent in the USA frequently are identified as Hispanic or Latino(a). Despite differences in meaning, both labels often are used interchangeably. *Hispanic*, a label derived from the Latin word 'Hispania' (Spain), is the official term coined to identify individuals of Spanish origin or descent. *Latino(a)* describes an origin from a Latin American country, including Portuguese-speaking Brazil and English-speaking Belize and the Guyanas (Marín & Marín, 1991). Nonetheless, as described later, because Hispanics or Latinos(as) in the USA represent a very diverse demographic profile, use of either label as an umbrella term can obscure specific differences among Hispanic/Latino(a) groups and among individuals in a Hispanic/Latino(a) group (also see Introduction to this volume for a related discussion). Particularly for research purposes, individual background characteristics need to be described.

The US Hispanic population is growing rapidly. Hispanics currently represent 42 million people or 14% of the total US population including both the continental territory and Puerto Rico (US Census Bureau, 2003). After African–Americans, Hispanics constitute the largest minority group in the US with an estimated increase to 25% of the overall population by 2050 (National Alliance for Hispanic Health, 2004). Moreover, important population trends among Hispanics have been reported (National Alliance for Hispanic Health, 2004). The Hispanic population is particularly young, with a median age of 25.8 years, compared with 38.6 years for non-Hispanics, and families are generally larger than among non-Hispanics in the USA. The majority of Hispanics are employed yet they are disproportionately likely to have low-paying uninsured jobs. Additionally, a high rate of high-school dropouts, at least since 1970, has also been reported for Hispanics.

Hispanics in the USA are a heterogeneous group who generally share language and aspects of Hispanic culture (Marín & Marín, 1991; National Alliance for Hispanic Health, 2004). They represent different countries of origin and varied educational and socioeconomic levels, and, linguistically speaking, a wide range of receptive and expressive skills in Spanish and English (Centeno & Obler, 2001; Roca & Lipsky, 1993; also see Introduction to this volume). As supported by the latest population reports, Mexican–Americans constitute the largest group followed by Central Americans and South Americans, Puerto Ricans, Cubans, and other Hispanics (US Census Bureau, 2002). In terms of annual earnings, Puerto Ricans are over-represented in the low-income bracket followed by Mexican–Americans, Cubans, Central and South Americans, and other Hispanics. Regarding educational attainments, Mexicans represent the largest group in the 'less than high school diploma' category followed by Central and South Americans, Puerto Ricans, and Cuban–Americans. Finally, regarding language, Hispanics employ a number of dialectal varieties of Spanish consistent with their countries and regions of origin. They also show different proficiency levels in Spanish and English, thus being identified as monolingual, when having minimal skills in either language, or bilingual, when having considerable skills in both languages (Centeno & Obler, 2001; Iglesias, 2002). Such discrepancies in socioeconomic, educational, and linguistic backgrounds among Hispanics need to be analyzed carefully when looking at each subgroup and individual because they have confounding effects on many other variables such as health risk, access to health care, and overall social achievements (Iglesias, 2002).

Cultural Factors in Research on Hispanic Populations

Characteristics of the target population must be understood for appropriate approaches to research and the collection of valid findings.

Particularly, formulation of the questions to be investigated, participant selection, research design, and data interpretation must realistically reflect the perspective of the individuals being studied (Burlew, 2003; Huer *et al.*, 2003; Kayser, 1995; Silverman, 1997).

Before turning to their ramifications for research, a number of culturally based characteristics of Hispanics in the USA need to be considered. It is important to bear in mind that the group or individual presence of these characteristics depends on a complex interaction of higher-level factors such as acculturation levels, generational factors, ancestry, and sociopolitical circumstances (Hidalgo, 1993; Matute-Bianchi, 1991; also see Brozgold & Centeno, ch. 5, this volume).

Acculturation refers to changes in the original culture experienced by an individual or group when contrasting cultural communities are in frequent contact (Marín *et al.*, 2003). Rather than being a unidimensional quantifiable phenomenon, acculturation involves multiple factors such as language preference, beliefs, group affiliation, gender roles, attitudes, and self-identity (Pontón, 2001b). Understanding the relationships, challenges, and outcomes in the interaction between ethnic identity formation and acculturation in minority–majority contexts is complex. Research has shown that both personal and societal factors need to be assessed as both minority group and individual separately experience their culture in the context of a larger majority society (Centeno, 2007; also see Brozgold & Centeno, ch. 5, this volume). Indeed, drawing from reports on Hispanics in the USA, cultural acceptance/rejection may vary according to gender, generation, urban versus rural locations, socio-economic circumstances, length of residence in the new country, and pressures from the majority society on the minority group and its members (see Hidalgo, 1993; Torres, 1997; Zentella, 1997).

For example, members of Hispanic groups who are born in the USA and are young tend to prefer English and more closely identify with American cultural values than foreign-born and older Hispanics (Matute-Bianchi, 1991; Zentella, 1997). Further, Hispanic individuals of any age may gravitate toward American norms, including the use of English, in situations of social pressure from the majority community (Hidalgo, 1993). Consequently, acculturation differences among Latinos(as) in the USA play an important role in defining heterogeneity within the group. Next, based on the extensive discussions provided by Marín and Marín (1991) and Pontón (2001a; 2001b), we summarize the most important variables pertinent to communication research on Hispanics, cautioning the reader to bear in mind that, due to acculturation levels, these factors may operate differently within the various Hispanic groups and its members.

Latinos(as) have been characterized as embracing certain attitudes in their social networks. Latino(a) communities tend to have a strong sense of collectivism, or *allocentrism*, in which, rather than stressing individuals' needs, the group's needs and objectives are emphasized. At the family level, Hispanics similarly show a strong identification with, and attachment to, their nuclear and extended families. This cultural phenomenon, labeled as *familialism* or *familism* (Marín & Marín, 1991), tends to involve strong loyalty and solidarity among members of the same family. Additionally, Hispanics also emphasize smooth and pleasant social interactions, or *simpatía*, hence showing empathy with the feelings of other people, minimizing conflict, and showing respect to others (Marín & Marín, 1991).

Distance – both metaphoric and literal – is another cultural phenomenon in Hispanic groups that requires attention. At a larger social level, power differentials play a role in determining the distance among individuals by promoting deference and respect toward certain groups or individuals (e.g. the rich, the educated, the aged). During conversation, Hispanic individuals have been shown to prefer shorter physical distances with their interlocutors than non-Hispanics do. Relative to non-Hispanics in the USA, Hispanics tend to have a flexible attitude to *time*, which often translates into being late for appointments or the misperception of length of time spent on tasks. Such a flexible orientation to time allows Hispanics to feel they are on time, even when they arrive late to an appointment by others' cultural norms (Marín & Marín, 1991).

Like all cultures, Hispanics have defined gender-related behaviors for both men and women. Cultural expectations for men relate to being strong, in control, as well as providers, protectors, and representatives of their families (*machismo*). In contrast, women have traditionally been viewed as caregivers devoted to the well-being and nurture of their family and living in sacred duty, self-sacrifice, and chastity; roles often associated with the special place that the Virgin Mary has in the largely Catholic Latin American culture (*marianism*) (Gil & Vazquez, 1996). Of course, not all Hispanics subscribe to these culturally stereotypic gender roles. In fact, as described later, because societal attitudes toward minority groups are generally based on stereotypes, researchers must be cautious with the possible effects of implicit attitudes and stereotyping on research with minorities (Khan, 2003.)

Finally, cultural phenomena in Hispanics in the USA cannot be examined without considering the concomitant linguistic heterogeneity in the group. As mentioned earlier in this section and elaborated on elsewhere in this book (see Anderson & Centeno, ch. 1, Brozgold & Centeno, ch. 5, and Centeno, Ch. 3, this volume), Hispanic individuals in the USA show considerable linguistic variability, representing different dialects of Spanish and varying degrees of proficiency in Spanish and English (Centeno & Obler, 2001; Iglesias, 2002). Such a linguistic scenario is a critical component when examining acculturation patterns and diversity in this community.

As with any participants in research studies, Hispanics' routine culturally determined behaviors and attitudes are likely to have an impact on their disposition, performance, and outcomes during clinical research investigations. We continue with a discussion of possible implications of the above cultural dynamics on the procedures employed in speech-language pathology research with Hispanic individuals.

Methodological Aspects in Research with Hispanic Speakers

Participant issues

Participants selected for research must be representative of the target group for valid and accurate generalization of the findings (Glattke, 2002; Mertens, 1998). An operational definition specifying the inclusion criteria used to identify the intended group of study is necessary. As described above, the Hispanic population in the USA is very diverse. On one hand, different levels of acculturation need to be understood. When differentiating among Hispanics, it is important to distinguish between race and ethnicity. While the former is a biologically determined condition resulting in physical characteristics, the latter is a complex pychoemotional phenomenon involving the interaction of acculturation levels, self-identity, language preference, social networks, and lifestyles (Marín & Marín, 1991; Mertens, 1998). In fact, in the last national census, Hispanics identified themselves with a variety of race categories, including white, Black or African–American, American Indian, Alaska Native, and Asian (US Census Bureau, 2000). On the other hand, other factors, such as different levels of bilingualism, countries of origins, and socioeconomic background, add to Hispanics' within-group heterogeneity. Yet, there are three ways Hispanic ethnicity may be operationalized: ancestry, cultural characteristics, and self-identification (Marín & Marín, 1991).

Once the target Hispanic participants have been defined, access to, recruitment, and retention of the sample follow (Burlew, 2003; Hammer, 2000; Huer *et al.*, 2003; Marín & Marín, 1991). Discussion of the numerous strategies suggested to minimize difficulties throughout such sampling steps in ethnic minorities is beyond this chapter. Most notably, minority individuals' healthy skepticism towards research and their resulting limited participation can effectively be addressed when the investigator becomes familiar with the community, establishes direct contact with potential participants, explains the legitimacy and benefits of the study to the group, obtains the sponsorship of local organizations and leaders, and provides compensation for participation in the study (Burlew, 2003; Hammer, 2000; Huer *et al.*, 2003; Marín & Marín, 1991).

The influence of cultural factors on the motivation, disposition, and interpersonal dynamics of Hispanic research participants deserves special attention. Simpatía may encourage an initial promise from the individuals to participate in the study which they may not fulfill later. Routine interactions with Hispanics who stand closer to the investigator may be misinterpreted by an investigator who is unfamiliar with the culture. On the other hand, the participant may perceive the investigator's need for more space as distant and cold, which may translate into feelings of exploitation. Additionally, as mentioned above, a flexible orientation to time may encourage Hispanics to feel they are on time even when they arrive late to their appointed times (see Marín & Marín, 1991, for an extensive discussion).

Measurement issues

Bias-free research in a multicultural environment requires instrument content, design, and administration to reflect the cultural assumptions, knowledge, and behaviors of the research participants (Bravo, 2003; Kayser, 1995; Marín & Marín, 1991). Differences in performance may not reflect a deficit but a culturally determined effect (Silverman, 1997). Particularly, measurement tools employed with ethnic minorities have to be grounded in realistic experiential, linguistic, socioeconomic, and metric principles if accurate cross-culture comparisons are to be made and realistic evidence-based clinical procedures are to be developed for the target group (Bravo, 2003; Kayser, 1995; Marín & Marín, 1991).

Linguistic content, behavioral requirements for administration, and numerical information to be obtained warrant special attention. Participants' linguistic background, be it monolingual Spanish or bilingual Spanish–English, as well as language stimuli, critically vocabulary and sentence structures, must be reflected in the stimuli and instructions used (also see Anderson, ch. 9, Anderson & Centeno, ch. 1, Centeno, ch. 3, Restrepo & Castilla, ch. 10, this volume for relevant discussions). In addition, behavioral test demands and familiarity with the test format may be in opposition to the individuals' typical routines (Bravo, 2003). For instance, a task measuring reaction time may yield inaccurate results if Hispanic research participants, based on a flexible attitude to time, provide pensive, articulate, and delayed responses to questions or other stimuli (Glattke, 2002). Additionally, some research contexts (e.g. interviews) might be seen as social occasions, rather than time-restricted sessions, by some Hispanics hence requiring the investigators to extend the length of the research activity to include social time (Huer *et al.*, 2003). Finally, if task administration employs the collection of scores, researchers must be aware of certain psychometric factors, such as available norms and content validity, that may not include or apply to the minority group in the study (Glattke, 2002; Marín & Marín, 1991).

Data interpretation issues

A number of cultural factors may have an impact on the participants' performance on tasks and, in turn, the validity of the data collected (Silverman, 1997). Marín and Marín (1991) discuss how some typical patterns in Hispanic culture, previously covered in this chapter, may affect the process and outcomes in a given study. For example, a tendency to favor respectful, nonconflictive interpersonal interactions may motivate Hispanic individuals to produce extreme, socially desirable, or acquiescent responses, or *yea-saying*, hence showing a tendency to agree in their answers. Similarly, the power/distance principle may result in exaggerated deference – by non-Hispanic standards – that Hispanic respondents may show for a researcher who comes from outside the community; a phenomenon requiring careful management to avoid extreme agreement responses during interviews. Such situations promoting extreme answers in Hispanic research participants warrant attention. These response trends impact data analysis and interpretation in a way that affects group variance and score correlations. In fact, investigators analyzing data obtained from Hispanics should examine actual score distributions rather than focusing on measures of central tendency as extreme response sets may provide inaccurate descriptions of a group's responses if only measures of central tendency are considered (Marín & Marín, 1991).

There is evidence suggesting over-reporting and under-reporting behaviors among Hispanics, like other minorities, in relating to investigators from outside the community, particularly when questions involve threatening or sensitive information. Based on an analysis of Hispanic informants' responses to health surveys, Aday *et al.* (1980) suggest that, relative to non-Hispanics in the USA, Hispanic individuals favored socially desirable responses hence over-reporting in their answers, and had a greater proportion of unanswered questions than non-Hispanics resulting in the under-reporting of information and incomplete data. Further, Hispanics may be more likely to under-report in situations of self-disclosure of personal information, such as talking about money, tastes, or when cultural gender dynamics make it difficult for the informant to speak freely to investigators of the opposite sex (Huer *et al.*, 2003; LeVine & Franco, 1981; Marín & Marín, 1991). Although there is limited evidence on such behaviors, researchers should exercise caution when administering instruments dealing with sensitive information to Hispanic research participants.

Future Directions

This chapter provided an overview of ethical, demographic, and cultural factors critical to the planning and implementation of clinical communication studies with Hispanics in the USA. Our discussion highlighted some special areas of concern relevant to participant selection and the collection of valid findings. Such logistical and methodological challenges can effectively be addressed with strategies grounded in the sound understanding of the different normative factors in Hispanic groups. Central to the research process is the realistic knowledge of typical cultural dynamics and their application throughout the conceptual, methodological, and analytical steps of the clinical communication study. Because working with Hispanic research participants, like other CLD populations, is complex, application of interdisciplinary research approaches should be helpful to enhance accuracy in the methods employed in clinical communication studies. For example, the use of acculturation measures, used in neuropsychological research (e.g. Pontón, 2001b), and multiple assessments of language identification and usage, used in sociolinguistic and neurolinguistic studies of child and adult bilingualism (e.g. De Houwer, 1995; Paradis, 2004; Torres, 1997; also see Centeno, ch. 3, this volume), would be useful tools to complement the existing battery employed in clinical communication investigations. The preceding instruments and methods would provide excellent complementary information to select and classify research participants, create appropriate tasks and stimuli, and interpret results.

Thus, training researchers to have in-depth knowledge of the different phenomena that impact communication skills in the heterogeneous Hispanic population in the USA is necessary. As Hispanics in the USA steadily increase in both numbers and diversity, the need for valid and accurate research to develop appropriate evidence-based clinical procedures for this population is imperative. Yet, in addition to the theoretical knowledge, such research must be grounded in appropriate ethical principles respecting Hispanic individuals' lives and considering their complex backgrounds. The principles discussed here, although primarily based on Hispanics in the USA, can be adapted to the unique sociocultural and linguistic contexts of Hispanic persons in other countries.

References

Aday, L.A., Chiu, G.Y. and Andersen, R. (1980) Methodological issues in health care surveys of the Hispanic heritage population. *American Journal of Public Health* 70, 367–374.

American Speech-Language-Hearing Association (2002) Ethics in research and professional practice. *ASHA Supplement* 22, 63–65.

Bravo, M. (2003) Instrument development: Cultural adaptations for ethnic minority research. In G. Bernal, J.E. Trimble, A.K. Burlew and F.T.L. Leong (eds) *Handbook of Racial and Ethnic Minority Psychology* (pp. 22–236). Thousand Oaks, CA: Sage.

108   *Part 1: Preliminary Considerations*

Burlew, A.K. (2003) Research with ethnic minorities: Conceptual, methodological, and analytical issues. In G. Bernal, J.E. Trimble, A.K. Burlew and F.T.L. Leong (eds) *Handbook of Racial and Ethnic Minority Psychology* (pp. 179–198). Thousand Oaks, CA: Sage.

Centeno, J.G. (2007) From theory to realistic praxis: Service-learning as a teaching method to enhance speech-language pathology services with minority populations. In A.J. Wurr and J. Hellebrandt (eds) *Learning the Language of Global Citizenship: Service-learning in Applied Linguistics*. Bolton, MA: Anker.

Centeno, J.G. and Obler, L.K. (2001) Principles of bilingualism. In M. Pontón and J.L. Carrión (eds) *Neuropsychology and the Hispanic Patient: A Clinical Handbook* (pp. 75–86). Mahwah, NJ: Lawrence Erlbaum.

De Houwer, A. (1995) Bilingual language acquisition. In P. Fletcher and B. MacWinney (eds) *The Handbook of Child Language* (pp. 219–250). London: Basil Blackwell.

Gil, R.M. and Vazquez, C.I. (1996) *The Maria Paradox: How Latinas Can Merge Old World Traditions with New World Self-Esteem*. New York: Berkley.

Glattke, T.J. (2002) Research involving multicultural populations. In D. Battle (ed.) *Communication Disorders in Multicultural Populations* (pp. 487–504). Boston: Butterworth-Heinemann.

Hammer, C.S. (2000) Strategies for recruiting African–American and Hispanic women as participants in research. *Contemporary Issues in Communication Science and Disorders* 27, 127–134.

Hidalgo, M. (1993) The dialectics of Spanish language loyalty and maintenance on the U.S.–Mexico border: A two-generation study. In A. Roca and J.M. Lipsky (eds) *Spanish in the United States: Linguistic Contact and Diversity* (pp. 47–74). Berlin: Mouton de Gruyter.

Huer, M.B. and Saenz, T.I. (2003) Challenges and strategies for conducting survey and focus group research with culturally diverse group. *American Journal of Speech-Language Pathology* 12, 209–220.

Iglesias, A. (2002) Latino culture. In D. Battle (ed.) *Communication Disorders in Multicultural Populations* (3rd edn, pp. 179–202). Boston: Butterworth-Heinemann.

Kayser, H. (1995). Research needs and conclusions. In H. Kayser (ed.) *Bilingual Speech-Language Pathology: An Hispanic Focus* (pp. 291–306). San Diego: Singular.

Khan, S.R. (2003) Implicit attitudes and stereotyping. In G. Bernal, J.E. Trimble, A.K. Burlew and F.T.L. Leong (eds) *Handbook of Racial and Ethnic Minority Psychology* (pp. 291–306). Thousand Oaks, CA: Sage.

LeVine, E. and Franco, J.N. (1981) A reassessment of self-disclosure patterns among Anglo Americans and Hispanics. *Journal of Counseling Psychology* 28, 522–524.

Marín, G. and Marín, B.V. (1991) *Research with Hispanic Populations*. Newbury Park, CA: Sage.

Marín, G., Organista, P.B. and Chun, R.M. (2003) Acculturation research: Current issues and findings. In G. Bernal, J.E. Trimble, A.K. Burlew and F.T.L. Leong (eds) *Handbook of Racial and Ethnic Minority Psychology* (pp. 208–219). Thousand Oaks, CA: Sage.

Matute-Bianchi, M. (1991) Situational ethnicity and patterns of school performance among immigrant Mexican-descent students. In M. Gibson and J. Ogbu (eds) *Minority Status and Schooling*. New York: Garland.

Mertens, D.M. (1998) *Research Methods in Education and Psychology: Integrating Diversity with Quantitative and Qualitative Approaches.* Thousand Oaks, CA: Sage Publications.

National Alliance for Hispanic Health (2004) *Delivering Health Care to Hispanics: A Manual for Providers.* Washington, DC: Estrella Press.

National Commission for Protection of Human Subjects of Biomedical and Behavioral Research (1979) *The Belmont Report: Ethical Principles and Guidelines for the Protection of Human Subjects of Research* (Department of Health, Education, and Welfare [DHEW] publication No. OS 78–0013). Washington, DC: Government Printing Office.

National Institutes of Health (1990) *NIH/ADAMHA Policy Concerning the Inclusion of Women and Minorities in Study Populations.* Bethesda, MD: NIH.

National Institutes of Health (1994) NIH guidelines on the inclusion of women and minorities as subjects of clinical research. *NIH Guide* 23 (11), March 18.

Paradis, M. (2004) *A Neurolinguistic Theory of Bilingualism.* Amsterdam: John Benjamins.

Pontón, M. (2001a) Hispanic culture in the United States. In M. Pontón and J.L. Carrión (eds) *Neuropsychology and the Hispanic Patient* (pp. 15–38). Mahwah, NJ: Lawrence Erlbaum.

Pontón, M. (2001b) Research and assessment issues with Hispanic populations. In M. Pontón and J.L. Carrión (eds) *Neuropsychology and the Hispanic Patient* (pp. 39–58). Mahwah, NJ: Lawrence Erlbaum.

Roca, A. and Lipsky, J.M. (1993) Introduction. In A. Roca and J.M. Lipsky (eds) *Spanish in the United States: Linguistic Contact and Diversity* (pp. 1–8). Berlin: Mouton de Gruyter.

Silverman, F.H. (1997) *Research Design and Evaluation in Speech-Language Pathology and Audiology* (4th edn). Boston: Allyn and Bacon.

Torres, L. (1997) *Puerto Rican Discourse: A Sociolinguistic Study of a New York Suburb.* Mahwah, NJ: Lawrence Erlbaum.

US Census Bureau (2000) *The Hispanic Population: Census 2000 Brief.* Washington, DC: US Census Bureau.

US Census Bureau (2002) *Annual Demographic Supplement to the March 2002 Current Population Survey.* Washington, DC: US Census Bureau.

US Census Bureau (2003) *Resident Population Estimates of the United Status by Sex, Race, and Hispanic or Latino origin* (released June 17, 2003). Washington, DC: US Census Bureau.

Zentella, A.C. (1997) Spanish. In O. Garcia and J.A. Fishman (eds) *The Multilingual Apple* (pp. 167–202). Berlin: Mouton de Gruyter.

Part 2

Research in Children: Conceptual, Methodological, Empirical, and Clinical Considerations

Chapter 9

Exploring the Grammar of Spanish-speaking Children with Specific Language Impairment

RAQUEL T. ANDERSON

Specific language impairment (SLI) is a diagnostic label for children who present with primary language learning disability in the absence of frank neurological, cognitive, and/or sensory deficits (Leonard, 1998). It has been studied extensively, as this population is well represented in speech-language caseloads. Theoretically, this clinical cohort informs us about how language is structured and how it can be impacted with other areas of cognition relatively spared. Although various areas of deficit have been noted, central to the disorder is the significant effect it has on children's grammatical skill.

Studies of this clinical group have been conducted primarily with monolingual English-speaking children, although recently there has been an increase in research with other monolingual populations such as Italian (e.g. Cipriani *et al.*, 1998), Swedish (e.g. Hansson & Nettelbladt, 1995), German (e.g. Clahsen *et al.*, 1997), and Hebrew (e.g. Leonard & Dromi, 1994). This increase in cross-linguistic examinations of SLI has been essential for the testing of various theoretical explanations concerning the nature of the disorder. Cross-linguistic research has also aided in describing how SLI is manifested across a variety of languages (see also Anderson, ch. 6, this volume).

In recent years, the study of SLI has been extended to Spanish-speaking populations, both in monolingual contexts (e.g. Anderson, 2001a) and in language contact situations (e.g. Jacobson & Schwartz, 2002). Such research has provided valuable information on how the disorder is manifested in this population and how different sociolinguistic environments may impact the language skills of Spanish-speaking children with SLI. The purpose of the present chapter is to summarize the data that have been obtained concerning the grammatical skill of Spanish-speaking children with SLI and to discuss potential areas of research with this population. Within this context, the importance of obtaining *cross-linguistic data* in the study of language disorders will be stressed. Included in this discussion are possible *methodological paradigms* that can aid us in understanding the nature of the deficit, its clinical symptoms, and the impact that sociolinguistic environment may have on its manifestation (also see Centeno & Gingerich, ch. 8, Restrepo & Castilla, ch. 10, for related discussion on research methodology with Hispanic children). The chapter will be divided into three major sections. In the first section, research on SLI with Spanish speakers is summarized and contrasted with what has been observed in other languages. The second section discusses how the observed patterns conform to the various theoretical explanations of the nature of SLI. The third section will present experimental paradigms that can provide important information concerning the nature of SLI in Spanish-speaking children, its general clinical expression, and how it can be identified in Spanish-speaking children from a variety of linguistic backgrounds and experiences.

The Nature of SLI in Spanish-speaking Children

Prior to summarizing the research on Spanish-speaking children, a brief review of the two main theoretical accounts of the nature of SLI is necessary. In general, explanations for the observed deficits noted in SLI have followed two different routes: (1) a processing/surface account, and (2) various linguistic accounts. The processing account has been formulated mainly by Leonard and colleagues (e.g. Leonard & Dromi, 1994). From this perspective, it is postulated that children with SLI have difficulty producing linguistic forms that are not perceptually salient, particularly those forms that have specific grammatical functions. Such difficulty is due to a limited processing capacity, which will result in children with SLI focusing more on salient characteristics of the input, and less on perceptually 'weaker' forms. Because of this limited processing capacity, children with SLI will have difficulty perceiving particular morphemes and identifying their grammatical function. Because languages differ as to what aspects are more salient for deriving meaning (e.g. English – word order, Spanish – inflectional morphemes), patterns of error may differ across languages (see also Anderson & Centeno, ch. 1, this volume).

The linguistic account takes one of two perspectives, one quite distinct from the other. The first, the *missing feature account*, posits that children with SLI have inherent deficits with particular grammatical phenomena (e.g. Clahsen *et al.*, 1997). These correspond to the more formal features of language, such as, for example, subject–verb agreement (as in *She walks* instead of *She walk* in Standard American English, or *Yo escucho* 'I listen to' instead of forms with alternate verb endings in Spanish). As a result, those formal features of the language that do not have a semantic interpretation, but that are primarily grammatical in nature, will be particularly difficult for children with SLI. The second linguistic account has been espoused by Wexler and Rice (e.g. Wexler, 2003). It proposes that children with SLI go through an *extended optional infinitive* (EOI) stage where use of agreement is not obligatory. As a result, children with SLI will produce both target and nontarget responses for a longer period, as contrasted to typically developing peers matched for both age and language ability. Nevertheless, the target forms, when produced, will be used correctly. In light of the existence of these three theoretical explanations of the nature of SLI, researchers have tended to study and contrast grammatical forms that vary with respect to perceptual saliency as well as with respect to the formal features of language.

Based on what has been reported in previous research with speakers of other languages (e.g. Leonard, 1998), investigators interested in describing the grammatical deficits of Spanish-speaking children with SLI have centered their study on specific linguistic features. In particular, they have addressed children's ability to produce noun phrases (NP) and to use a variety of verbal inflections. The following areas have been studied: (1) NP structure, (2) use of direct object pronouns (i.e. clitics), and (3) verb tense and agreement (see Anderson & Centeno, ch. 1, this volume for a review of pertinent linguistic features). Other research has focused on the ability of children with SLI to learn new grammatical rules via invented morpheme tasks (Anderson, 2001a; Roseberry & Connell, 1991). Although small in number, such studies have provided a broad view of the language learning abilities of Spanish-speaking children with SLI.

Noun phrase use in Spanish

Various researchers have studied the use of NP constituents, specifically articles, by Spanish-speaking children with SLI (Anderson, 2003; Anderson & Souto, 2005; Bedore & Leonard, 2001; Bosch & Serra, 1997; Restrepo & Gutiérrez-Clellen, 2001). Articles have been the focus of such research because they have been noted as being potential areas of deficits in other languages, for example English (Leonard, 1998) and Italian (Bortoloni *et al.*, 1997). Because Spanish articles provide two potential areas of difficulty (i.e. actual production of these nonsalient forms and agreement for both number and gender between them and the noun they modify), attention to children's use of these forms can, moreover, help account for the deficits observed in children with SLI.

Results from studies on children's use of articles suggest that these forms may be particularly difficult for Spanish-speaking children with SLI. Comparisons with same-age peers (Anderson, 2003; Anderson & Souto, 2005; Restrepo & Gutiérrez-Clellen, 2001) and MLU-word matched controls (Bedore & Leonard, 2001; Bosch & Serra, 1997) present a pattern whereby children with SLI are significantly less accurate in their production of articles. This trend has been noted in both spontaneous samples as well as in experimental probes, both in preschool and early elementary school-age children. Nevertheless, there is disagreement with respect to the particular pattern of error noted. Most studies indicate that the most frequent error pattern observed in the children is that of omission, particularly in the use of definite articles (e.g. *el*, *la* 'the'). This pattern corresponds to that reported for monolingual English-speaking children and monolingual Italian-speaking children with SLI (Bortoloni *et al.*, 1998), the latter being a language that is similar to Spanish with respect to NP agreement. Data reported by Restrepo and Gutiérrez-Clellen (2001), on the other hand, indicate that the main error noted in children with SLI was that of gender agreement.

Several differences in participant characteristics may explain the conflicting results with respect to the type of error. First, differences in performance may be ascribed to the participants' phonological skill. Anderson and Souto (2005) and Bosch and Serra (1997) included children with mild to significant phonological deficits in their participant sample. On the other hand, Restrepo and Gutiérrez-Clellen (2001) included only children with typical phonological skill. The former two studies reported that the children who presented with phonological deficits also pre-sented with higher incidence of article errors, mainly omission. If children omit articles altogether, then the opportunity for nontarget responses, such as gender substitution, is reduced, as one cannot see substitutions in the absence of attempted production. While relative phonological skill, thus, would appear to impact incidence of errors, differences in relative phonological skill across the studies cannot completely explain the diverging results. For example, in both Anderson and Souto's (2005) and Bosch and Serra's (1997) studies, there were children with typical phonological skill who did not present with gender substitution errors, as noted by Restrepo and Gutiérrez-Clellen (2001), even though these children had ample opportunity to produce this type of nontarget response.

A second factor that may explain the observed cross-study differences is the sociolinguistic environment in which the children were using Spanish. The children who presented with omission as the main error pattern, with the exception of those who participated in Bedore and Leonard's (2001) study, were living in countries where Spanish was the majority language. On the other hand, the children who participated in Restrepo and Gutiérrez-Clellen's (2001) study and who presented mainly gender agreement errors lived in the USA, and, thus, in an English–Spanish language contact situation. In a language contact situation, such as the one in the USA, Spanish can be considered a marginalized language or one with a lower 'status', at least for many of the communities in the country (Anderson, 2001b, 2003, 2004; Silva-Corvalán, 1991; also see Brozgold & Centeno, ch. 5, this volume). A usual consequence of this unequal status is that Spanish is restricted to particular situations, usually interactions at home and with adults, not with children. As the use of English increases, via schooling and peer interaction, the amount of time children spend listening to and using Spanish decreases. This has been shown to impact productive use of both lexical and morphosyntactic aspects of the language that are intertwined in NP gender agreement (e.g. Fillmore, 1991; Gutiérrez, 1990; Lipski, 1993; Ocampo, 1990; Silva-Corvalán, 1991). In this American context, researchers have noted that NP gender agreement is problematic for adults (Lipski, 1993) and for children (Anderson, 2001b; Brisk, 1974). Why, then, did Bedore and Leonard's (2001) study not find the same pattern as Restrepo and Gutiérrez-Clellen (2001), even though their participants were also Spanish–English bilinguals in a situation where Spanish was a minority language? It is plausible that, because in Bedore and Leonard's study children were younger, they were perhaps less affected by the language contact situation than the older children studied by Restrepo and Gutiérrez-Clellen.

Spanish direct object clitics

To date, three studies have addressed the use of object clitic pronouns, specifically third person forms, in Spanish-speaking children with SLI. Two of these investigations gathered data from preschoolers via experimental probes in a Spanish-as-a-minority-language context (Bedore & Leonard, 2001; Jacobson & Schwartz, 2002) while the other study examined older children via analysis of spontaneous speech samples in a Spanish-speaking country (Bosch & Serra, 1997). Results from these studies agree in that clitic object pronouns are particularly difficult for Spanish-speaking children with SLI, in comparison with language-matched and/or age-matched peers. Such results are in consonance with those reported for speakers of Italian and French (Cipriani *et al.*, 1998; Paradis *et al.*, 2003). They also coincide in that omissions were the most frequent error pattern. In addition, a small number of gender-agreement errors were reported (Jacobson & Schwartz, 2002). These errors consisted of the use of the masculine form *lo* for the feminine form *la* (e.g. *Lo ví* 'I saw him' – where the referent is *la niña* 'the girl'). It is plausible that, in the case of clitic productions, the type of procedure used to elicit children's use of these forms may impact error production. Studies based on spontaneous data, for example, report minimal, if any, gender errors in the use of the direct object clitics *lo* and *la* (Bosch & Serra, 1997). On the other hand, Jacobson and Schwartz (2002), who report a higher incidence of gender errors, used an experimental probe procedure that aimed at obligating the use of these forms. Although it could be argued that language contact could explain the incidence of gender errors reported by Jacobson and Schwartz (2002), a recent study with monolingual Spanish-speaking children in a Spanish-as-the-majority-language context (i.e. Puerto Rico) and using a similar experimental procedure, also reported gender errors in children's productions (Vargas, 2005). In fact, most of the children's errors were of this type, while typical age-matched peers did not evidence this pattern of nontarget production. Unlike articles, where differences in specific error patterns were noted across studies that relied on the same methodology, but where the children were either in a language contact or monolingual context, clitic production appears to be influenced more by how the data are collected (also see pertinent discussion on methodological issues in Jackson-Maldonado & Conboy, ch. 11, Restrepo & Castilla, ch. 10, this volume).

Spanish verbal inflection

Examination of verb phrase (VP) use in Spanish-speaking children with SLI, especially verbal inflection, has been neglected in research. Although some studies have looked at verb inflectional morphology in Spanish-speaking children (e.g. Bedore & Leonard, 2001), the focus has been on a limited number of inflections. This is unfortunate, as the inflectional system in Spanish verbs provides ample opportunity to evaluate areas of deficit in SLI and to test the various theoretical constructs proposed to explain this disorder. Available data suggest that verbal inflection, at least with respect to person agreement (first and third) and some tenses (perfect preterite and present indicative) does not appear to be problematic for Spanish-speaking children with SLI. This is in contrast with the exceptional difficulty that English-speaking children with SLI demonstrate in the use of person (i.e. third person singular /-s/, /-z/ /-ɪz/) and tense (i.e. past) inflections.

As part of a larger study, Bedore and Leonard (2001) studied verbal inflection in preschool-age Spanish-speaking children with SLI. Via a picture description elicitation task, they compared these children to age-matched and MLU-word-matched peers on the following verbal inflections: (1) present first (*camino* 'I walk') and third (*camina* 'he/she walks') person singular; (2) present first (*caminamos* 'we walk') and third (*caminan* 'they walk') person plural; (3) past first (*caminé* 'I walked') and third (*caminó* 'he/she walked') singular; (4) past first (*caminamos* 'we walked') and third (*caminaron* 'they walked') person plural; and (5) infinitive forms (*caminar* 'to walk'). All Spanish infinitive endings (i.e. -ar/*caminar* 'to walk'; -er/*comer* 'to eat'; -ir/*vivir* 'to live') were targeted. While for some inflections the children with SLI performed significantly worse than same-age peers, they did not differ in accuracy of use of the various inflections from their MLU-word-matched peers. Bedore and Leonard concluded that, at least for the targeted items, Spanish-speaking children with SLI do not present with significant difficulties in the production of verbal inflection.

Verb inflection was also studied in a longitudinal case study of a Spanish-speaking child with SLI who was acquiring English as a second language and was experiencing first language (L1) loss (i.e. a reduction in productive skill in Spanish, Restrepo & Kruth, 2000) (also see Centeno, ch. 3, this volume for related discussion on expressive features in bilingual speakers). The child's language skills were assessed via two spontaneous speech samples and contrasted to those of a typically developing child who was also in a similar language contact situation. Although detailed analysis of verb forms was not conducted, Restrepo and Kruth reported that the child with SLI presented with a limited use of verb tenses in her speech samples, as compared to her typical peer. This was especially noted in the later sample, thus suggesting that Spanish-speaking children with SLI in a language contact situation, where the native language (i.e. L1) is used less frequently than the majority language (hence reducing quantity and variety of L1 exposure), verbal inflection – especially for tense – may be vulnerable to loss or attrition. Further research with more children in a similar sociolinguistic context is needed in order to ascertain if language contact situations differentially impact productive use of inflectional morphemes in Spanish verbs.

The Nature of SLI in Spanish: What the Data Suggest

The studies reviewed all coincide in reporting that Spanish-speaking children with SLI, as observed in children from other language groups, do present with significant deficits in grammatical skill. These restrictions appear to be evidenced more dramatically in children's NP use while VP tense and person distinctions, at least those studied, are not problematic. Such a pattern is consistent with what has been observed in other Romance languages, such as Italian and French (e.g. Bortoloni *et al.*, 1998; Cipriani *et al.*, 1998; Paradis *et al.*, 2003). Cross-study differences, however, have been noted, especially with respect to the specific error patterns in the production of certain target forms.

How do the data inform us of the nature of SLI? Recall that there are two main theoretical views of the inherent problem of SLI: a processing view and a linguistic view. NP constituents investigated in research (i.e. definite articles) have been described as being unstressed (Alarcos Llorach, 1994) and, thus, having low perceptual saliency. These constituents, in turn, have been consistently noted as being problematic for Spanish-speaking children with SLI. In addition, because tense and person appear to not be areas of deficit, many of the researchers who have studied SLI in this population adhere to the processing account as the best explanation for the observed difficulties with Spanish NPs. Because the most consistent pattern observed was one of omission and correct production when produced, inherent deficits in grammatical knowledge (i.e. knowing where to place clitics and articles) cannot be the explanation for these difficulties. It can be argued, consistent with the linguistic view of SLI proposed by Wexler and Rice for SLI (Wexler, 2003), that perhaps the problem is not one of processing deficits *per se*, but, rather, one of establishing that the use of these NP constituents is not optional, but obligatory. In fact, Wexler (2003) has argued that the pattern of clitic omission and lack of use of uninflected forms should be expected in languages such as Spanish, as its characteristic grammatical features, such as the use of null subjects, would predict the patterns one sees, which would then be explained by the EOI account.

What other information do the Spanish data provide? First, they provide information for clinicians regarding potential areas of difficulty in morphosyntactic skill. Utilizing these data, clinicians can devise more linguistically appropriate assessment procedures that target those aspects that are problematic (e.g. articles and clitic forms), hence obtaining a more comprehensive and true picture of the Spanish-speaking child's grammatical skill. In addition, by addressing those aspects that are more problematic, effective intervention decisions can be made. For example, the use of clitic pronouns is an important aspect of Spanish, as it is central to its grammar. Children with deficits in the use of these forms will certainly present with significant problems when attempting to communicate with others. From a functional perspective, then, these grammatical forms should be targeted.

Secondly, the data discussed in this chapter suggest that two main child-specific factors appear to influence children's language skills: (1) relative phonological skill and (2) sociolinguistic environment. As mentioned previously, studies focusing on the use of articles by children with SLI point to an interaction between phonological skill and article use. In both Bosch and Serra's (1997) and Anderson and Souto's (2005) investigations, children with concomitant phonological deficits pre-sented with a higher incidence of article omission. On the other hand, children who did not present phonological deficits were more accurate in their use of these forms. Although they did present with omissions, the incidence was much lower than in those children with phonological disorders. At least for articles, the data do point to phonological skill as a variable impacting children's accuracy in producing certain grammatical forms. Because relative phonological skill was not comprehensively addressed in studies evaluating other grammatical structures, for example clitics, it is unclear if this factor can also influence other Spanish grammatical forms in children with SLI.

Sociolinguistic environment similarly appears to influence how SLI is manifested in Spanish-speaking children (also see Restrepo & Castilla, ch. 10, this volume). Recall that in the studies on article use, the pattern of error reported differed across studies. In research with Spanish-speaking children from countries where Spanish is the majority language, error patterns were consistently those of omission (Anderson & Souto, 2005; Bosch & Serra, 1997). In contrast, the study that reported a significant amount of gender errors in the use of articles was conducted with children from a sociolinguistic environment where Spanish is not the language of the nation, but a minority language whose restricted use results in lower linguistic quantity and diversity relative to the majority language (Restrepo & Gutiérrez-Clellen, 2001). It is plausible, then, that depending on the sociolinguistic context, particularly those resulting in attrition in the minority language, Spanish-speaking children with SLI may present with different patterns of deficit, although similar aspects of grammar are affected (i.e. articles). Previous studies with typically developing Spanish-speaking children and adults in language contact situations have reported a high incidence of gender-agreement errors (Anderson, 2001b; Brisk, 1974; Lipski, 1993). These types of errors have been reported as rare in monolingual developmental data (Hernández-Pina, 1984; Idiazabal, 1995; López-Ornat, 1997). It is plausible, then, that the language contact situation influenced the use of NP gender agreement in the children with SLI as it has also influenced that of typical learners.

Further evidence of the impact of sociolinguistic environment on Spanish-speaking children with SLI was provided by Restrepo and Kruth (2000). In their case study of a Spanish-speaking child with SLI who was in a language contact situation, as compared to a peer in a similar linguistic context, a rapid decline in Spanish-speaking skills was noted. In particular, significant reductions were apparent in sentence complexity, use of a variety of verbal inflections, and production of articles and prepositions. The researchers suggest that, in language contact situations where L1 loss can occur, children with SLI are particularly vulnerable to this phenomenon, more so than their typically developing peers. Thus, sociolinguistic environment is certainly a variable that needs to be considered when studying the language abilities of Spanish-speaking children with SLI.

Methodological Considerations and Directions for Further Study

The study of Spanish-speaking children with SLI is in its infancy. At the present time, research has provided initial data for understanding the disability and for developing sound assessment and intervention methodologies. Due to the multiple factors that may influence how the disorder is characterized and how it progresses, research with this population needs to consider all of these factors, including those that are child-specific (e.g. phonological skill) and those that pertain to the sociolinguistic environment (e.g. restricted communication contexts,

amount and diversity of linguistic input) in which the child is communicating. In addition, in order to collect data that would assess the
adequacy of the theoretical models to explain the nature of SLI in
Spanish-speaking children, research needs to expand both in scope and
in methodology (also see Centeno & Gingerich, ch. 8, this volume).

Participant selection

Because both child-specific and environment-specific factors may
affect how SLI is manifested, careful attention should be given to the
particular characteristics of the children who will be participants.
Aspects such as phonological skill and comprehension abilities should
be controlled. Comparison across subgroups of children can, thus, be
made following similar methodologies for data collection. In this way,
the relative influence of other aspects of language skill on children with
SLI can be ascertained. It has been suggested that there may be
subgroups of SLI children who differ on how the disorder is manifested
in their language production (e.g. Van der Lely, 2003). Including children
with SLI with various linguistic profiles may help in discerning if such
subgroups do exist in Spanish. These data will be of clinical relevance, as
clinicians can, therefore, modify their assessment and intervention to
accommodate these individual differences.

One of the main characteristics of the research with Spanish-speaking
children with SLI is that the population studied has been recruited from
different sociolinguistic environments. Children studied have included
monolinguals from diverse Spanish-speaking countries and, primarily,
Spanish speakers in an English-Spanish bilingual context. These data, in
turn, suggest that these differing environments, in particular monolingual
versus bilingual contexts, may impact how SLI is manifested. Research
should, thus, aim to address how context interacts with language skill in
these children. Methodologies should, in turn, be developed where
children in both monolingual and bilingual environments are followed,
controlling for the other participant characteristics mentioned previously.
In this way, the relative influence of sociolinguistic context on language
skill on such children can be identified.

Linguistic aspects to study

Because it is in its infancy, research with Spanish-speaking children
with SLI has focused on a rather narrow component of grammar. This
narrow focus is mainly the result of initial attempts to address how
structures that have been previously identified as problematic in SLI in
other languages apply to Spanish speakers. Although essential for our
understanding of SLI, this approach has failed to provide a comprehensive view of the grammatical deficits that characterize Spanish SLI.
Future studies should expand to include other important areas of

Spanish grammar to determine if and how these are problematic in Spanish-speaking children with SLI. In particular, aspects of verb inflection that include the full person-inflection paradigm, as well as mood, aspect, and tense, should be evaluated. In addition, SLI research needs to address the use of both direct object and indirect object clitics that include both reflexive and nonreflexive forms and all person distinctions (see Anderson & Centeno, ch. 1, for other grammatical areas for possible research). Children's comprehension of all grammatical features that have been mentioned should be addressed. Furthermore, in order to study the inter-relationship among different grammatical features as well as the explanatory power of various theoretical models of SLI, a variety of grammatical features should be studied in the same group of children.

A potentially useful research paradigm that can also be incorporated in the study of Spanish-speaking children with SLI is one that has been used previously with typically developing children from various language groups and English-speaking children with SLI. In this paradigm, children are either taught an invented morpheme (Connell & Stone, 1992), one that is not part of the target language's adult system, or invented words are used to assess how children apply particular language rules (Pérez-Pereira, 1991). The former task has been used to identify the language learning patterns of children with SLI but its applications to Spanish-speaking children with SLI have been limited (e.g. Anderson, 2001a; Roseberry & Connell, 1991). The significance of this research paradigm is that it has all children, both typical and atypical, at the same level of knowledge for the new language rule that is introduced. In the case of using invented words, the children will have equivalent exposure to the targets and specific aspects of the items can be controlled to identify factors that impact language skill. Both can be applied to SLI research and can serve two main purposes. First, typical and SLI comparisons can potentially pinpoint differences in performance that, perhaps, can be used to identify SLI in Spanish-speaking children (Roseberry & Connell, 1991). Second, because particular characteristics of the target items can be controlled, such an approach can potentially inform us on the factors that may influence performance in these children. Features such as stress pattern, phonology, meaning represented in the morpheme, grammatical complexity, and pragmatic demands, can be controlled, hence providing valuable resources for testing both linguistic and processing accounts of SLI.

Conclusions

This overview of SLI manifestations in Spanish underscores the need for continued research with this clinical population. Nevertheless, the body of work that has been conducted provides viable venues for further research. It has indicated potential areas of deficit (e.g. articles, clitics, and certain verb forms) that can be studied in more detail and via a variety of experimental methods. It has also suggested potential factors that may impact how SLI is manifested in Spanish thus providing researchers with information that can aid them in securing potential participants and in establishing other areas of inquiry pertinent to Spanish (e.g. monolingual versus various language contact situations). From a clinical perspective, the research conducted thus far does present with important evidence for designing better assessment tools and for identifying potential intervention targets for Spanish-speaking children with SLI. More importantly, the continued study of SLI in Spanish-speaking children will provide the much-needed cross-linguistic data for testing the various theoretical accounts espoused for explaining SLI and, in turn, for explaining how language, in general, is structured, processed, and represented in the brain.

References

Alarcos Llorach, E. (1994) *Gramática de la Lengua Española*. Madrid: Espasa Calpe.

Anderson, R.T. (2001a) Learning an invented inflectional morpheme in Spanish by children with typical language skills and with specific language impairment. *International Journal of Language and Communication Disorders* 36, 1–20.

Anderson, R.T. (2001b) Loss of gender agreement in L1 attrition: Preliminary results. *Bilingual Research Journal* 23, 389–408.

Anderson, R.T. (2003) Article use in Spanish-speaking children from varied backgrounds and abilities. Paper presented at the Fourth International Symposium on Bilingualism, Arizona State University, Tempe, AZ.

Anderson, R.T. (2004) First language loss in Spanish-speaking children: Patterns of loss and implications for clinical practice. In B.A. Goldstein (ed.) *Bilingual Language Development and Disorders in Spanish–English Speakers* (pp. 187–212). Baltimore, MD: Brookes.

Anderson, R.T. and Souto, S.M. (2005) The use of articles by monolingual Puerto Rican Spanish-speaking children with specific language impairment. *Applied Psycholinguistics* 26, 621–647.

Bedore, L.M. and Leonard, L.B. (2001) Grammatical morphology deficits in Spanish-speaking children with specific language impairment. *Journal of Speech, Language, and Hearing Research* 44, 905–924.

Bortoloni, U., Leonard, L.B. and Caselli, M.C. (1998) Specific language impairment in Italian and English: Evaluating alternative accounts of grammatical deficits. *Language and Cognitive Processes* 13, 1–20.

Bosch, L. and Serra, M. (1997) Grammatical morphology deficits of Spanish-speaking children with specific language impairment. *Proceedings of the Fourth Symposium of the European Group on Child Language Disorders* 6, 33–45.

Brisk, M.E. (1974) A preliminary study of the syntax of the five year-old Spanish speakers of New Mexico. *International Journal of the Sociology of Language* 1, 69–78.

Cipriani, P., Bottari, P., Chilosi, A.M. and Pfanner, L. (1998) A longitudinal perspective on the study of specific language impairment: The long term follow-up of an Italian child. *International Journal of Language and Communication Disorders* 33, 245–280.

Clahsen, H., Bartke, S. and Göllner, S. (1997) Formal features of impaired grammars: A comparison of English and German SLI children. *Journal of Neurolinguistics* 10, 151–171.

Connell, P.J. and Stone, C.A. (1992) Morpheme learning of children with specific language impairment under controlled instructional conditions. *Journal of Speech and Hearing Research* 35, 844–852.

Fillmore, L.W. (1991) When learning a second language means losing the first. *Early Childhood Research Quarterly* 6, 323–346.

Gutiérrez, M. (1990) Sobre el mantenimiento de las cláusulas subordinadas en el español de Los Angeles. In J.J. Bergen (ed.) *Spanish in the United States: Sociolinguistic Issues* (pp. 31–38). Washington, DC: Georgetown University Press.

Hansson, K. and Nettelbladt, U. (1995) Grammatical characteristics of Swedish children with SLI. *Journal of Speech and Hearing Research* 38, 589–598.

Hernández-Pina, F. (1984) Teorías Psicolingüísticas y su Aplicación a la Adquisición del Español como Lengua Materna. Madrid, Spain: Siglo XXI.

Idiazabal, I. (1995) First stages in the acquisition of noun phrase determiners by a Basque–Spanish bilingual child. In C. Silva-Corvalán (ed.) *Spanish in Four Continents: Studies in Language Contact and Bilingualism* (pp. 260–278). Washington, DC: Georgetown University Press.

Jacobson, P.F. and Schwartz, R.G. (2002) Morphology of incipient bilingual Spanish-speaking preschool children with specific language impairment. *Applied Psycholinguistics* 23, 23–41.

Leonard, L.B. (1998) *Children with Specific Language Impairment*. Cambridge, MA: MIT Press.

Leonard, L.B. and Dromi, E. (1994) The use of Hebrew verb morphology by children with specific language impairment and children developing language normally. *First Language* 14, 283–304.

Lipski, J.M. (1993) Creolid phenomena in the Spanish of transitional bilinguals. In A. Roca and J.M. Lipski (eds) *Spanish in the United States: Linguistic Contact and Diversity* (pp. 155–182). NY: Mouton de Gruyter.

López-Ornat, S. (1997) What lies between a pre-grammatical and a grammatical representation? Evidence on nominal and verbal form-function mappings in Spanish from 1;7 to 2;1. In A. Pérez-Leroux and W.R. Glass (eds) *Contemporary Perspectives on the Acquisition of Spanish, Vol. 1: Developing Grammars* (pp. 3–20). Sommerville, MD: Cascadilla Press.

Ocampo, F. (1990) El subjuntivo en tres generaciones de hablantes bilingües. In J.J. Bergen (ed.) *Spanish in the United States: Sociolinguistic Issues* (pp. 39–48). Washington, DC: Georgetown University Press.

Paradis, J., Crago, M. and Genesee, F. (2003) Object clitics as a clinical marker of SLI in French: Evidence from French–English bilingual children. *Proceedings of the Annual Boston University Conference on Language Development* 27, 638–649.

Pérez-Pereira, M. (1991) The acquisition of gender: What Spanish children tell us. *Journal of Child Language* 18, 571–590.

Restrepo, M.A. and Gutiérrez-Clellen, V.F. (2001) Article use in Spanish-speaking children with specific-language impairment. *Journal of Child Language* 28, 433–452.

Restrepo, M.A. and Kruth, K. (2000) Grammatical characteristics of a Spanish–English bilingual child with specific language impairment. *Communication Disorders Quarterly* 21, 66–76.

Roseberry, C. and Connell, P.J. (1991) The use of an invented language rule in the differentiation of normal and language impaired Spanish-speaking children. *Journal of Speech and Hearing Research* 34, 596–603.

Silva-Corvalán, C. (1991) Spanish language attrition in a contact situation with English. In H.W. Seliger and R.M. Vago (eds) *First Language Attrition* (pp. 151–171). Cambridge, UK: Cambridge University Press.

Van der Lely, H.K.J. (2003) Do heterogeneous deficits require heterogeneous theories? SLI subgroups and the RDDR hypothesis. In Y. Levy and J. Schaeffer (eds) *Language Competence Across Populations: Towards a Definition of Specific Language Impairment* (pp. 109–134). Mahwah, NJ: Lawrence Erlbaum.

Vargas, S.M. (2005) Definite articles and direct object clitic pronouns used by Puerto Rican Spanish-speaking children with specific language impairment. Paper presented at ASHA National Convention, San Diego, CA.

Wexler, K. (2003) Lenneberg's dream: Learning, normal language development, and specific language impairment. In Y. Levy and J. Schaeffer (eds) *Language Competence Across Populations: Towards a Definition of Specific Language Impairment* (pp. 11–62). Mahwah, NJ: Lawrence Erlbaum.

Chapter 10

Language Elicitation and Analysis as a Research and Clinical Tool for Latino Children

MARÍA ADELAIDA RESTREPO and ANNY PATRICIA CASTILLA

The analysis of spontaneous language samples produced by children is a critical tool for both research and clinical/educational services. The examination of children's conversational utterances allows investigators in clinical communication to study linguistic processing in young language learners. It also allows speech-language practitioners to identify and diagnose children at risk of language disorders, and to implement and monitor intervention procedures (McCabe & Bliss, 2003; Miller & Chapman, 1984). Identifying language elicitation techniques that maximize children's linguistic productions is, therefore, critical. Although a number of studies have focused on identifying elicitation techniques that are appropriate for a variety of purposes and contexts with children in the USA, further research in this area is still needed, especially with monolingual Spanish-speaking children and bilingual Spanish–English-speaking children with typical and atypical language skills. The considerable presence of these populations in educational and clinical settings makes such research imperative.

The purpose of this chapter is to review the literature on effective techniques for the elicitation and analysis of children's language samples with particular emphasis on methods with Latino children in both monolingual Spanish and bilingual Spanish–English contexts in the USA. Specifically, this chapter will discuss elicitation procedures employed with children in general, and summarize useful procedures for eliciting and analyzing language samples in Latino children in the USA (also see Anderson, ch. 6 and 9, Jackson-Maldonado & Conboy, ch. 11, this volume for related discussions). Throughout the chapter, we similarly address both strengths and weaknesses of proposed language analysis techniques, and highlight possible directions to improve current procedures. Because Latino children in the USA may be monolingual Spanish or bilingual Spanish–English speakers, we use the term Latino in our discussions to refer to those two language contexts.

Elicitation Techniques

Anderson (ch. 9, this volume) describes some factors, such as socio-linguistic contexts and phonological skills of children, that impact grammatical analysis of children's utterances. Additionally, language elicitation techniques influence the expressive outcomes in the language produced by children. Therefore, the purpose of the language analysis[1] should guide the selection of the elicitation techniques. Yet, speech-language service providers often use a limited repertoire, if any, of language collection methods and analyses for educational and clinical purposes. For example, research has demonstrated that, in English-speaking children in the USA, conversational contexts tend to result in more fluent language than narratives, although narration can lead to longer mean length of utterance (MLU) in words (Wagner *et al.*, 2002). Further, interviewing children, that is, having an adult ask children questions, can lead to more utterances in children's productions than a free-play format (Hadley, 1998).

Several studies have addressed different modalities to elicit stories whereas other studies have addressed whether the format, in the form of conversations, interviews, or stories, leads to increased sentence com-plexity or lexical diversity. Gummersall and Strong (1999), for instance, investigated three conditions to determine which one would elicit more complex sentences during narrative tasks with third-grade, typically developing children. In condition 1, children listened to a story, imitated each sentence, and retold the story. In condition 2, children listened to a story twice, and retold the story. In condition 3, children listened to a story once and, then, retold the story. The researchers found that total number of words, number of minimal terminal units (T-units), words per T-units, and mean number of subordinate (dependent) clauses for conditions 1 and 2 were significantly greater than the ones in condition 3. However, the authors found no significant differences between conditions 1 and 2, in which the amount of exposure was similar between conditions. In addition, the authors found that condition 1 led to a greater variability of clause connectors and left branching (use of embedding elements in the subject) than conditions 2 and 3. These findings suggest that increasing the number of exposures to a story improves a child's recall, fluency, and syntactic length and complexity.

Using story retelling, in contrast to asking questions about a story, also leads to different language products. Gazella and Stockman (2003) studied whether modality of presentation and task conditions influenced the length, lexical diversity, and sentence complexity of language samples in a group of 29 preschool English-speaking children. They investigated the effects distinguishing a story retelling task and a story questioning task, and found that the story-retelling task yielded greater productivity in terms of grammatical complexity, length, and complete-ness than the story questioning task. On the other hand, the story questioning task yielded a greater number of utterances and a larger number of different words than story retelling. In addition, Gazella and Stockman evaluated any performance differences in grammatical mea-sures when comparing the presentation of a story in the auditory-only modality relative to the auditory-visual modality. They found no differences according to task modality, although their study participants seemed to be more attentive in the auditory-visual modality.

Although story retelling is an appropriate technique to elicit complex utterances, other formats, such as conversations, interviews, and stories, can lead to different expressive outcomes. In general, conversations seem to lead to more fluency and to greater number of utterances than stories, while stories lead to more complex sentences than conversations. Wagner *et al.* (2002) compared two elicitation techniques, conversation and narration, to determine which one led to greater intelligibility, fluency, MLU, and grammatical skills in a group of 28 Swedish-speaking children with language impairments. They found that conversation led to increased intelligibility and fluency (as measured by number of utterances with mazes), and narration enhanced MLU in number of words. In addition, the investigators reported that narrative tasks resulted in more grammatical morphemes and greater sentence complexity as measured by the number of phrasal expansions, whereas conversation led to more complex verb forms.

The preceding studies support that, for some cultural groups, story retelling leads to greater utterance complexity than conversation or story generation. However, similar results may not be found across cultures. Southwood and Russell (2004) studied language samples from 10 five year-old Afrikaans-speaking boys. They investigated the possible effects of conversation, free play, and story generation on the number of utterances, variety of syntactic structures, MLU, number of syntactic errors, and proportion of complex syntactic structures. Findings suggest that free play led to more utterances than story generation; story generation led to shorter MLUs than free play and conversation; and story generation and conversation led to higher proportions of complex utterances than free play. The investigators, however, did not find any differences in syntactic structures and number of syntactic errors among the three tasks. Interest-ingly, these results are inconsistent with the studies discussed above which also employed conversations or stories. Hence, before we generalize this type of research across cultures, researchers and practitioners in clinical communication need to evaluate how children from different cultures respond to different elicitation tasks.

Elicitation across Groups with Different Language Ability

Given that the studies discussed have mostly evaluated children with typical language, it is possible that elicitation techniques may impact children differently depending on the integrity of their language abilities. Evans and Craig (1992) studied structural and conversational behaviors in the language samples of ten children with specific language impairment (SLI) (mean age 8;5) produced during free play and in an interview. The samples were evaluated using the developmental-sentence-score analysis, MLU, type-token ratio (TTR), advanced semantic and syntactic features, and conversational behaviors, such as intentions, turn-taking, and responsiveness. Evans and Craig found that, with the interview, children produced greater number of utterances, longer MLUs, and higher frequencies of advanced syntactic and semantic features than free play. Further, interviews led to greater responsiveness and simultaneity, but free play led to more child requests. There were no differences between interview and free play on developmental sentence scores and TTR.

Masterson and Kamhi (1991) studied three different sampling conditions in three groups of children: ten children with typical language, ten children with deficits in oral and written language, and ten children with only written language deficits. They examined contextual support (referent present versus referent absent), discourse genre (story retelling versus explanation versus description), and listener's knowledge of information being provided (shared knowledge versus unshared knowledge). Findings suggested that children produced more complex and accurate sentences when the referent was absent and the information was unshared. Additionally, syntactic complexity and grammatical and phonemic accuracy increased when the context was unshared. In discourse genre, story telling yielded longer utterances than explanations, and retelling stories and explanations yielded longer utterances than descriptions. Descriptions elicited more lexical errors than explanations and story retellings. Finally, they found no differences in responses between children with typical and atypical oral or written language skills. Similarly, Botting (2002) investigated whether story generation and story retelling were useful to assess the language of five eight-year old children with pragmatic language impairments and five eight-year-old children with SLI. Using a descriptive analysis, the investigator concluded that story generation differentiated between groups, but story retelling did not. Children with SLI produced shorter stories than children with pragmatic impairments when generating a story.

In summary, research with English-speaking children with different language abilities suggests that children with language disorders will produce more utterances with an interview format, although some children may produce more complex sentences with a story retelling task. In addition, having unshared information and contexts with absent referents leads to greater complexity in different language ability groups. Yet, research evaluating which techniques result in greater grammatical errors is limited; such evidence would, in turn, enhance the sensitivity in the identification of language disorders, such as SLI (Leonard, 1998). The above studies, nonetheless, suggest that using at least *two different elicitation techniques* may be best to capture a range of language skills.

Given that children from home environments with limitations in parental educational backgrounds and literacy experiences, or from different cultural scenarios, may show compromised performance in narrative tasks, language elicitation and analysis measures must be carefully chosen to determine actual learning and academic potential in these children realistically (also see Kayser & Centeno, ch. 2, this volume). However, current methods in the literature provide some limited evidence concerning how children's narratives may differ across cultures and educational levels. Determining the benefits from different elicitation techniques across a variety of children and groups is still necessary, especially for clinical and educational purposes.

Research with Latino Children

Latino children in the USA represent various linguistic and cultural backgrounds, which translate into considerable variability in discourse styles, cultural norms, Spanish dialects, and levels of bilingualism (McCabe & Bliss, 2003; also see Anderson, ch. 9, Centeno, ch. 3, this volume). Hence, research with a specific group of Latino children, whether these children are developing in the USA or in another country, cannot be generalized to different Latino children from other linguistic and cultural developmental experiences. In general, the study of language elicitation techniques with Latino children is still in its early stages, and its generalizability across children from various Latino cultures remains to be assessed.

Discourse characteristics in Latino children

Understanding discourse characteristics in Latino children is important to develop appropriate elicitation procedures, accurate analysis methods, and appropriate interpretations. For example, McCabe and Bliss (2003) suggest that Latino children tend to talk more about families in their narratives than any other topics. This is particularly noticeable in Mexican–American families, although other Latin American cultures have been found to do so as well. In addition, McCabe and Bliss reported that one of the primary roles of narratives in Mexican–American families is to entertain the listener or to participate in discourse rather than to provide a specific sequence of events. Further, the authors report that European–American children tend to use stories as part of a repertoire of language skills in which children are socialized in preschool. In contrast, African–American children use oral styles of stories similar to those of Mexican–Americans, i.e. to entertain the listener rather than demonstrate the skill of story telling. Hence, using family-related topics as possible conversational themes with Latino children may lead to greater expressive output. Similarly, it is possible that, across cultures, the purpose of discourse in children may vary when telling stories or personal narratives, and this, in turn, may have consequences for whether a discourse's structure is deemed typical or not.

Interpreting discourse in Latino children requires the examination of the *conversational routines* to which they are exposed in their communities (also see Anderson, ch. 9, this volume). Latino children may vary in relation to how they are socialized in their conversations, stories, and personal narratives, which may also impact how we should elicit and analyze their language samples. For instance, studies with Puerto Rican adults have found that they tend to favor the use of topic-association styles in their narratives and conversations, which contrasts with the topic-centered narratives in European–American English-speaking adults (Pérez, 1998, as cited in McCabe & Bliss, 2003). Therefore, if Latino children have the same narrative style as the adults in their community, this may present a cultural mismatch with European–American educators, researchers, and clinicians, who have different narrative style and expectations (McCabe & Bliss, 2003).

Variations in individual expressive styles may also be due to differences in specific adult–child socialization practices. Melzi (2000), for example, found that Central American mothers asked their children for more reported speech and used more generic narrative prompts such as *¿qué más?* 'what else?' than European–American mothers who used more content-specific prompts in eliciting personal narratives. Further, European–American mothers used more closed-ended questions than Central American mothers, who used more open-ended questions in both shared and unshared experience conversations. These observations suggest that the interaction routines used by Central American mothers seem to place more responsibility on the child to organize and control conversation, which contrasts with those activities that clinicians and teachers ask children to do in more structured settings. Therefore, the effect of adult–child communication dynamics in language elicitation may need to be investigated further to ensure that realistic language samples are collected from Latino children.

Narration may also vary at the level of linguistic forms used in the stories and conversations. Sebastián and Slobin (1994) investigated how children use verb tense in their narratives and found that children from monolingual Spanish-speaking backgrounds (i.e. Chile, Spain, and Peru) tended to include present progressive and present tense in narratives, instead of past tense. In addition, they found that some of the children switched between past and present tenses with no clear justification of the change of tense. Sebastián and Slobin also investigated the use of the progressive aspect. They found that younger children (i.e. preschool and early school age) used this verb form more frequently than adults and older children when they retold stories. These results are important in language analysis. The use of present tense in a story retelling task is an appropriate form to retell stories, and the absence of past tense should not be interpreted as a difficulty in using past tense. Further research may evaluate whether the high frequency of the progressive form is also seen in bilingual Spanish–English children, where verb usage trends in the two languages may influence each other.

Additional studies with monolingual Spanish-speaking children have also found some differences in how Latino children express some *concepts*, such as movement and location, in relation to English-speaking children (see Slobin, 1996). Slobin and Bocaz (1988), for instance, found that monolingual Spanish-speaking children in Argentina expressed the path of motion (location) through the verbs that express motion and direction, like *subir* 'to go up'. On the other hand, in English, children expressed location of movement more specifically through verb particles such as *up* in *go up*. For instance, in English, speech-language pathologists may focus on eliciting production and comprehension of prepositions, and on having children describe setting, motion, and location in their stories. However, expecting Latino children's stories to do the same may lead to inappropriate generalizations concerning their language ability and story-telling skills when they are not routinely socialized to do so. In terms of expressing action, the opposite occurs. English has several ways to describe motion, when Spanish may have just one verb that describes this concept. Therefore, when researchers or clinicians try to determine how bilingual Spanish–English children express themselves in two languages, these children may not have a comparable range of verb repertories in Spanish and English to express motion events at their disposal. For example, when describing *running*, English provides a variety of verbs like *run*, *scurry*, and *sprint*, whereas Spanish only has one verb *correr* 'run'. Hence, to specify the meaning of the verb, other elements, such as adverbs, may be employed in the sentence context. This difference in the expression of motion, therefore, can lead to differences in how this concept is detailed in stories produced in each language, and may contrast with the expectations that educators, speech-language pathologists, and researchers may have.

Despite differences across languages, there are some similarities, as well. For example, children develop *causal relationships* and *reference cohesion* in a similar manner in English and Spanish. Gutiérrez-Clellen and Heinrichs-Ramos (1993) found that Spanish-speaking Puerto Rican children improved their ability to include the referents in a movie retelling task as they got older. Similarly, Gutiérrez-Clellen and Iglesias (1992) found that, as children's age increased, so did the complexity of the causal chains they produced when retelling a movie. Therefore, it seems that, cross-linguistically, children increase their narrative complexity in terms of reference and causal relationships. These studies further demonstrate that some of the language analyses used in English may be appropriate for Spanish, although whenever this approach is taken, we should first evaluate if that is the case.

Language elicitation techniques with Latino children

Although there is a paucity of research on language elicitation techniques with Latino children, some studies have described successful methods (Castilla & Restrepo, 2004; Fiestas & Peña, 2004; Gutiérrez-Clellen & Heinrichs-Ramos, 1993; Restrepo, 1998). Latino children can be successful story tellers from an early preschool age, especially if they have some training or models (Castilla & Restrepo, 2004; Fiestas & Peña, 2004; Gutiérrez-Clellen, 1998; Restrepo, 1998). In fact, when comparing story retelling and spontaneous story production, the former task seems to be more fruitful to elicit language than the latter in both preschool and school-age populations of Latino children (Castilla & Restrepo, 2004). Gutiérrez-Clellen and colleagues (Gutiérrez-Clellen, 2002; Gutiérrez-Clellen *et al.*, 1995, 2000; Gutiérrez-Clellen & Hofstetter, 1994; Gutiérrez-Clellen & Iglesias, 1992; Restrepo & Gutiérrez-Clellen, 2001) have used a variety of methods as well, including retelling of silent movies and story formulation from wordless picture books, similarly supporting that eliciting stories is more productive than spontaneous story generation for most Latino children.

In order to address whether different elicitation techniques resulted in different grammatical profiles and, therefore, might compromise the accurate identification of language disorders in Latino children, Restrepo *et al.* (2005) examined whether Mexican–American children with typical and atypical language differed on three elicitation techniques: interview or adult-led conversation, picture description, and story retelling. The study included 15 children in each group between the ages of 5 and 7 years of age (mean age 5 years 11 months) whose primary language spoken at home and school was Spanish. Results showed that groups differed in the number of grammatical sentences in their samples (number of grammatical errors per sentence) and in MLU, as expected. In addition, they found that picture description led to longer utterances than interview or adult-led conversation and story retelling, but that the stories resulted in more errors than interview or adult-led conversation and picture description. Moreover, the interview yielded the fewest errors and the most utterances, at least in the typically developing group.

These results suggest that, in order to best identify children with language disorders, at least in elementary school years, story retelling may serve as the most sensitive procedure to identify language disorders, despite being the context that may lead to the fewest utterances. For a representative sample, then, researchers, clinicians, and educators should use at least two contexts to elicit the samples.

Other studies evaluating different elicitation formats have found no differences across tasks. Gutiérrez-Clellen (1998) compared narrative samples from 28 Spanish-speaking children with average achievement (mean age 8;1) and 29 Spanish-speaking children with low achievement (mean age 7.7). The narrative samples were elicited with book and movie retelling tasks. Gutiérrez-Clellen found no differences between narration elicited with a book and narration elicited with a movie in terms of syntactic measures. However, she found differences between low-achieving and typically achieving children in sentence complexity (i.e. nominal clauses, relative clauses, prepositional phrases, subordination index, and mean length of T-units) and number of mazes. These results suggest that either the book or the movie elicitation technique was appropriate to encourage children to produce language.

Similarly, Fiestas and Peña (2004) examined the effects of elicitation tasks and language of elicitation on narrative samples from 12 Spanish–English bilingual children. Children were asked to generate narratives from a wordless picture book and a picture. To analyze the complexity of narratives, the investigators measured the story structure and number of C-units of each language sample. They found that children produced equally complex stories in Spanish and English with the wordless picture book. Some children generated descriptions and scripts rather than narratives with the picture stimulus in both languages. Due to this difference in task interpretation, the results from the narratives based on the picture were considered inconclusive. Children produced more attempts at initiating events in Spanish, but more consequences of story structure in English.

In summary, in terms of eliciting language samples with Latino children, it is recommended that at least *two contexts* be used for a representative sample. Story retelling seems to yield more errors but fewer utterances; interviews seem to yield more utterances but fewer errors, and picture description leads to longer utterances. Moreover, stories elicited through movies, books, or pictures seem to yield similar types of information, thus suggesting that ease of administration and availability of the materials may be what determines which technique to use. However, as will be discussed below, the type of analysis may need to be selected carefully.

Language Analyses as a Clinical and Research Tool

Narrative studies, therefore, support that story retelling is a technique that can have important diagnostic uses with Latino children in clinical and educational settings. Particularly, story retelling seems to be sensitive to distinguishing between children with typical and atypical language skills and identifying children at risk of academic difficulties. To date, the use of language sample analyses continues to be part of the best practices in the assessment of Spanish-speaking and bilingual Latino children for the purpose of identifying language disorders (Gutiérrez-Clellen *et al.*, 2000; Restrepo, 1998). However, language sample analyses require *well-designed elicitation techniques* to ensure that the samples reflect the child's true language skills while simultaneously stressing the language system enough to identify language disorders (Lahey, 1990).

Restrepo (1998) found that analyses using the combined samples obtained with three different elicitation tasks were critical in obtaining information to identify children with language disorders. She found that language sample analyses, used in conjunction with parent interviews, yielded very good *sensitivity and specificity* in the identification of Mexican–American children with language disorders. Specifically, Restrepo found that the number of grammatical errors per sentence and sentence length were sensitive to language ability status if jointly used with *family history and parental report*. Similarly, Gutiérrez-Clellen (1998) found that Spanish-speaking low-achieving children produced less complex sentences than their peers with typical achievement.

Because measures of grammatical errors per sentence can be good identifiers of language disorders in Spanish-speaking children (Gutiérrez-Clellen *et al.*, 2000; Restrepo, 1998), further studies are necessary to determine what error rates are considered typical across tasks, ages, and linguistic groups. For example, based on Restrepo's (1998) study on 5- and 6-year-old children, typical Spanish-speaking children obtained a mean of 0.09 error per sentence (SD = 0.05), indicating that, at least for this age and dialectal group, a rate of 0.15 errors per sentence or below may be considered typical. Because this research involved children who were primarily Spanish-speaking and the disordered children had moderate to severe language difficulties, additional research in this area is imperative. For example, these numbers may change when children are bilingual, younger, have milder language disorders, or speak different Spanish dialects. As discussed earlier, the different tasks may also yield different error rates. Hence, in order for this elicitation technique and analysis to be useful clinically, future studies may want to standardize the task to obtain the error rate for a variety of children in order for this measure to be used broadly.

The use of language sample analysis is also an important research and clinical tool in the prediction of *second language acquisition* and in the assessment of effectiveness of *language education and intervention*. Castilla and Restrepo (2004) found that Spanish MLU in words and subordination index (number of dependent clauses per sentence) obtained from story retellings are sensitive to language growth in preschool Spanish-speaking children. They also found that preschool children receiving bilingual intervention demonstrated significant productivity in these two measures across time within a school year, compared to children in English-only language interventions. This type of research is critical to demonstrate possible differences in language skills between children attending bilingual or English-only school programs, and the effectiveness of language intervention in Latino children with language disorders.

Language sample analysis similarly has critical value in assessing and understanding *developmental linguistic changes* in situations of language contact. Restrepo (2003) found, for example, that two bilingual Spanish–English children with language disorders, attending English-only schools, demonstrated different attrition (loss) patterns in Spanish, their first language. Upon examination of both MLU and grammatical errors per sentence in Spanish, one child demonstrated growth in MLU while his utterances increased in errors. The other child exhibited a decrease in MLU and a decrease in errors per utterance. This type of research, when conducted on a large scale in various communication contexts (e.g. home, school, with different interlocutors, and so forth), may allow investigators to interpret how different communication environments impact bilingual children's language development, especially young bilinguals with more limited language-processing capacities, such as those with SLI (see Evans, 2002; Weismer *et al.*, 1999; also see Anderson, ch. 9, this volume).

Further, grammatical skills in the first language may have a *cross-linguistic effect* on the acquisition of the second language. Castilla and Restrepo (2004) found that Spanish mean length of sentence prior to the acquisition of English was a significant predictor of acquisition of grammar in English as a second language in preschool Spanish-speaking children. Castilla and Restrepo suggest that this type of research is important in understanding the true impact of native language skills in second language acquisition, given that current research using structured and standardized tasks does not seem to indicate that skills in the first language have any impact on second language skills. The issue may be a measurement problem rather than the lack of a relationship between languages. That is, language sample analyses may be able to detect relationships and variables that standardized measures, such as the *Peabody Picture Vocabulary Test* (Dunn & Dunn, 1997) and the *Test de Vocabulario en Imágenes* (Dunn *et al.*, 1997), do not identify.

Conclusions

In summary, to identify children with language disorders and children at risk of academic failure, sentence-length measures from story retelling, such as syntactic complexity and grammaticality, may be valuable. However, standardization of these measures across Latino groups, ages, and tasks are needed before they can be used as a reliable clinical tool. In addition, some of these measures are also significant predictors of English grammatical development in children who are learning English as a second language (Castilla & Restrepo, 2004). Further research in this area will lead to better understanding of how the two languages in bilingual children interact, how typical children develop when there is limited native language stimulation, and how children with language disorders perform under a variety of conditions and stressors to their linguistic system. Language elicitation and spontaneous language analysis will only become a critical tool in the evaluation of treatment effects, relative to structured tasks or measures, as their validity is enhanced. Thus, research in the area of language sample elicitation and analysis across groups of Latino children is needed. This research has great potential to help speech-language practitioners and educators interpret and analyze language performance and, in turn, help develop valid and reliable clinical and educational tools with Latino children in both monolingual Spanish and bilingual Spanish–English contexts.

Notes

1. This glossary includes important terminology employed in this chapter:-
    Communication Units (C-unit): each independent clause plus its modifiers. Elliptical answers are also considered C-units (Loban, 1976).
    Developmental Sentence Score Analysis: speech-sample analysis method which evaluates eight syntactic categories: indefinite pronouns, personal pronouns, main verbs, embedded verbs, negative markers, conjunctions, interrogative reversals, and wh-question forms (Lee, 1974).
    Mazes: pauses and self-repairs found in speech (Navarro-Ruiz & Rallo-Fabran, 2001).
    Minimal Terminable Unit (T-units): one main clause plus its subordinate clauses. Elliptical answers and sentence fragments are not considered T-units (Hunt, 1965). We use T-units because they are representative of the language children can produce, although they originally were designed for written language.
    Subordination Index: number of complex sentences divided by total number of sentences (Paul, 2001).
    Type-Token Ratio (TTR): measure of lexical diversity. It is the ratio of the number of different words compared to the total number of words (Richards, 1987).

References

Botting, N. (2002) Narrative as a tool for the assessment of linguistic and pragmatic impairments. *Child Language Teaching and Therapy* 18, 1–21.

Castilla, A.P. and Restrepo, M.A. (2004) L1 predictors of semantic and morphosyntactic development in English as a second language. Unpublished manuscript.

Dunn, L.M. and Dunn, L.M (1997) *Examiner's Manual for The PPVT-3* (3rd edn). Circle Pines: American Guidance Service.

Dunn, L.M., Lugo, D.E., Padilla, E.R. and Dunn, L.M. (1997) *Test de Vocabulario en Imágenes Peabody.* Circle Pines: American Guidance Service.

Evans, J. (2002) Variability in comprehension strategy use in children with SLI. *International Journal of Language and Communication Disorders* 37, 95–116.

Evans, J. and Craig, H.K. (1992) Language sample collection and analysis: Interview compared to free play assessment context. *Journal of Speech and Hearing Research* 35, 343–353.

Fiestas, C.E. and Peña, E. (2004) Narrative discourse in bilingual children: Language and task effects. *Language, Speech, and Hearing Services in Schools* 35, 155–166.

Gazella, J. and Stockman, I.J. (2003) Children's story retelling under different modality and task conditions: Implications for standardizing language sampling procedures. *American Journal of Speech-Language Pathology* 12, 61–72.

Gummersall, D.M. and Strong, C.J. (1999) Assessment of complex sentence production in a narrative context. *Language, Speech, and Hearing Services in Schools* 30, 152–164.

Gutiérrez-Clellen, V.F. (1998) Syntactic skills of Spanish-speaking children with low school achievement. *Language, Speech, and Hearing Services in Schools* 29, 207–315.

Gutiérrez-Clellen, V.F. (2002) Narratives in two languages: Assessing performance of bilingual children. *Linguistics and Education* 13, 175–197.

Gutiérrez-Clellen, V.F. and Heinrichs-Ramos, L. (1993) Referential cohesion in the narratives of Spanish-speaking children: A developmental study. *Journal of Speech and Hearing Research* 36, 559–567.

Gutiérrez-Clellen, V.F. and Hofstetter, R. (1994) Syntactic complexity in Spanish narratives: A developmental study. *Journal of Speech and Hearing Research* 37, 645–654.

Gutiérrez-Clellen, V.F. and Iglesias, A. (1992) Causal coherence in the oral narratives of Spanish-speaking children. *Journal of Speech and Hearing Research* 35, 363–372.

Gutiérrez-Clellen, V.F., Peña, E. and Quinn, R. (1995) Accommodating cultural differences in narrative style: A multicultural perspective. *Topics in Language Disorders* 15, 54–67.

Gutiérrez-Clellen, V.F., Restrepo, M.A., Bedore, L., Peña, E. and Anderson, R.T. (2000) Language sample analysis: Methodological considerations. *Language, Speech, and Hearing Services in Schools* 31, 88–98.

Hadley, P.A. (1998) Language sampling protocols for eliciting text-level discourse. *Language, Speech, and Hearing Services in Schools* 29, 132–147.

Hunt, K. (1965) *Grammatical Structures Written at Three Grade Levels* (Rep. No. 3). Champaign, IL: National Council of Teachers of English.

Lahey, M. (1990) Who shall be called language disordered? Some reflections and one perspective. *Journal of Speech and Hearing Research* 55, 612–620.

Lee, L. (1974) *Developmental Sentence Analysis*. Evanston: Northwestern University Press.

Leonard, L.B. (1998) *Children with Specific Language Impairment*. Cambridge, MA: The MIT Press.

Loban, W. (1976) *Language Development: Kindergarten through Grade Twelve*. Urban, IL: National Council of Teachers.

Masterson, J.J. and Kamhi, A.G. (1991) The effects of sampling conditions on sentence production in normal, reading-disabled, and language-learning-disabled children. *Journal of Speech, Language, and Hearing Research* 34, 549–558.

McCabe, A. and Bliss, L.S. (2003) *Patterns of Narrative Discourse*. Boston: Pearson Education.

Melzi, G. (2000) Cultural variations in the construction of personal narratives: Central American and European American mothers' elicitation styles. *Discourse Processes* 30, 153–177.

Miller, J.F. and Chapman, R.S. (1984) Disorders of communication: Investigating the development of language of mentally retarded children. *American Journal of Mental Deficiencies* 88, 536–545.

Navarro-Ruiz, I. and Rallo-Fabran, L. (2001) Characteristics of mazes produced by SLI children. *Clinical Linguistics and Phonetics* 15, 63–66.

Paul, R. (2001) *Language Disorders from Infancy Through Adolescence* (2nd edn). St Louis, MO: Mosby.

Pérez, C. (1998) The language of native Spanish and English speaking schizotypal college students. Unpublished dissertation, University of Massachusetts, Boston.

Restrepo, M.A. (1998) Identifiers of predominantly Spanish-speaking children with language impairment. *Journal of Speech, Language, and Hearing Research* 41, 1398–1411.

Restrepo, M.A. (2003) *PAVED for Success: A Biliteracy Program for Bilingual Children*. Paper presented at the American Speech-Language-Hearing Annual Convention, Chicago.

Restrepo, M.A. and Gutiérrez-Clellen, V.F. (2001) Article production in bilingual children with specific language impairment. *Journal of Child Language* 28, 433–452.

Restrepo, M.A., Youngs, C. and Castilla, A.P. (2005) Evaluation of three language elicitation techniques with Spanish-speaking children. Manuscript in preparation.

Richards, B. (1987) Type-token ratios: What do they really tell us? *Journal of Child Language* 14, 201–209.

Sebastián, E. and Slobin, D.I. (1994) Development of linguistic forms: Spanish. In R.A. Berman and D.I. Slobin (eds) *Relating Events in Narrative: A Crosslinguistic Developmental Study* (pp. 239–284). Hillsdale, NJ: Erlbaum.

Slobin, D.I. (1996) Two ways to travel: Verbs of motion in English and Spanish. In M. Shibitani and S.A. Thompson (eds) *Essays in Semantics* (pp. 46–58). Oxford: Oxford University Press.

Slobin, D.I. and Bocaz, A. (1988) Learning to talk about movement trough time and space: The development of narrative abilities in Spanish and English. *Lenguas Modernas* 15, 5–24.

Southwood, F. and Russell, A.F. (2004) Comparison of conversation, free play, and story generation as methods of language sample elicitation. *Journal of Speech, Language, and Hearing Research* 47, 366–376.

Wagner, C.R., Nettelbladt, U., Sahlen, B. and Nilholm, C. (2002) Conversation versus narration in pre-school children with language impairment. *International Journal of Communication Disorders* 35, 83–93.

Weismer, S.E., Evans, J. and Hesketh, L. (1999) An examination of verbal working memory capacity in children with specific language impairment. *Journal of Speech, Language, and Hearing Research* 42, 1249–1260.

Chapter 11

Utterance Length Measures for Spanish-speaking Toddlers: The Morpheme versus Word Issue Revisited

DONNA JACKSON-MALDONADO and BARBARA T. CONBOY

Amongst her many contributions as a child language researcher, the late Elizabeth Bates emphasized the limitations of generalizing information about language development from studies conducted only in English, a language whose sparse morphology and strict word order set it apart from many of the world's languages (e.g. Bates *et al.*, 2001; Devescovi *et al.*, 2003). In this chapter we continue this legacy by focusing on the issue of adapting the widely accepted metric known as *Mean Length of Utterance* (MLU) for use in Spanish, a language with rich morphology and flexible word order (see Anderson & Centeno, ch. 1, for pertinent discussion).

Roger Brown (1973) was the first to propose the use of MLU in morphemes as a means for determining stages of language development in English. The impact of MLU on the field of child language development has been immense. Adaptations of MLU have been used in multiple languages for comparing experimental and control groups in research, for determining stages of language development and assessing impairment, and for suggesting intervention strategies in clinical practice (also see Anderson, ch. 9, and Restrepo & Castilla, ch. 10, for related discussions). Still, criticisms of Brown's (1973) proposal began to appear shortly after its publication and have continued until the present time. For example, in a review of Brown's book, Crystal (1974) stated that the concept of what constitutes a morpheme was not well defined, and that this could lead to problems with reliability. Arlman-Rupp *et al.* (1976) pointed out the limitations of the MLU measure for Dutch due to that language's morphology. More recently, other authors have called into question the use of MLU as an index of language development (Eisenberg *et al.*, 2001; Johnston, 2001; Leonard & Finneran, 2003; Rollins *et al.*, 1996). Although no one doubts the usefulness of measuring the length of children's utterances, what is being discussed is the extent to which MLU should be employed, the need for further definition of its constructs, and the way in which it is calculated. What must be considered, as well, is that MLU is a broad measure of expressive language development and, therefore, does not offer detailed enough information for establishing treatment targets in language intervention.

We begin this chapter by reviewing previous research on the utility of MLU as a clinical marker and for determining developmental milestones. We discuss how word and morpheme counts have been calculated in previous research, the drawbacks and/or advantages of these methods, and how discourse factors during language sampling influence the utterance types elicited and, subsequently, MLU scores. We then present data from a study in which we evaluated the effectiveness of two different MLU measures with typically developing Spanish-speaking 20–30-month-old children. We end by discussing the implications of using these MLU measures in clinical practice. Based on our results, we propose that an MLU word count based on parental reports of children's utterances may be useful in clinical practice as well as in research with Spanish-speaking children under the age of 3 years.

Definition and Measurement of MLU

Words or morphemes?

One important and basic issue related to the use of MLU deals with how it is calculated. For English, Brown (1973) proposed using a measure of morphemes; however, there are many problems with this method. Reliability in scoring can be hindered by the lack of a solid definition of what constitutes a morpheme in early child language (Crystal, 1974). This problem is further compounded when obligatory contexts have not been well defined, and when morpheme counts are applied to languages in which information regarding typical morphological development in children is lacking. Several authors have addressed the difficulties involved in applying morpheme counts to morpheme-rich languages such as Spanish, Dutch, Italian, Hebrew, Irish, and Icelandic (Aguado Alonso, 1989; Arlmann-Rupp *et al.*, 1976; Devescovi *et al.*, 2003; Dromi & Berman, 1982; Echeverría, 1979; Gutiérrez-Clellen *et al.*, 2000; Hickey, 1991; Leonard *et al.*, 1988; Linares-Orama & Sanders, 1977; Rom & Leonard, 1990; Thordardottir & Weismer, 1998). For example, Dromi and Berman (1982) cautioned that morpheme counts in languages with synthetic morphology, that is, in which grammatical distinctions are marked through inflections, are highly complex, though not impossible. Hickey (1991) and Thordardottir and Weismer (1998) also proposed morpheme counts for Irish and Icelandic, respectively, not withstanding caveats about how the procedure should be applied. Researchers studying development in these languages have all raised similar issues regarding what is to be considered a root, whether gender and number are to be marked on all grammatical categories, what cases are to be counted, and what is productive in the early stages of language development. Clearly, the answers to such questions require knowledge of the acquisition of morphology in the relevant language. Hickey, and Thordardottir and Weismer discussed the difficulties of obtaining accurate data from morpheme counts and proposed that more developmental data, based on stringent productivity criteria, need to be considered for these languages. Because the criteria for determining what should be considered a morpheme tend to be arbitrary or too complex and, hence, unreliable, many researchers have suggested the use of a *word (MLU-w)* rather than a *morpheme (MLU-m)* count for synthetic languages.

Devescovi and colleagues (2003) compared word-based and several morpheme-based measures of utterance length in English- and Italian-speaking monolingual toddlers using data obtained from parental reports of children's *mean of the three longest utterances* (M3L) from the MacArthur Communicative Development Inventories (Caselli & Casadio, 1995; Fenson *et al.*, 1993). For both languages, all of the measures were similarly related to children's vocabulary size, suggesting that, regardless of how it is measured, the use of longer utterances is paced by increasing vocabulary skills. Gutiérrez-Clellen and colleagues (2000) analyzed Spanish data from preschool children using four different methods of MLU-m analysis. They found large inconsistencies in morpheme counts across procedures due to differing criteria regarding which morphemes should be counted. For instance, irregular verbs and morphological inflections reflecting person and number agreement were counted differently across procedures. Gutiérrez-Clellen and colleagues suggest that these methodological problems cannot be solved without further information about morphological acquisition in Spanish. They, therefore, suggest that word counts, which produce more reliable results, should be used as an overall measure of Spanish utterance length. Similar conclusions have been reached for Dutch, Irish, Hebrew, and Icelandic (Arlmann-Rupp *et al.*, 1976; Hickey, 1991; Rom & Leonard, 1990; and Thordardottir & Weismer, 1998, respectively).

To summarize, there is general agreement that, although MLU-m may provide more detail than MLU-w, MLU-m is less reliable and more time consuming to calculate than MLU-w, primarily because the lack of an adequate developmental frame of reference in morpheme-rich languages leads to difficulty establishing which morphemes to count. Moreover, MLU-w measures seem to capture developmental phenomena as well as MLU-m in such languages. MLU-w has therefore become widely accepted for languages other than English.

Contexts for counting MLU

Whether morphemes or words are counted, choices regarding which utterances to use for analysis must be made carefully. Several researchers (e.g. Eisenberg *et al.*, 2001; Johnston, 2001; Miller & Chapman, 1981) have shown that MLU varies considerably depending on the types of utterances included in the language sample. Brown (1973) excluded imitations and unintelligible forms, and other researchers have additionally excluded single-word utterances and answers to yes/no questions, elliptical wh- questions, or questions that constrain the response (Johnston, 2001; Klee, 1992); exact repetitions, routines and self-repetitions (Scarborough *et al.*, 1991); and frozen phrases such as songs, prayers, and counting (Devescovi *et al.*, 2003).

Sampling procedures and discourse factors may affect MLU more than a child's true ability. For example, MLU tends to decrease with an increase in adult questioning. Johnston (2001), therefore, suggested that the MLU calculation be modified if question–answer ratios exceed 38% of the utterances in language samples. Another discourse factor that affects MLU is the interlocutor with whom the child is interacting at the time the sample is collected. Bornstein *et al.* (2000) found differences in MLU depending on whether children interacted with a stranger or family member. In sum, context, type of discourse, interlocutors, and communicative intentions may all have an effect on MLU scores and should be considered whenever language samples are analyzed (also see Restrepo & Castilla, ch. 10, this volume). Therefore, parental reports of children's expressive language, rather than spontaneous speech or structured elicitation methods, may be better suited for ensuring the highest score possible.

MLU as a Developmental Milestone and Clinical Marker

One of the primary ways MLU counts have been used is for determining developmental stages in order to identify language delays and/or disorders. Miller and Chapman (1981) established that MLU is a better predictor of syntactic development than age. Klee and colleagues (1989) and Scarborough and colleagues (1991) found significant linear relationships between MLU and age. The age limit for which MLU is still useful has been questioned. It is generally agreed that for typically developing children MLU is no longer an effective language measure after 48 months of age (Klee & Fitzgerald, 1985; Scarborough *et al.*, 1991). Other authors have suggested that MLU is useful only up to 3 years of age (Eisenberg *et al.*, 2001; Rondal *et al.*, 1987). For children with language disorders, MLU may also be useful at older ages.

The validity of MLU as an index of grammatical development is still in question. One way to determine concurrent validity is to compare MLU with other measures of grammatical development in the same children. Several studies conducted in English have shown strong relations between MLU and other morphosyntactic measures. Rollins and colleagues (1996) found a strong positive correlation between MLU-m and a measure of noun structures in 14–32-month-old children. In contrast, Scarborough and colleagues (1991) compared MLU-m to performance on a test of syntax in typically developing children and children with various language disorders (i.e. Fragile X, Down Syndrome, and autism). They found that MLU-m overestimated the syntactic ability of children with language disorders, and that MLU-m and syntactic ability were less strongly associated when MLU-m exceeded 3.0. Similarly, Klee and Fitzgerald (1985) found that MLU-m was positively correlated with another measure of syntax but only up to Stage II, or an MLU of 2.5. Thus, MLU-m may be a valid measure of only certain aspects of grammatical development and only at specific developmental stages.

In order for MLU to be used as a means of identifying language impairment, specificity and sensitivity must first be shown (Eisenberg *et al.*, 2001). In fact, some authors have questioned the use of MLU as a clinical tool because it obscures individual differences (Leonard & Finneran, 2003; Plante *et al.*, 1993; Rollins *et al.*, 1996). For example, in a comparison of typically developing children and those with specific language impairment (SLI), Leonard and Finneran (2003) demonstrated that *same can be less*: children with similar MLUs may use different structures. While one child might use many utterances with prepositions, another child with the same MLU might use more finite verb forms. Similarly, Rollins and colleagues (1996) found that MLU-m could not account for semantic content and morphological sophistication. One of the children in their study had achieved 90% mastery of morphological markers in noun phrases whereas another child who was at a similar MLU level made many errors such as deletion of morphological markers in noun phrases. They suggested that a standard MLU measure cannot account for such differences in developmental levels and, therefore, a variety of linguistic skills need to be assessed in studies of children with language impairment.

Miller and Chapman (1981) cautioned years ago that MLU not be used alone for a clinical decision, but, rather, that it could indicate the need for further assessment. Other recent research has suggested that utterance length is not always an accurate clinical marker of language impairment. Scarborough and colleagues (1991) found that MLU overestimated the complexity of language of children with SLI. In contrast, Eisenberg and colleagues (2001) found that a very low MLU in children with normal language could be erroneously interpreted as a sign of a language disorder. Leonard and Finneran (2003) compared typically developing children to children with SLI and found that a difference of as little as 0.2 morphemes could make children of one group look like those of the other. Thus, the use of MLU to differentiate groups could lead to bias. In contrast, Klee and colleagues (1989) found that MLUs were significantly higher in typically developing children than in those with SLI at the same age, and concluded that MLU has diagnostic potential for differentiating populations.

As noted earlier, the use of MLU measures with children who speak languages other than English may have different implications. The clinical utility of MLU must be established for the languages in which it is to be used. For Icelandic, Thordardottir and Weismer (1998) proposed that the MLU-w measure is more appropriate for clinical purposes than MLU-m because it is more reliable, although a measure of complex sentence use was strongly correlated to both MLU-w and MLU-m. For school-age speakers of Spanish, Restrepo (1998) used an alternative measure, the mean number of *morphemes per T-unit* (MLT), which differentiated children with SLI from a typically developing control group. Also in Spanish, Linares-Orama and Sanders (1977) found that MLU-m and a grammar test identified language differences in children aged 3;0– 3;11.

In sum, more research is needed in languages other than English to determine how utterance-level measures should be used clinically, including the upper limits, in both age and MLU score, at which such measures are valid and reliable. It has been suggested that MLU be used as a stage delimiter and not to describe morphological development. Even within stages, care must be taken to determine individual differences in how children arrive at the same MLU, and multiple assessment instruments should always be used to ensure accurate diagnosis.

MLU Data and Analysis in Spanish-speaking Children

The studies reviewed above have established that MLU is correlated with other measures of grammatical development and with age. As noted above, many researchers have discussed the effects of context, types of utterances, and interlocutors on MLU scores. One way to reduce such effects is by using an utterance length count from parental report, such as the M3L, mentioned earlier. Parental report measures of language bypass the performance limitations inherent in spontaneous and structured language sampling, and they are obtained more efficiently. Devescovi and colleagues (2003) demonstrated that, for Italian and English, M3Ls calculated from parental report were strongly correlated with age. In a study of typically developing Spanish-speaking children, Thal *et al.* (2000) found high correlations between M3L count at the word level (M3L-w), based on parental report, and MLU-w, based on spontaneous speech. Furthermore, both measures were related to other measures of grammatical complexity. Based on these findings, the analyses we present in the next sections have been done using the parental report of M3L measure rather than the more traditional MLU calculated on a sample of 50 or 100 utterances (e.g. Brown, 1973). We explored the association of the M3L measure at word and morpheme levels (i.e. M3L-w and M3L-m, respectively) with other measures of grammatical development. Our hypothesis was that the two measures would be equally good predictors of grammatical development in this age range, but that M3L-w would yield higher reliability and require less time and skill in linguistic analysis to score.

The data set

Data were obtained from 195 typically developing children between the ages of 20 and 30 months, who participated in two larger studies of language development. Children were from monolingual Spanish homes living in Central Mexico and in a border city in Northern Mexico. Parents were asked to fill out the *MacArthur Inventario del Desarrollo de Habilidades Comunicativas-Palabras y Enunciados* (also known as *Inventario 2*; Jackson-Maldonado *et al.*, 2003; Thal *et al.*, 2000). Based on parental report, this inventory includes information on word production, word combinations, verbal inflection, M3L measures, and sentence complexity. For the M3L section, parents were asked to write down the three longest utterances they had heard their child use in the recent past. For this study, M3L was calculated using both M3L-m and M3L-w. Both measures were compared to the total number of verbal inflections (out of a total of 26), and the number of complex sentence forms (total of 37) reported by the parents.

Rules for calculating M3L in words and morphemes

For both the word and morpheme counts, we followed the general criteria established in the User's Manual of the *Inventarios* (see Jackson-Maldonado *et al.*, 2003, for scoring procedures). A summary of the most pertinent rules is given here. Utterances were excluded if they were completely unintelligible. A maximum of three utterances was included for each child and utterances were segmented according to the guidelines in the User's Manual. *Words* were operationally defined as any string of letters appearing between spaces, with some exceptions, as follows (see, also, Jackson-Maldonado *et al.*, 2003, for a complete list and Table 11.1 for more examples):

(1) Utterances that were clearly *routines* (e.g. segments of songs, nursery rhymes, or poems) were counted as one word if they were part of a longer utterance. If they stood alone, they were not counted.

(2) Frozen phrases like *akitá* [aquí está] 'here it is' and *por favor* 'please', and combined words such as *cepillo de dientes* 'toothbrush' were counted as single words.

Table 11.1 Rules for counting words

Phrase	Count	Explanation
Akita bebé	2	'akita' + bebé
Am ti baco .	3	Child words
Quíta-te maña, ve-te	3 2	2 utterances: 1. 'quíta-te' (clitic) is 2 words + maña 2. 've-te' 2 counts
Te acuerdas venimos **al** parque con Jude, Fer y Bety	11	the contraction 'al' counts as 2 words: a + el
Había una vez una familia de osos que vivían en una casa en medio del bosque	15	'Había una vez' is a routine (1 word), 'del' is 2 words
Fui a México, fui a casa de abuela y a mi casa de mis primas	3 12	Expresses two ideas. Fui a México Fui a casa de abuela y a mi casa de mis primas

Adapted from: Jackson-Maldonado *et al.* (2003)

(3) Children's word forms, even when misarticulated, were each given a separate count.

(4) In verbs with attached clitics, such as *sientate* 'sit down', the clitic (i.e. *te*) was counted as a separate word and in prepositions contracted with articles (e.g. *del*), each segment was counted as a separate word (*de* and *él*).

Morphemes were counted following the procedures proposed by Linares-Orama and Sanders (1977) and García (1978), with a few modifications. Briefly, an initial count of 1 was given for each root, and inflections beyond the root were added on. Decisions regarding these criteria were based on multiple published and unpublished studies of the acquisition of Spanish morphology (also see Anderson & Centeno, ch. 1, for pertinent discussion on Spanish morphology). The basic principle followed was to give credit for forms that are contrastive and not routine-like in the language of children in this age range.

The relation between words and morphemes

Given that both the M3L-w and M3L-m scores have word counts at their core, we expected that the two measures would be strongly correlated with each other, and this was the case ($r = 0.94$, $p < 0.01$).

We also assessed the association of each M3L score with age and other measures of grammar to determine whether both measures accounted for development in a similar way. As Figure 11.1 illustrates, there was a steady increase in both measures across ages.

Children were then divided based on a median split of vocabulary size from the *Inventario* (44–273 words in the lower group and 278–646 words in the higher group), and by age group (20–24 months and 25–30 months). In this sample of children, as with most samples in this age range, vocabulary size is highly variable across ages. Although mean vocabulary size was larger in the older than the younger age group, the ranges of vocabulary sizes were similar for each group (44–642 words in the younger group and 49–646 words in the older group). Separate ANOVAs indicated that the way in which M3L was scored interacted with age ($F[1,193] = 16.46$, $p < 0.0001$, $\eta_p^2 = 0.079$) and with vocabulary size ($F[1,193] = 11.92$, $p < 0.001$, $\eta_p^2 = 0.058$). The difference between M3L-w and M3L-m was larger for the older group ($M = 3.96$ versus 6.61) than for the younger group ($M = 2.96$ versus 4.65), and it was larger for the higher vocabulary group ($M = 3.87$ versus 6.47) than for the lower group ($M = 3.12$ versus 4.92). Furthermore, the difference between each age and vocabulary group was greater when the morpheme score was used.

We then explored the relationships between each M3L score and other measures of grammatical development. In the first analysis we looked at how each measure related to the measure of verbal inflection from the *Inventario*. Results showed that both scores were good predictors of the mean verbal inflection score ($r^2 = 0.15$ for M3L-w and $r^2 = 0.18$ for M3L-m). M3L-m predicted a significant 3% of the variance in verbal

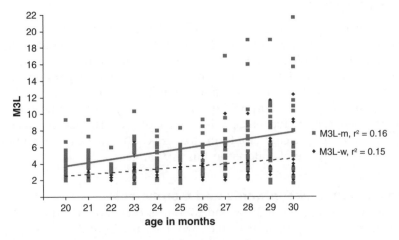

Figure 11.1 Relation of M3L words and morphemes to age

inflection above and beyond M3L-w ($p < 0.01$). However, when regressions were conducted separately for each age and vocabulary group, it was discovered that this 'advantage' for M3L-m was only found for the younger children, or for those who had lower vocabulary levels. This finding likely reflects the widely reported observation that Spanish finite verbs do not have zero forms. When children use Spanish verbs, they use inflectional morphemes on those verbs, never just the root of the verb. Decisions regarding when to count verb inflections as *true* morphemes for the child can only be made based on evidence of contrastive use of such morphemes from larger language samples, not from counts of morphemes. Thus, when Spanish utterance length is measured in terms of morphemes, it will necessarily be inflated by verb inflections during the earliest periods of development. This is a clear example of the limitations of using measures of utterance length to tap into grammatical development in a highly inflected language such as Spanish. There was even less of a difference in the relationships between each M3L score and the sentence complexity score. In this case, an additional 1% of the variance was accounted for by the morpheme versus the word score ($r^2 = 0.45$ and 0.44, respectively, $p = 0.05$), and, again, this advantage was limited to the younger group. From these results, it is clear that M3L-w and M3L-m are both good predictors of two other parent-report measures of grammatical ability in 20–30-month-old Spanish-speaking children. Even when the morpheme count does account for additional variance in another measure of grammar, this effect is small and its benefit may not outweigh the additional costs involved in counting morphemes, in terms of time and reliability.

Conclusions

Research across several languages has questioned the validity of MLU measures and the relevance of using a morpheme versus word count, particularly in morpheme-rich languages such as Spanish. In this chapter, we addressed this issue by presenting data from Spanish-speaking toddlers that were analyzed using both types of counts. Given the poor reliability and time cost of computing M3L-m in Spanish, and the fact that M3L-w is as good a measure for determining development, there may be little benefit to using M3L-m as a gross measure of language ability in this age range. *We acknowledge that a parental report measure is not a substitute for other sampling or assessment procedures.* Still, the use of the *Inventario* M3L measure does provide a window into developing language skills, hence allowing us to measure children's ability to produce multiword utterances without the confounds resulting from the use of spontaneous speech samples.

Our results also shed light on the theoretical question of whether measures of utterance length reflect children's grammatical development. Specifically, there was a clear relationship between utterance length and two aspects of Spanish morphosyntax: verbal inflection and sentence complexity.

Clinical Implications

We close this chapter with a brief note on the clinical implications of our findings and the other findings reviewed in this chapter. An important factor that affects language data is the context or situation in which the data are collected, as discussed by Anderson, ch. 9, and Restrepo and Castilla, ch. 10, in this volume. As noted above, MLU varies considerably depending on the types of utterances used in the calculation, the interlocutors present when those utterances are recorded, and whether the recordings are collected during a child-directed or adult-directed conversation. An ideal situation for obtaining MLU information may run contrary to the nature of many clinical interactions. Clinician–child interactions tend to be characterized by high frequencies of imitations, self-repetitions, and didactic question–answer sequences, which can deflate MLU scores. If optimal MLU scores are desired, these practices should be avoided during the language sampling interaction. However, some children may be used to expecting interactions with adults to be adult-centered, and may not display their true abilities during more child-centered interactions. Therefore, we propose that a viable alternative for obtaining an estimate of a child's ability to use multiword utterances is a parental report instrument such as the *MacArthur Inventario*.

We have presented data showing that both M3L-w and M3L-m are valid measures that correlate similarly with age and with other measures of grammatical development in the 20–30-month age range. Based on our findings, as well as the findings of other studies reviewed in this chapter, we suggest that a word count rather than a morpheme count be used in calculating utterance length in Spanish because the latter may be unreliable and highly time consuming. A word count can provide similar results regarding a child's developmental status compared to peers. For information about a child's morphological development, we suggest that clinicians use measures that were created for the purpose of assessing morphological development in the language of interest. We have shown that there are significant relationships between M3L-w and the use of verb inflections as well as complex utterances. By promoting learning in any of these areas, clinicians are likely to promote the development of the grammatical system.

MLU-w and M3L-w counts might be used for making cross-linguistic comparisons, matching clinical cases with control groups in research studies, and for diagnostic purposes. Although these measures have been shown to broadly reflect levels of grammatical development, it should be emphasized that they should never be used as the sole means for determining development, especially in the case of clinical diagnosis. Multiple measures should always be administered in order to provide a complete picture of a child's language development. It is also important to remember that the present results were obtained with children in the earliest stages of grammatical development (under 3 years of age) and might not apply to older children. As children advance into higher levels of grammatical development, utterance length measures may not be sufficient measures of development. Finally, our results were obtained with typically developing children. Further research with Spanish-speaking toddlers who are at risk for language impairment is needed to determine whether the present findings may be generalized to that population.

Acknowledgements

This work was supported, in part, by a grant from the Consejo Nacional de Ciencia y Tecnología (CONACYT) to the first author and a grant from the John D. and Catherine T. MacArthur Foundation to Donna Thal, San Diego State University. We would like to thank Jennifer Alargunsoro for her aid in data analysis and José G. Centeno and Raquel T. Anderson for their detailed suggestions and comments.

References

Aguado Alonso, G. (1989) *TSA: El Desarrollo de la Morfosintáxis en el Niño.* Madrid, Spain: Ciencias de la Educación Preescolar y Especial.

Arlman-Rupp, A.J.L., van Niekerk de Haan, D. and van de Sandt-Koenderman, M. (1976) Brown's early stages: Some evidence from Dutch. *Journal of Child Language* 3, 267–274.

Bates, E., Devescovi, A. and Wulfeck, B. (2001) Psycholinguistics: A cross-language perspective. *Annual Review of Psychology* 52, 369–398.

Bornstein, M.H., Haynes, O., Painter, K. and Genevro, J. (2000) Child language with mother and with stranger at home and in the laboratory: A methodological study. *Journal of Child Language* 27, 407–420.

Brown, R. (1973) *A First Language: The Early Stages.* Cambridge: Harvard University Press.

Caselli, M.C. and Casadio, P. (1995) *Il Primo Vocabolario del Bambino: Guida all'uso del Questionario MacArthur.* Milan, Italy: Franco Angeli.

Crystal, D. (1974) Review of R. Brown, A first language: The early stages. *Journal of Child Language* 1, 289–307.

Devescovi, A., Caselli, M.C., Marchione, D., Reilly, J. and Bates, E. (2003) A cross-linguistic study of the relationship between grammar and lexical development (Topic area: Grammar) [Tech. Rep. No. CND-0301]. La Jolla: University of

California, San Diego, Project in Cognitive and Neural Development, Center for Research in Language.

Dromi, E. and Berman, R.A. (1982) A morphemic measure of early language development: Data from modern Hebrew. *Journal of Child Language* 9, 403–424.

Echeverría, M.S. (1979) Longitud del enunciado infantil: Factores ambientales e individuales. In *Estudios Generales 1. Actas del 5o Seminario de Investigación y Enseñanza de la Lingüística* (pp. 56–68). Santiago, Chile: Sociedad Chilena de Lingüística y Universidad Técnica del Estado.

Eisenberg, A., Fersko, T.M. and Lundgren, C. (2001) The use of MLU for identifying language impairment in preschool children: A review. *American Journal of Speech-Language Pathology* 10, 323–342.

Fenson, L., Dale, P.S., Reznick, J.S., Thal, D., Bates, E., Hartung, J.P., Pethick, S. and Reilly, J.S. (1993) *The MacArthur Communicative Development Inventories: User's Guide and Technical Manual*. San Diego: Singular.

García, E. (1978) *Early Childhood Bilingualism With Special Reference to the Mexican American Child*. Albuquerque, NM: University of New Mexico.

Gutiérrez-Clellen, V., Restrepo, M.A., Bedore, L., Peña, E. and Anderson, R. (2000) Language sample analysis in Spanish-speaking children: Methodological considerations. *Language, Speech, and Hearing Services in Schools* 31, 88–98.

Hickey, T. (1991) Mean length of utterance and the acquisition of Irish. *Journal of Child Language* 18, 553–569.

Jackson-Maldonado, D., Thal, D., Marchman, V., Fenson, L, Newton, T. and Conboy, B. (2003) *Inventarios del Desarrollo de Habilidades Comunicativas: User's Guide and Technical Manual*. Baltimore, MD: Paul H. Brookes.

Johnston, J. (2001) An alternate MLU calculation: Magnitude and variability of effects. *Journal Speech Language and Hearing Research* 44, 156–164.

Klee, T. (1992) Developmental and diagnostic characteristics of quantitative measures of children's language production. *Topics in Language Disorders* 12, 28–41.

Klee, T. and Fitzgerald, M.D. (1985) The relation between grammatical development and mean length of utterance in morphemes. *Journal of Child Language* 12, 251–269.

Klee, T., Schaffer, M., May, S., Membrino, I. and Mougery, K. (1989) A comparison of the age-MLU relation in normal and specifically language-impaired preschool children. *Journal Speech and Hearing Disorders* 54, 226–233.

Leonard, L.B. and Finneran, D. (2003) Grammatical morpheme effect on MLU: "The same can be less" revisited. *Journal Speech Language and Hearing Research* 46, 878–888.

Leonard, L.B., Sabbadini, L., Volterra, V. and Leonard, J. (1988) Some influences on the grammar of English and Italian-speaking children with specific language impairment. *Applied Psycholinguistics* 9, 39–57.

Linares-Orama, N. and Sanders, L.J. (1977) Evaluation of syntax in three-year-old Spanish-speaking Puerto Rican children. *Journal of Speech and Hearing Research* 20, 350–357.

Miller, J.F. and Chapman, R.S. (1981) The relation between age and mean length of utterance in morphemes. *Journal of Speech and Hearing Research* 24, 154–161.

Plante, E., Swisher, L., Kiernan, B. and Restrepo, M.A. (1993) Language matches: Illuminating or confounding? *Journal of Speech, Language and Hearing Research* 36, 772–776.

Restrepo, M.A. (1998) Identifiers of predominantly Spanish-speaking children with language impairment. *Journal of Speech, Language and Hearing Research* 41, 1398–1411.

Rollins, P.R., Snow, C.E. and Willett, J. (1996) Predictors of MLU: Semantic and morphological developments. *First Language* 16, 243–259.

Rom, A. and Leonard, L.B. (1990) Interpreting deficits in grammatical morphology in specifically language-impaired children: Preliminary evidence from Hebrew. *Clinical Linguistics and Phonetics* 4, 93–105.

Rondal, J.A., Ghiotto, M., Bredart, S. and Bachelet, J. (1987) Age-relation, reliability and grammatical validity of measures of utterance length. *Journal of Child Language* 14, 433–446.

Scarborough, H.S., Rescorla, L., Tager-Flusberg, H., Fowler, A. and Sudhalter, V. (1991) The relation of utterance length to grammatical complexity in normal and language-disordered groups. *Applied Psycholinguistics* 12, 23–45.

Thal, D., Jackson-Maldonado, D. and Acosta, D. (2000) Validity of a parental report measure of vocabulary and grammar for Spanish-speaking toddlers. *Journal of Speech Language and Hearing Research* 43, 1087–1100.

Thordardottir, E.T. and Weismer, S.E. (1998) Mean length of utterance and other language sample measures in early Icelandic. *First Language* 18, 001–032.

Chapter 12

Lexical Skills in Young Children Learning a Second Language: Methods, Results, and Clinical Applications

KATHRYN KOHNERT and PUI FONG KAN

In this chapter, we focus on the measurement of lexical skills in early sequential bilinguals – specifically, those children who learn a single language at home (i.e. their first language, L1) from birth, and begin learning a second language (L2) sometime between the ages of 3 and 6 years (also see Centeno, ch. 3, for related discussion on bilingualism in children). Sufficient lexical knowledge (in terms of breadth and depth of vocabulary) as well as efficient access to this knowledge is fundamental to overall language proficiency. On the flip side, deficits at the lexical level have been documented in a broad range of developmental language disorders. Therefore, the measurement of lexical skills is a fundamental component in clinical assessment of children with suspected language impairments. This chapter has four sections. We begin with an overview of lexical knowledge and processing development in a first language. In the second section, we describe young children learning a second language. In the third section, we review studies that have systematically investigated lexical skills in children learning a second language. We conclude by discussing the implications these studies have for the clinical assessment of lexical skills in young second language learners with suspected language delays or deficits.

Lexical Knowledge and Processing in a First Language

The rapid acquisition of word forms for objects, events, actions, and attributes is a core feature of child language learning, achieved through the complex interactions of cognitive, social, and linguistic systems (Bloom, 2000; Tomasello, 2003). Typically, developing children learning a single language know several hundred words at age 2;0, and several thousand words by age 5;0 (Bloom, 2000). Word learning remains robust throughout childhood and beyond, with approximately 300 additional words added to children's lexicons during each year they attend school (Clark, 1995). The understanding of words typically precedes and exceeds the ability to generate words, although there is a strong relationship between lexical comprehension and production (Tomasello, 2003). In addition to knowing large numbers of words and their meanings, language proficiency also requires the ability to use this lexical-semantic knowledge efficiently during the fast-paced communicative interactions that characterize real-time language use. Consider that conversational speech among adult native speakers of any language takes place at a rate of approximately 125–225 words per minute (e.g. Foss & Hakes, 1978). While working at this speed, proficient speakers of a language must select and produce an intended word from many thousands of alternatives. On the receiving end, listeners first perceive the signal, then retrieve the speaker's intended meaning from a stream of sounds that are exceedingly fast (i.e. an average of 5–8 syllables per second) with overlapping borders between meaningful units (Fowler, 1980; Liberman, 1970). In order to process linguistic information in real-time, conversational participants need to do so automatically, resisting interference from either internal or external distractions. The ability to quickly learn, recall, access, and deploy known lexical information in real-time continues to develop throughout adolescence (Kohnert, 2004).

The measurement of lexical knowledge and processing skills is important in the assessment of developmental language impairment. When compared to their typically developing peers, children with language delays may have smaller vocabularies, slower rates in acquiring new words, relatively limited meanings attached to known lexical forms, or longer response times for recognizing or producing previously acquired word forms (see Windsor & Kohnert, 2004). In addition, empirical evidence points to a core role for the lexicon in grammatical organization in general (Bates & Goodman, 1997; Caselli *et al.*, 1999). Strong, positive correlations between lexical and grammatical development in young monolingual children suggest that a clear understanding of lexical-semantic skills across development is critical to understanding deficits in grammar, which are often considered a hallmark of primary language impairment in English-speaking preschool-aged children (Leonard, 1998). Therefore, it is important that all comprehensive assessments of language include different measures of lexical-semantic skills.

The adequacy of a particular child's lexical-semantic system is typically determined by comparing his or her performance on a combination of knowledge and processing-based measures to the performance of other children of the same age, with similar cultural, social, and language-learning experiences (Kohnert, 2004). Knowledge-based lexical measures are designed to index the number or type of words children recognize or produce, the depth of meanings attached to these words, or the conceptual frameworks in which this lexical-semantic information is embedded. Examples of tasks that emphasize lexical knowledge include standardized measures of vocabulary breadth, such as Spanish and English versions of the *Peabody Picture Vocabulary Test* (Dunn & Dunn, 1997; Dunn *et al.*, 1986), and the *Expressive Vocabulary Test* (Brownell, 2000; 2001), as well as tasks that require a child to provide the definitions of words or identify similarities or differences between two words.

In contrast to knowledge-dependent measures, processing-dependent measures of the lexicon are concerned with the efficiency with which individuals can either learn new lexical forms, or access and deploy previously acquired forms. The linguistic units included in these tasks are intended to be equally familiar to all children (e.g. high-frequency vocabulary words or concepts with which individuals have substantial experience) or equally unfamiliar to children (e.g. nonsense words that do not exist in the language). The idea is to minimize the role that prior language-specific experience may have on performance. In this way, experimental processing-dependent measures attempt to measure the integrity of the underlying language learning system. Examples of tasks that emphasize lexical processing include novel word learning or fast mapping paradigms, and rapid color, digit, or object naming. Other tasks that emphasize processing at the interface of lexical and phonological levels include the repetition of nonsense words (e.g. Campbell *et al.*, 1997) or the identification of cross-linguistic cognate words in another language where there is some overlap (Kohnert *et al.*, 2004).

Young Children Learning a Second Language

As mentioned earlier, children who are early sequential bilinguals learn one language at home from birth (L1), then begin to learn an L2 (typically the majority language of the community) before they can read or write in L1. This includes, for example, children living with their Spanish-speaking parents in the USA, who attend preschool or elementary educational programs in English. Prior to the introduction of the L2, we can reasonably expect that early sequential bilinguals will develop their home language (i.e. L1) at a similar rate and to similar levels as typically developing monolingual children, provided other factors known to influence language, such as socioeconomic circumstances and literacy levels, are comparable (also see Centeno, ch. 3, this volume). It is what happens after the systematic introduction of the L2 that separates these early sequential bilinguals from single-language learners, simultaneous bilinguals (children who learn two languages from birth), and older L2 learners.

For early sequential bilinguals, at some point, the development of the L1 is affected by regular experience in the L2. When this L2 is the majority language of the community and the primary language of instruction in preschool or elementary school settings, the minority L1 may no longer be the primary vehicle for learning or social interactions. Under these conditions (sometimes referred to as *subtractive bilingualism*), it is possible that the L1 may regress, plateau, or develop at a rate slower than would be expected based on research with monolingual children. It is also possible that different lexical skills are developed in L1 and L2, consistent with the different uses of language required by home and school environments. Consider, for example, that the typically developing 3-year-old child from a predominantly Spanish-speaking family produces several hundred words in Spanish, and comprehends even more. These words include names, attributes and actions associated with familiar people, places, objects, and events. This child then enters an English-speaking preschool program. Although there will be some overlap between home and school experiences and corresponding vocabulary items, there may also be experiences that are unique to each setting. When languages serve different social functions, young children may develop skills in each language consistent with these different purposes (also see Centeno, ch. 3, this volume). As such, measuring skills in only one of the early sequential bilingual's two languages may not adequately reveal the child's full repertoire of lexical skills. If the goal is to determine the integrity or extent of the child's language system, in order to separate typical learners from those children with language impairments, skills in both the L1 and L2 must be measured, using parallel tasks (e.g. Oller & Pearson, 2002). In the following section we review studies that have investigated lexical skills in both L1 and L2 of early sequential bilinguals.

Lexical Skills in L1 and L2 of Typical Early Sequential Bilinguals

Performance by *typical learners* in both the L1 and L2 provides a critical reference point for comparing the performance of those sequential bilingual children with suspected language delays/deficits. The relatively few studies that have investigated lexical skills in both the L1 and L2 of typically developing sequential bilinguals have relied on picture naming and picture identification tasks. Picture naming and picture identification tasks have a long history of use in educational, clinical, and research settings, with monolingual and bilingual individuals (e.g. see Kohnert *et al.*, 1999; Rice, 1996, for reviews). Variations of the picture naming task are used to measure lexical production, and different types of picture identification tasks are used to measure lexical comprehension. The response variables of interest on these tasks are accuracy (reflecting lexical knowledge), response speed (reflecting processing efficiency), or both. Lexical stimuli selected for these tasks vary along a number of different features, including word class or type (such as nouns, verbs, or adjectives) as well as the presumed frequency or familiarity of these target words (consider high frequency words such as *ball*, *eat*, and *slow* as compared to lower frequency words such as *sphere*, *digest*, and *sluggish*).

Leseman (2000) used response accuracy on picture naming and picture identification tasks to investigate vocabulary knowledge in the L1 and L2 of Turkish preschool children in the Netherlands. The majority of these children were second or third generation immigrants from low-income families, living in a subtractive bilingual language environment. Turkish was spoken in their homes and they attended a preschool program in Dutch beginning at age 3;0. Both receptive and expressive vocabulary measures revealed significant and positive growth in Dutch (L2). In contrast, performance in Turkish (L1) did not change and, over time, lagged behind that of monolingual Turkish peers from the same community who did not attend preschool. Similar findings of reduced L1 skills alongside positive gains in L2 for preschool children were found by Schaerlaekens *et al.* (1995). This study investigated vocabulary skills in 3–5-year old children who spoke French (L1) and attended a Dutch preschool (L2). In this study, both L1 and L2 had high social status and families represented the range of income levels. Nonetheless, outcomes were similar in that L1 lexical performance declined at the same time performance on the lexical task in L2 improved. Specifically, Schaerlaekens *et al.* reported a 40% increase in L2 scores between the ages of 3 and 5 years, alongside a 30% decrease in L1.

Results from two other studies, however, indicate that early introduction of L2 need not result in a regression of L1 (Rodríguez *et al.*, 1995; Winsler *et al.*, 1999). In these studies, children from low-income Spanish-speaking families attended bilingual preschool programs, five full days per week. Instructional activities were in both Spanish (L1) and English (L2). Performance on standardized language measures in Spanish and English were compared with a control group of children who did not attend preschool. On all measures, both between-group and longitudinal, there were significant positive gains in L1 and L2 for children attending the bilingual preschool. Discrepant findings across studies may be traced to differences in the populations studied, to differences in data collection procedures, as well as to fundamental differences in the types of educational programs children attended. Children who attended bilingual educational programs and lived in bilingual communities showed improved lexical skills in both L1 and L2 (Rodríguez *et al.*, 1995; Winsler *et al.*, 1999). In contrast, for children who received little or no support for L1 in the educational setting and broader community, lexical gains were restricted to only L2 (Leseman, 2000; Schaerlackens *et al.*, 1995).

Kan and Kohnert (2005) used picture naming and picture identification tasks to investigate lexical knowledge in 3–5-year-old children learning Hmong as their L1, and English as their L2. All children were from homes in which Hmong was the primary language spoken, and attended a bilingual Hmong–English preschool. The mean age for the younger group was 3;11, with an average of six months of preschool attendance. The mean age for the older group was 5;0 years, with an average of 16 months of preschool attendance. On the Hmong (L1) tasks, there were no differences in either receptive or expressive lexical skills between younger and older groups. In contrast, in English (L2), the older children named and identified significantly more items than the younger children. These findings of significant differences in L2 between younger and older participants highlight the robust and efficient nature of lexical learning in preschool age children. At the same time, the relative stagnation of Hmong (L1) skills across age during the same period underscores the overall vulnerability of L1. Perhaps the L1 system is even more vulnerable when differences between home and community cultures and languages are great, as is the case with Hmong and English (cf. Genesee *et al.*, 2004). Although one of the goals of the early childhood educational program that Hmong participants attended was to support and develop the home language, observation of classroom interactions indicated that instructional activities were primarily in English, while classroom management took place primarily in Hmong. Findings here suggest that if a goal of the early childhood education program is to develop the home language (along with L2) to maintain family links and cultural identity, educational and enrichment activities should be provided in L1 (see Kohnert *et al.*, 2005).

As noted in the previous section, children learning two languages may develop and use words in L1 and L2, in different settings, and for different purposes. That is, a child may have some concepts, including those for household objects or family-related activities, lexicalized only in L1; other concepts, including those associated with academic tasks may be lexicalized only in the L2, and still other concepts may have a linguistic form in L1 as well as L2. Pearson *et al.* (1993) introduced a method that compares the total lexicalized concepts distributed across both languages (composite vocabulary score) to the number of lexicalized concepts in a single language (conventional score in each language). In order to obtain a composite score, parallel tasks are administered in both the child's L1 and L2, then a single point is awarded for any items named or identified, independent of language. For example, if *dog* and its Hmong equivalent *aub* are both used to name a pictured dog, only one point is awarded in the composite scoring method; similarly, if a picture of a hand is named in English, but not Hmong, the item is also scored as correct. Kan and Kohnert (2005) found that composite scores were significantly greater than either single language for both expressive and receptive lexical tasks for all preschool children in their study. This finding of conceptual knowledge distributed across two lexical systems also seems to hold for Spanish–English preschool children. Peña *et al.* (2002) found that 68% of the items produced in a scripted word-generation task by 4–7-year-old bilingual children were unique to either Spanish or English. These results indicate that one language does not simply form a subset of information encoded in the other language, or that semantic information from one language is automatically transferred to the other.

Other studies have emphasized the processing of lexical information in L1 and L2 in an attempt to identify patterns of skill development and use in typical early sequential bilingual children. In a series of cross-sectional and longitudinal studies, Kohnert and colleagues measured the processing of lexical skills during picture naming and picture-word verification tasks (Jia *et al.*, 2006; Kohnert, 2002; Kohnert & Bates, 2002; Kohnert *et al.*, 1999). The experimental tasks used in these studies emphasized processing efficiency over breadth of vocabulary knowledge by measuring how quickly participants could accurately retrieve the names of high-frequency nouns or verbs, in low-demand and high-demand response conditions. All participants lived in the USA, and had learned Spanish as L1 at home and English as L2 in the educational system, beginning at about five years of age. At the time of testing, participants ranged in age from 5 to 22 years. For both comprehension and production, there were gains in lexical processing efficiency across age, such that older participants outperformed younger participants in both Spanish and English. Importantly, however, across time these gains in processing efficiency were greater in L2 (English) than in L1 (Spanish). The end result of these different growth rates between Spanish and English was a shift across age/experience from greater processing efficiency in L1 to L2, evident first on the comprehension task, and later on the production task – a finding that may reflect differences in task demands.

Gains in processing efficiency in picture naming after a 1-year interval were obtained for a subgroup of these typically developing children (Kohnert, 2002). All participants demonstrated positive change on at least one of the response variables measured (speed or accuracy in L1 and L2 in low-demand and high-demand processing conditions). However, none of these typically developing children demonstrated gains on all of the response variables measured. In some cases, performance on a given measure improved, in other cases it remained the same, and in some cases performance actually declined. Importantly, children showed gains in lexical skill in different ways – either in improved accuracy or response speed, sometimes in only one language, and sometimes in both the L1 and L2. This variability was present not only in absolute terms, but also in individual performance relative to that of peers with similar language and cultural experiences. Thus, in addition to the significant variability that exists between children learning two languages, we see that there is also considerable variability within each child. The overall trajectory, however, was upward, with gains in speed, accuracy, or control of the lexical system in at least one of the child's two languages evident across development.

In summary, at the group level, studies consistently reported significant gains in lexical knowledge or processing in L2 across age and corresponding experience with the community language. Results for L1 were much more variable. Some studies found that children's lexical skills in L1 decline (Leseman, 2000; Schaerlackens *et al.*, 1995), other studies found a relative stabilization of L1 skills (Kan & Kohnert, 2005; Kohnert & Bates, 2002; Kohnert *et al.*, 1999), and still other studies reported increased abilities on lexical measures in L1 (Kohnert, 2002; Rodríguez *et al.*, 1995; Winsler *et al.*, 1999). Differences in both the direction and rate of language change may be the result of a number of different factors, including the types of tasks used to measure lexical abilities, differences between home and community cultures and languages, the children's ages and level of L1 development when consistent experience in L2 begins, the level of continued support for the development of L1 lexical skills in the home and in other environments, and individual differences in children's learning rates and styles. Importantly, it seems that even when quantitative measures seem to point to one language as 'dominant' or stronger, qualitative measures may reveal that lexical knowledge is distributed across L1 and L2 and, as such, unique lexical-semantic information is present even in the so-called 'weaker' language (Kohnert & Derr, 2004). The implications of these collective findings for the clinical assessment of lexical skills in linguistically diverse learners are discussed in the following section.

Implications for the Clinical Assessment of Lexical Skills in Young L2 Learners

Regular exposure to two (or more) languages does not cause language delays or disorders (e.g. Genesee *et al.*, 2004). However, as with monolingual children, we can reasonably anticipate that approximately 5–10% of children learning two languages will have a primary impairment in language (cf. Reed, 2005). Deficits at the lexical-semantic level, such as limited vocabularies, slower rates of word learning, and difficulty in the timely retrieval of previously acquired words, are common in children with language delays or deficiencies. A fundamental goal of speech-language pathologists is to identify children whose language skills lag significantly behind those of their peers, who may need specialized instruction to ameliorate the long-term consequences that accompany such delays.

The task of identifying potential lexical deficiencies in linguistically diverse learners is complicated by a number of factors, including the limited normative data available for children learning two languages sequentially as well as the tremendous amount of normal variation in skill development that is characteristic of this population. Despite these formidable complications, combined results from the studies reviewed in the previous section provide some basic guidelines for assessing lexical skills in young children learning an L2. These basic guidelines are that: (1) measures of lexical skills should be obtained in both the L1 and L2, although comparisons with monolingual speakers may not be valid for either; (2) performance on lexical measures administered in each language should be scored in different ways, considering each language separately as well as the composite or total lexical-semantic system, (3) processing-dependent measures are an important complement to more traditional knowledge-based measures of lexical abilities, and (4) measures of lexical performance at different points in time are needed in order to index both rate and direction of change. Each of these general guiding principles for lexical assessment is discussed in the following paragraphs.

The first guiding principle is that lexical skills should be measured in both the child's L1 and L2. Although it is sometimes assumed that the first language the child learns will be the strongest, this is often not the case. As shown by the studies reviewed in the previous section, lexical skills in L1 may be vulnerable in typically developing young children who begin attending educational programs in which the primary language of instruction is L2 (e.g. Kan & Kohnert, 2005; Leseman, 2000; Schaerlackens *et al.*, 1995). It is possible that for children with language impairments, this L1 vulnerability is even greater (Kohnert *et al.*, 2005; Restrepo & Kruth, 2000). The clinical implication is that, in the absence of direct measurements, we cannot assume that the child's current level of lexical skill in L1 is greater than that of L2. Also, because the rate and course of development of the L1 may vary considerably following the introduction of L2, normative data based on the performance of monolingual speakers of either of the child's two languages may not provide valid comparisons. Although this point is generally acknowledged for the L2, it is often assumed that, if normative data on monolingual speakers of the L1 are available, these data somehow would provide a valid comparison for early sequential bilinguals. This is not necessarily the case (e.g. Grosjean, 1998; Kohnert, 2004). The language experiences of early sequential bilinguals are fundamentally different from those of their monolingual age peers, so it is not surprising that on many measures lexical performance will also differ (also see

Centeno, ch. 3, this volume). The exception here is that monolingual normative data may be used as a reference point to *rule out* a deficit at the lexical level. Such comparisons, however, are not sufficient to *rule in* a disorder, as they tend to underestimate the bilingual child's lexical skills. Alternative comparison groups, including local norms, siblings, or classmates with similar language experiences, may be more appropriate.

Although it is important to document performance separately in each language of the developing bilingual, the resulting cross-linguistic profile may fail to capture the full extent of the child's lexical-semantic skills. This is true even when one of the languages appears to be dominant or stronger in terms of the overall number of lexical items accurately produced or understood. It is, therefore, important to complement traditional single language scoring procedures with composite scores to obtain a measure of the total number of concept-form mappings present in the bilingual child's combined lexical-semantic system. In composite scoring, as mentioned previously, a single point is awarded for any items named or identified, independent of language. The comparison of composite to single-language scores provides a measure of the total number of concept-form mappings present in the bilingual child's collective lexical-semantic system. This is possible using both standardized lexical measures, such as the Spanish and English versions of the *Expressive One-Word Picture Vocabulary Test* (Brownell, 2000; 2001), as well as through clinician created criterion-referenced tasks. The distribution of lexical skills across languages also indicates that both the L1 and L2 should be systematically addressed in clinical intervention for those children who are found to have more general language impairments (Kohnert & Derr, 2004; Kohnert *et al.*, 2005).

A third general guideline for increasing the validity of assessment with young L2 learners is to include processing-dependent lexical measures. The collective results from studies on sequential bilingual learners, interpreted within the broader literature on language development in young children, clearly indicate that tasks that tap the efficiency with which lexical information is processed are an important complement to more traditional measures of vocabulary breadth or depth. This is true not only for assessments with linguistically diverse children, but for all children. However, the point is underscored here because tasks that emphasize processing, in terms of learning or response efficiency, may reduce the bias inherent in more knowledge or experience-dependent language tasks (Campbell *et al.*, 1997; Kohnert, 2004; Kohnert & Windsor, 2004). Processing-dependent measures of lexical skills include rapid naming or novel word learning paradigms. Although there are no published studies investigating rapid naming or fast-mapping in both L1 and L2 of sequential bilinguals, clinicians may adapt tasks that have previously been used in a single language to create criterion-referenced measures of lexical processing skills for young L2 learners.

The fourth general assessment guideline is to document the child's lexical knowledge and processing skills in both L1 and L2 across time. Assessments at a single point in time may provide important information regarding the child's current level of lexical ability. However, they do not provide information about the child's rate or direction of learning. This information about the direction and rate of lexical development is critical to separating typical learners from those at risk for persistent delays in language acquisition. For typically developing bilingual children, we anticipate that there will be gains on some lexical measures, in at least one of the child's languages, across relatively short time intervals. It is not clear that this would be the case for children with language impairments. It is also important here to use peer comparisons at different test points so that the amount of relative change across children with similar experiences may be compared.

In summary, current research on lexical development in typical second language learners has a number of important implications for increasing the effectiveness of clinical assessments with young children learning an L2. It will be important for future studies to investigate lexical skills in both languages of typical as well as atypical sequential bilinguals with a much broader range of tasks to support and extend these preliminary recommendations.

References

Bates, E. and Goodman, J. (1997) On the inseparability of grammar and the lexicon: Evidence from acquisition, aphasia, and real-time processing. *Language and Cognitive Processes* 12, 507–584.

Bloom, P. (2000) *How Children Learn the Meaning of Words*. Cambridge, MA: MIT Press.

Brownell, R. (2000) *Expressive One-Word Picture Vocabulary Test* (3rd edn). Novato, CA: Academic Therapy Publications.

Brownell, R. (2001) *Expressive One-Word Picture Vocabulary Test: Spanish-English edition*. Novato, CA: Academic Therapy Publications.

Campbell, T., Dollagan, C., Needleman, H. and Janosky, J. (1997) Reducing bias in language testing: Processing-dependent measures. *Journal of Speech, Language, and Hearing Research* 40, 519–525.

Caselli, C., Casadio, P. and Bates, E. (1999) A comparison of the transition from first words to grammar in English and Italian. *Journal of Child Language* 26, 69–111.

Clark, E. (1995) Later lexical development and word formation. In P. Fletcher and B. MacWhinney (eds) *The Handbook of Child Language* (pp. 393–412). Oxford: Basil Blackwell.

Dunn, L.M. and Dunn, L.M. (1997) *Peabody Picture Vocabulary Test-Revised* (3rd edn). Circle Pines, MN: American Guidance Service.

Dunn, L.M., Padilla, E.R., Lugo, D.E. and Dunn, L.M. (1986) *Test de Vocabulario en Imagenes Peabody*. Circle Pines, MN: American Guidance Service.

Foss, D.J. and Hakes, D.T. (1978) *Psycholinguistics: An Introduction to the Psychology of Language*. Englewood Cliffs, NJ: Prentice-Hall.

Fowler, C. (1980) Coarticulations and theories of extrinsic timing. *Journal of Phonetics* 8, 113–133.

Genesee, F., Paradis, J. and Crago, M.B. (2004) *Dual Language Development and Disorders*. Baltimore: Paul H. Brookes.

Grosjean, F. (1998) Studying bilinguals: Methodological and conceptual issues. *Bilingualism: Language and Cognition* 1, 131–149.

Jia, G., Kohnert, K., Collado, J. and Gracia, F.A. (2006) Action naming in Spanish and English by sequential bilingual children and adolescents. *Journal of Speech, Language, and Hearing Research* 49, 588–602.

Kan, P.F. and Kohnert, K. (2005) Preschoolers learning Hmong and English: Lexical-semantic skills in L1 and L2. *Journal of Speech, Language, and Hearing Research* 48, 1–12.

Kohnert, K. (2002) Picture naming in early sequential bilinguals: A 1-Year Follow-up. *Journal of Speech, Language, and Hearing Research* 45, 759–771.

Kohnert, K. (2004) Processing skills in early sequential bilinguals: Children learning a second language. In B. Goldstein (ed.) *Bilingual Language Development and Disorders in Spanish-English Speakers* (pp. 53–76). Baltimore: Paul. H. Brookes.

Kohnert, K. and Bates, E. (2002) Balancing bilinguals II: Lexical comprehension and cognitive processing in children learning Spanish and English. *Journal of Speech, Language, and Hearing Research* 45, 347–359.

Kohnert, K., Bates, E. and Hernández, A.E. (1999) Balancing bilinguals: Lexical-semantic production and cognitive processing in children learning Spanish and English. *Journal of Speech, Language, and Hearing Research* 42, 1400–1413.

Kohnert, K. and Derr, A. (2004) Language intervention with bilingual children. In B. Goldstein (ed.) *Bilingual Language Development and Disorders in Spanish-English Speakers* (pp. 315–343). Baltimore: Paul. H. Brookes.

Kohnert, K., Yim, D., Nett, K., Kan, P.F. and Duran, L. (2005) Planning and implementing intervention with linguistically diverse children: Critical questions and tentative answers. *Language, Speech, and Hearing Services in School* 36, 251–263.

Kohnert, K. and Windsor, J. (2004) In search of common ground – Part II: Nonlinguistic performance by linguistically diverse learners. *Journal of Speech, Language, and Hearing Research* 47, 891–903.

Kohnert, K., Windsor, J. and Miller, R. (2004) Crossing borders: Recognition of Spanish words by English-speaking children with and without language impairment. *Journal of Applied Psycholinguistics* 25, 543–564.

Leonard, L.B. (1998) *Children with Specific Language Impairment*. Cambridge, MA: MIT Press.

Leseman, P. (2000) Bilingual vocabulary development of Turkish preschoolers in the Netherlands. *Journal of Multilingual and Multicultural Development* 21, 93–112.

Liberman, A.M. (1970) The grammars of speech and language. *Cognitive Psychology* 1, 301–323.

Oller, D.K. and Pearson, B.Z. (2002) Assessing the effects of bilingualism: A background. In D.K. Oller and R.E. Eilers (eds.) *Language and Literacy in Bilingual Children* (pp. 3–40). Clevedon, UK: Multingual Matters.

Pearson, B.Z., Fernández, S.C. and Oller, D.K. (1993) Lexical development in bilingual infants and toddlers: Comparison to monolingual norms. *Language and Learning* 43, 93–120.

Peña, E., Bedore, L.M. and Zlatic-Giunta, R. (2002) Category-generation performance of bilingual children: The influence of condition, category, and language. *Journal of Speech, Language, and Hearing Research* 45, 938–947.

Reed, V. (2005) *An Introduction to Children with Language Disorders* (3rd edn). Boston: Pearson Education.

Restrepo, M.A. and Kruth, K. (2000) Grammatical characteristics of a bilingual student with specific language impairment. *Disorders Quarterly Communication Journal* 21, 66–76.

Rice, M. (1996) "Show me X": New views of an old assessment technique. In K. Cole, P. Dale and D. Thal (eds) *Assessment of Communication and Language* (pp. 183–206). Baltimore: Paul. H. Brookes.

Rodríguez, J., Díaz, R., Duran, D. and Espinosa, L. (1995) The impact of bilingual preschool education on the language development of Spanish-speaking children. *Early Childhood Research Quarterly* 10, 475–490.

Schaerlackens, A., Zink, J. and Verheyden, L. (1995) Comparative vocabulary development in kindergarten classes with a mixed population of monolinguals, simultaneous and successive bilinguals. *Journal of Multilingual and Multicultural Development* 16, 477–495.

Tomasello, M. (2003) *Constructing a Language: A Usage-based Theory of Language Acquisition*. Cambridge, MA: Harvard University Press.

Windsor, J. and Kohnert, K. (2004) In search of common ground – Part I: Lexical performance by linguistically diverse learners. *Journal of Speech, Language, and Hearing Research* 47, 877–890.

Winsler, A., Díaz, R., Espinosa, L. and Rodríguez, J. (1999) When learning a second language does not mean losing the first: Bilingual language development in low-income Spanish-speaking children attending bilingual preschool. *Child Development* 70, 349–362.

Chapter 13

Measuring Phonological Skills in Bilingual Children: Methodology and Clinical Applications

BRIAN A. GOLDSTEIN

Phonological disorders are among the most prevalent communication disorders in preschool and school-age children affecting about 10% of this population, and for about 80% of children with phonological disorders, the severity is high enough to require clinical services. Furthermore, 50–70% of school-age children with phonological disorders exhibit general academic difficulty and often require other types of remedial services (Gierut, 1998). There is also an observed relationship between early phonological disorder and subsequent reading, writing, spelling, and mathematical abilities (Stackhouse, 1997). Thus, phonological disorders are prevalent, usually require intervention, and impact academic achievement.

In the USA, children with phonological disorders account for 28% of the caseload of school-based speech-language pathologists (SLPs) (Peters-Johnson, 1998), and 91.8% of school-based SLPs indicate having children with articulation/phonological disorders on their caseloads (American Speech-Language-Hearing Association [ASHA], 2003). Many of those children are from culturally and linguistically diverse populations and are likely to be bilingual (often referred to as *English Language Learners* (ELLs)). According to the US Census Bureau (2000), there are almost 47 million individuals (17.9% of the population) who speak a language other than English at home. Of those 47 million individuals, almost 6.8 million are children between the ages of 5 and 17 (US Census, 2000). The number of 2–5-year-olds (the age when SLPs often begin to assess children with nonorganic phonological disorders) who speak a language other than or in addition to English is unknown. If, however, the prevalence figure of 10% cited previously is applied to 5–17-year-olds who speak a language other than or in addition to English, then some 680,000 children are affected by a phonological disorder and likely would require services in a language other than, or in addition to, English. Given that the bilingual population of the USA is increasing, the practice of using approaches to measure phonological skills that have been developed for monolingual children may not provide an adequate picture of phonological skills in bilingual children.

Providing clinical services to bilingual children with phonological disorders is usually difficult because of the limited information on typical and atypical phonological development, the lack of valid and reliable assessment methods, and the absence of guidelines for the selection of appropriate intervention goals. Although the research base related to these issues has been increasing steadily over the last decades, the number of studies related to bilingual children is relatively limited. Without information from well designed research studies, the decision process used by SLPs to determine appropriate assessment and intervention for bilingual children with phonological disorders may be flawed. As a result, a number of unwanted outcomes may occur: bilingual children may be overidentified or underidentified; their diagnostic and intervention services might be delayed; and their phonological skills may be incorrectly characterized. The present state-of-the-art requires an increase in well controlled studies that would enhance the knowledge base of phonological skills in bilingual children and account for their linguistic variation.

Examining the phonological skills of bilingual children and subsequently informing assessment and intervention requires consideration of factors not usually associated with phonological research in monolingual children. First, in the context of the USA, how should descriptive information be gathered for languages other than English, especially understudied languages spoken in the country (e.g. Haitian Creole, Hmong, Russian)? For better studied languages like Spanish, researchers can use already-developed assessment protocols to reliably and validly measure children's phonological skills. Second, should phonological skills be examined in the child's first language (L1) or second language (L2), or both? Although some studies have examined phonological skills in both languages (e.g. Goldstein & Washington, 2001), some have examined the children's skills only in English (e.g. Gildersleeve *et al.*, 1996). Third, how can researchers and practicing SLPs disentangle within-language versus cross-language effects? That is, it is necessary to establish sound changes specific to each ambient language versus those that are the result of the influence of one language on the other (Barlow, 2001). Fourth, what sociolinguistic factors might be important to consider in identifying participants in bilingual phonological research? These factors might include issues such as the dialect(s) of the participants (Goldstein & Iglesias, 2001), language history (i.e. when the languages were acquired), relative levels of input/output in each language, and how well each participant understands and uses each language (Restrepo, 1998; also see Yavaş & Goldstein, 1998). Finally, what measures should be used to analyze the data from bilingual children? How can standard measures of phonological skill (e.g. consonant accuracy and percentage-of-occurrence of phonological patterns) be combined with relatively new ones (e.g. phonological MLU; Ingram, 2002) to inform phonological development and disorders in bilingual children?

It is beyond the scope of this chapter to answer all these questions. Beginning to answer these questions, however, requires, at a minimum, attention to the heterogeneity of bilingual phonological development (including within- versus cross-language characteristics) and variation within this group (i.e. dialect). The purpose of this chapter is to highlight the methodological issues required to measure phonological skills in bilingual children and relate those methods to clinical practice. Specifically, we will emphasize methodological and clinical issues related to bilingual phonological development, sociolinguistic considerations, and dialect. Because of the relative paucity of research related to bilingual speakers, information from studies examining monolingual speakers will be recounted. These studies, however, will be used to underscore issues related to bilingual speakers. Although the focus is on bilingual Spanish–English children in the USA, principles predicated in this chapter should be adapted to bilingual children developing speech in other sociolinguistic scenarios.

Bilingual Phonological Development

Because bilingual children are acquiring two phonological systems, it is likely that phonological acquisition in each language is different for bilingual children than it is for monolingual children. There is increasing evidence that the phonological system (i.e. both segment- and pattern-based aspects of speech sound production) of bilingual speakers develops somewhat differently from monolingual speakers of either language. Gildersleeve *et al.* (1996) examined the English phonological skills of typically developing, bilingual (English–Spanish) 3-year-olds. The results indicated that the bilingual children showed an overall lower intelligibility rating, made more consonant and vowel errors, and produced more uncommon error patterns than either monolingual English or monolingual Spanish speakers. The bilingual children also exhibited error patterns found in both languages (e.g. cluster reduction) and patterns that were not exhibited by either monolingual Spanish speakers (e.g. final consonant devoicing) or monolingual English speakers (e.g. initial consonant deletion).

Gildersleeve-Neumann and Davis (1998) examined the English phonological skills at the beginning of the school year of 27 typically developing, 3-year-old bilingual (English–Spanish) children and compared them to the phonological skills of 14 typically developing, monolingual 3-year-old English speakers and 6 typically developing, 3-year-old monolingual Spanish speakers. The bilingual children exhibited, on average, a higher percentage of occurrence for six of the ten phonological processes analyzed (i.e. cluster reduction, backing, final consonant deletion, final devoicing, initial voicing, and stopping) than either the monolingual English or monolingual Spanish speakers. These results indicated that the bilingual children demonstrated different developmental patterns than their monolingual counterparts and also exhibited more errors initially than monolingual speakers. However, these differences decreased over time. When the bilingual children were tested at the end of the school year, again in English, their phonological skills were commensurate with their monolingual peers.

Goldstein and Washington (2001) examined the English and Spanish phonological skills of typically developing, 4-year-old bilingual (Spanish–English) children and found that there were no significant differences between the two languages on percentage of correct consonants; percentage of correct consonants for sound classes; or percentages of occurrence for phonological processes. The results also indicated that the overall phonological skills of these bilingual 4-years-olds were similar to monolingual children. The bilingual children, however, were much less accurate than monolingual speakers on a few sound classes (i.e. fricatives, flap, and trill in Spanish). Thus, examining types of errors might shed light on the relative similarities and difference between monolingual and bilingual children.

Arnold *et al.* (2004) longitudinally examined the consonant production of 18 Spanish–English typically developing, bilingual children (nine sequential learners and nine simultaneous learners). At the onset of the study, the average age of the children acquiring the two languages simultaneously and sequentially was 3;9 and 3;7, respectively. The children's consonant production skills were sampled at eight time periods over four years. The results indicated that based on independent analyses, the pattern of sound acquisition for the bilingual children was similar to monolingual children. Accuracy (i.e. percent correct consonants) between sequential and simultaneous learners was similar in English but was slightly higher in Spanish for sequential learners.

Some researchers have claimed that bilingual children exhibit *atypical error patterns* (i.e. those not usually exhibited by monolingual children). Dodd *et al.* (1996) examined the phonological skills of 16 typically developing, Cantonese-speaking children who were acquiring English in preschool. They found that the bilingual children's error patterns were atypical for monolingual speakers of either language. Specifically, the bilingual children produced a number of atypical error patterns (e.g. initial consonant deletion) that are usually associated with children with phonological disorders. Not all studies of bilingual children, however, have found a similar result.

In a group of Spanish–English 5-year-olds, Goldstein *et al.* (2005) found that bilingual children largely produced substitutions that also have been attested in monolingual children. These Spanish–English bilingual children did not exhibit a large proportion of atypical error patterns, producing few substitution types in Spanish or English that were not attested in monolingual Spanish- (Goldstein, 2005) or monolingual English-speaking children (Smit, 1993). Thus, studies to date indicate that bilingual children will exhibit atypical errors, although it should be noted that monolingual children also exhibit these types of errors (e.g. initial consonant deletion). Future studies, including cohorts of bilingual and monolingual children, are needed to examine error patterns specifically to determine if bilingual children are more likely than monolingual children to produce atypical errors. Such studies also will aid in disentangling *within-language and cross-linguistic patterns.*

Languages vary with respect to segmental, syllabic, and prosodic features. Consideration of these differences is necessary to differentiate within-language versus cross-linguistic patterns. The studies summarized previously indicate that phonological skills in bilingual children are both similar to and different from monolingual speakers. The results of these studies also indicate that typically developing bilingual children show many of the same acquisition patterns that are exhibited by monolingual children. For example, anterior sounds (e.g. bilabials) tend to be acquired before posterior sound (e.g. velars) and stops typically are acquired before liquids (Locke, 1983). Although there are common cross-linguistic tendencies, this commonality of acquisition is tempered by constraints of the specific language (for monolingual children) or languages (for bilingual children) being acquired.

Children are attuned to the specific language (or languages) they are acquiring. Studies of monolingual and bilingual children show this trend. For example, children acquiring Putonghua (Modern Standard Chinese) showed high rates of deaspiration (e.g. $/t^h/ \rightarrow [t]$), a pattern that was exhibited less commonly in children speaking other languages (Zhu & Dodd, 2000). Putonghua-speaking children exhibited this tendency because that language contains many aspirated sounds. Spanish-speaking children tended to exhibit less final consonant deletion than English-speaking children because there are relatively few final consonants in Spanish, at least in comparison to English (Goldstein & Iglesias, 1996). Bilingual children also evidence this phenomenon. Anderson (2004) examined the first and second language phonological skills in five children acquiring English as their second language. The first language of the children was Korean (three children), Russian (one child), and French (one child). Anderson found that all five children were sensitive to the sounds common to both languages and unique to each language. With rare exceptions, sounds shared by both languages were indeed produced in both languages, whereas sounds unique to one language were produced only in that language.

Despite the fact that children seem to be attuned to the *phonotactic structure* (i.e. segmental, syllabic, and prosodic structure) of the language or languages they are acquiring, there is the possibility that the interaction between the two languages may result in cross-linguistic effects. *Cross-linguistic effects* are defined as the use of nonambient sounds in the other language (e.g. use of the Spanish trill in an English production). The presence of cross-linguistic effects is one of the attested hallmarks of bilingual language development. Many bilingual researchers have indicated that cross-linguistic effects are a unique aspect of bilingual phonological development (Watson, 1991). Fantini (1985) found that his preschool son acquiring Spanish and English aspirated voiceless stops in Spanish (/tet∫o/ 'roof' → [tʰet∫o]) even though stops in Spanish typically are described as unaspirated (Hammond, 2001). In studies of their two sons acquiring Spanish and English, Schnitzer and Krasinski (1994; 1996) found that their older son showed a low frequency of cross-linguistic effects, but their younger son exhibited a high proportion of cross-linguistic effects. In a group of 12 Spanish–English bilingual children aged 5;0–7;0, Goldstein *et al.* (2003) noted a low frequency (< 1%) of cross-linguistic effects, although they were bidirectional, affecting the children's English and Spanish productions.

The results from these studies indicate that bilingual phonological development is both similar to and different from monolingual speakers of either language. As a result, researchers (and practitioners for clinical purposes) must use the appropriate comparison database when discussing how the results of their studies compare to those in the literature. That is, data from bilingual children should be compared to bilingual children who are in similar *sociolinguistic situations*. For example, the results of a research study focusing on the phonological skills of 5-year-olds whose parents adopted the *one-person-one-language model* (i.e. where one parent speaks L1 exclusively and the other parent speaks L2 exclusively) would need to be compared to results from other studies that have examined same-aged children undergoing the same linguistic experience. Comparing the children whose parents used the one-person-one-language model with children whose parents regularly used both languages and codeswitched extensively likely would not be valid. This type of variability needs to be taken into account in research with bilingual children (also see Centeno, ch. 3, this volume for pertinent discussion on the role of sociolinguistic contexts in childhood bilingualism.)

Variability in the Phonological Skills of Bilinguals

Despite the similarities in phonological skills between monolingual and bilingual children, considerable heterogeneity exists among bilingual speakers. That heterogeneity is due, at least in part, to the sociolinguistic circumstances under which the two languages were acquired (see Centeno, ch. 3, this volume). That is, to effectively measure phonological skills in bilingual children, it might be important to examine their phonological development in light of how proficient the children are in each language in light of the dialect(s) they are acquiring. Although it is unlikely that there will be standardized measures of these sociolinguistic variables (they are often gleaned from teacher and/or parent report; e.g. Gutiérrez-Clellen & Heinrichs-Ramos, 1993; Restrepo, 1998), they need to be considered. Unfortunately, there are few studies examining phonological development in bilingual children in which these variables have been examined. Goldstein *et al.* (2005) examined the relationship between the amount of output (i.e. percentage of the time each language was spoken) and phonological skills (i.e. consonant accuracy, syllable accuracy, and percentage of occurrence of phonological patterns) in a group of five Spanish–English bilingual children, five predominantly Spanish-speaking children, and five predominantly English-speaking children. The results indicated that there was no significant correlation between amount of output and phonological skills. The results were limited, however, by a relatively small sample size and the use of parental report only as the measure of output as opposed to using more objective measures of output such as grammaticality (Gutiérrez-Clellen & Kreiter, 2003). Despite these limitations, the results indicate that the relationship between sociolinguistic variables and phonological skills should continue to be explored.

The studies recounted here highlight the need to take *variation* into account. No population, not even subgroups within a population, is homogeneous. As such, research conducted with any population or subpopulation must account for this existing variation. One other important aspect of this variation is *dialect* (i.e. the rule-governed variants of a language). All speakers of a language utilize some dialect of that language, although not all speakers use all features of the dialect they are acquiring. The specific dialect features that speakers do use are *not* applied indiscriminately; they are rule-governed and show regular patterns (Wolfram & Schilling-Estes, 1998). Phonetic context and dialectal density (i.e. the frequency with which dialect features occur) may influence the evidence of specific patterns.

Rules sometimes apply across all segments and, similarly, they sometimes apply across a subset of segments. From both a clinical and research perspective, it is important to determine the *phonological environment* in which the rule applies. There is a tendency to assume that rules apply across all environments when in reality the context in which the rule applies is much more specific. For example, deletion of syllable final /s/ in Caribbean Spanish is a well attested feature of the dialect. Deletion of that segment, however, is not indiscriminate and is governed mainly by two factors: word length and position in the noun phrase (Terrell, 1981). Terrell indicates that /s/ is more likely to be preserved in monosyllabic words (e.g. /es/ 'is') than in multisyllabic words (e.g. /nosotʃos/ 'we'). Moreover, /s/ tends to be preserved when it is in words that precede the head of the noun phrase and deleted when it occurs in other positions; so, for example, the most common production of /los libʃos/ 'the books' would be [los libʃo]. Data like these indicate that in describing phonological patterns, the contexts in which these patterns take place and the specific segments being affected need to be vigilantly described.

Not all speakers of a particular dialect use features of the dialect to the same extent. Some speakers will simply use more features of the dialect than other speakers (i.e. they are high dialect users; Washington & Craig, 1994). Thus, Speaker A may exhibit a higher dialect density than Speaker B although they speak the same dialect. *Dialect density* has been shown to vary by age, geographic location, task, and socioeconomic status (SES). In a study of 3- and 4-year-old Puerto Rican Spanish-speaking children, Goldstein and Iglesias (2001) found that 3-year-olds exhibited a significantly higher dialect density than did 4-year-olds. Moreover, the results indicated that the number of consonant errors, the number of errors within individual sound classes, and the percentages of occurrence for phonological processes all decreased after accounting for Puerto Rican dialect features. Finally, the results indicated that some typically developing children would have been misclassified as phonologically disordered had dialect features not been taken into account.

In addition to varying by age, dialect density also varies by geographical location. Terrell (1981) found such an effect on the phonology of Spanish speakers, particularly with dialectal differences that existed between speakers of urban/rural and coastal/inland Puerto Rican Spanish. Thus, researchers and SLPs need to identify the general geographic location of those they examine and then attempt to discern if dialect density might vary because of their geographic location.

Speaking contexts also seem to affect dialect density. Poplack (1980) found that, in Puerto Rican Spanish speakers, the use of dialect features varied based on speaking situations. In more informal speaking situations, dialect density was higher, in that participants tended to use more dialect features. In formal situations, however, dialect density was lower; participants tended to use fewer dialect features. Thus, results of any study might be affected by the way in which participants view the speaking task. If children interpret the task as a more formal one, they may use fewer features of the dialect. Given that the nature of the data collection task may influence the number of dialect features exhibited, the methodology used to elicit samples must be clearly specified and the results need to be interpreted in light of possible task effects on children's output.

The SES of study participants influences dialect density. Specific dialect features might be stratified by SES, with some subgroups using the feature and others not using it or using it less often. For example, Cal Varela (1998) found that educational level and occupation had a significant effect on Spanish–English adults' production of /i/ and /I/ in English. A number of studies on Spanish dialects have indicated that individuals from higher socioeconomic groups tend to preserve segments more commonly than do individuals from lower socioeconomic groups (e.g. Hammond, 1978). It is important also to note that, in terms of general phonological acquisition, there seems to be little effect of SES on long-term phonological development for either English- (Smit *et al.*, 1990) or Spanish-speaking children (Pandolfi & Herrera, 1990). This suggests that, regardless of the speaker's dialectal density, all speakers will acquire the phonology of their speech community and be competent speakers of the language.

So far, the discussion has centered on speakers who use only one dialect; however, many speakers may have more than one variety in common, as happens when two different speech communities coexist in close proximity. For example, Poplack (1978) and Wolfram (1974) found that speakers of Puerto Rican Spanish who were acquiring English used features of both Spanish-influenced English (e.g. /ʃɛvi/ 'Chevy' → [tʃɛvi]) and African–American English (AAE) (e.g. /bæθ/ 'bath' → [bæf]) because of their close contact with their AAE-speaking neighbors. Not taking into consideration the potential for multiple dialect use might cause examiners to mistakenly attribute specific dialect features observed as those of one dialect (e.g. Spanish-influenced English) when in reality they are features of another dialect (e.g. AAE).

The issue of dialect becomes critical in clinical decision-making, and several studies have been conducted in order to evaluate the extent to which taking dialect into account affects the *sensitivity and specificity* of phonological assessment. Goldstein and Iglesias (2001) examined the effect that dialect had on the phonology of 108 Puerto Rican Spanish-speaking children (54 typically developing and 54 with phonological disorders). Results indicated that, after taking into account the features of Puerto Rican Spanish, there was a reduction in the number of consonant errors, number of errors within individual sound classes and percentage-of-occurrence for phonological processes, and an increase in consonant accuracy. Approximately half the typically developing children would have been characterized with, at least, a mild phonological disorder had dialect features not been considered in the analysis. In addition, three phonological processes – final consonant deletion, liquid simplification, and weak syllable deletion – might have been considered incorrectly, as intervention targets for many children with phonological disorders, had the features of Puerto Rican Spanish not been taken into account.

Researchers and SLPs obviously need to specify the dialect of bilingual children, gauge their dialect density, and consider dialect in completing phonological analyses. However, no study could ever be expected to sample all members of a speech community. Thus, researchers select members who are deemed to be representative of the population to be studied. Based on the evidence presented, this selection process must take into account dialectal features used by the speakers selected. Consideration must be given to the extent to which the use of these features might vary as a function of context, speakers' dialectal density, SES, and perception as to the formality of the task.

Summary

Given the relative paucity of phonology studies related to bilingual speakers, existing studies must be evaluated for their attention to variation. Variation might be related to language (specifically, language status and/or cross-linguistic versus ambient language effects), socio-linguistic factors, and dialect. It is important to determine the effect of these variables on all aspects of research related to bilingual phonological development. Not doing so calls into question the implications of the findings and makes it difficult to determine whether the results might generalize to all individuals within that group or across speakers of different groups. In addition, from a clinical perspective, SLPs' knowledge of these issues will help to ensure less-biased assessment and more appropriate selection of intervention goals to bilingual children with phonological disorders.

Acknowledgements

The writing of this chapter was funded in part by National Institute of Deafness and Other Communication Disorders contract #N01-DC-8-2100.

References

American Speech-Language-Hearing Association (2003) *2003 Omnibus Survey Caseload Report: SLP.* Rockville, MD: American Speech-Language-Hearing Association. .

Anderson, R.T. (2004) Phonological acquisition in preschoolers learning a second language via immersion: A longitudinal study. *Clinical Linguistics and Phonetics* 18, 183–210.

Arnold, E., Curran, C., Miccio, A. and Hammer, C. (2004) Sequential and simultaneous acquisition of Spanish and English consonants. Poster presented at the annual convention of the American Speech-Language-Hearing Association, Philadelphia, PA.

Barlow, J. (2001) Error patterns and transfer in Spanish–English bilingual phonological production. Paper presented at the 26th Annual Boston University Conference on Language Development, Boston, MA.

Cal Varela, M. (1998) /I/ and /i/ in Gibraltarian English: A sociolinguistic analysis of interference from Spanish. In J. Fontana, L. McNally, M. Turell and E. Vallduví (eds) *Proceedings of the First International Conference on Language Variation in Europe* (pp. 34–42). Universitat Pompeu Fabra: Unitat de Recerca de Variació Lingüistica.

Dodd, B., So., L. and Li, W. (1996) Symptoms of disorder without impairment: The written and spoken errors of bilinguals. In B. Dodd, R. Campbell and L. Worrall (eds) *Evaluating Theories of Language: Evidence from Disorder* (pp. 119–136). London: Whurr Publishers.

Fantini, A. (1985) *Language Acquisition of a Bilingual Child: A Sociolinguistic Perspective (to Age 10)*. San Diego: College Hill Press.

Gierut, J. (1998) Treatment efficacy: Functional phonological disorders in children. *Journal of Speech, Language and Hearing Research* 41, S85–S100.

Gildersleeve, C., Davis, B. and Stubbe, E. (1996) When monolingual rules don't apply: Speech development in a bilingual environment. Paper presented at the annual convention of the American Speech-Language-Hearing Association, Seattle, WA.

Gildersleeve-Neumann, C. and Davis, B. (1998) Learning English in a bilingual preschool environment: Change over time. Paper presented at the annual convention of the American Speech-Language-Hearing Association, San Antonio, TX.

Goldstein, B. (2005) Substitutions in the phonology of Spanish-speaking children. *Journal of Multilingual Communication Disorders* 3, 56–63.

Goldstein, B., Fabiano, L. and Iglesias, A. (2003) The representation of phonology in sequential Spanish–English bilingual children. Poster session presented at the 4th Annual International Symposium on Bilingualism, Tempe, AZ.

Goldstein, B., Fabiano, L. and Washington, P. (2005) Phonological skills in predominantly English, predominantly Spanish, and Spanish–English bilingual children. *Language, Speech, and Hearing Services in the Schools* 36, 201–218.

Goldstein, B. and Iglesias, A. (1996) Phonological patterns in normally developing Spanish-speaking 3- and 4-year-olds of Puerto Rican descent. *Language, Speech, and Hearing Services in the Schools* 27, 82–90.

Goldstein, B. and Iglesias, A. (2001) The effect of dialect on phonological analysis: Evidence from Spanish-speaking children. *American Journal of Speech-Language Pathology* 10, 394–406.

Goldstein, B. and Washington, P. (2001) An initial investigation of phonological patterns in 4-year-old typically developing Spanish-English bilingual children. *Language, Speech, and Hearing Services in the Schools* 32, 153–164.

Gutiérrez-Clellen, V. and Heinrichs-Ramos, L. (1993) Referential cohesion in the narratives of Spanish-speaking children: A developmental study. *Journal of Speech and Hearing Research* 36, 559–567.

Gutiérrez-Clellen, V.F. and Krieter, J. (2003) Understanding child bilingual acquisition using parent and teacher reports. *Applied Psycholinguistics* 24, 267–288.

Hammond, R. (1978) The velar nasal in Miami Cuban speech. In J. Lantolf, F. Frank and J. Guitart (eds) *Proceedings from the Third Colloquium in Hispanic and Luso Brazilian Linguistics* (pp. 19–36). Washington, DC: Georgetown University Press.

Hammond, R. (2001) *The Sounds of Spanish: Analysis and Application (with Special Reference to American English)*. Somerville, MA: Cascadilla Press.

Ingram, D. (2002) The measurement of whole-word productions. *Journal of Child Language* 29, 713–733.

Locke, J. (1983) *Phonological Acquisition and Change.* NY: Academic Press.

Pandolfi, A.M. and Herrera, M.O. (1990) Producción fonológica de niños menores de tres años. *Revista Teórica y Aplicada* 28, 101–122.

Peters-Johnson, C. (1998) Action: School services. *Language, Speech, and Hearing Services in the Schools* 29, 120–126.

Poplack, S. (1978) Dialect acquisition among Puerto Rican bilinguals. *Language in Society* 7, 89–103.

Poplack, S. (1980) Deletion and disambiguation in Puerto Rican Spanish. *Language* 56, 371–385.

Restrepo, M.A. (1998) Identifiers of predominantly Spanish-speaking children with specific language impairment. *Journal of Speech, Language, and Hearing Research* 41, 1398–1411.

Schnitzer, M.L. and Krasinski, E. (1994) The development of segmental phonological production in a bilingual child. *Journal of Child Language* 21, 585–622.

Schnitzer, M. and Krasinski, E. (1996) The development of segmental phonological production in a bilingual child: A contrasting second case. *Journal of Child Language* 23, 547–571.

Smit, A. (1993) Phonologic error distributions in the Iowa-Nebraska articulation norms project: Consonant singletons. *Journal of Speech and Hearing Research* 36, 533–547.

Smit, A., Hand, L., Freilinger, J., Bernthal, J., and Bird, A. (1990) The Iowa articulation norms project and its Nebraska replication. *Journal of Speech and Hearing Disorders* 55, 779–798.

Stackhouse, J. (1997) Phonological awareness: Connecting speech and literacy problems. In B. Hodson and M.L. Edwards (eds) *Perspectives in Applied Phonology* (pp. 157–196). Gaithersburg, MD: Aspen.

Terrell, T. (1981) Current trends in the investigation of Cuban and Puerto Rican phonology. In J. Amastae and L. Elías-Olivares (eds) *Spanish in the United States: Sociolinguistic Aspects* (pp. 47–70). Cambridge, UK: Cambridge University Press.

US Bureau of the Census (2000) Language use. On WWW at http://www.census.gov. Accessed 12.4.04.

Washington, J. and Craig, H.K. (1994) Dialect forms during discourse of poor, urban African American preschoolers. *Journal of Speech and Hearing Research* 37, 816–823.

Watson, I. (1991) Phonological processing in two languages. In E. Bialystock (ed.) *Language Processing in Bilingual Children* (pp. 25–48). Cambridge: Cambridge University Press.

Wolfram, W. (1974) *Sociolinguistic Aspects of Assimilation: Puerto Rican English in New York City.* Arlington, VA: Center for Applied Linguistics.

Wolfram, W., and Schilling-Estes, N. (1998) *American English: Dialects and Variation.* Oxford, UK: Blackwell.

Yavaş, M. and Goldstein, B. (1998) Phonological assessment and treatment of bilingual speakers. *American Journal of Speech-Language Pathology* 7, 49–60.

Zhu, H. and Dodd, B. (2000) The phonological acquisition of Putonghua (Modern Standard Chinese). *Journal of Child Language* 27, 3–42.

Part 3

Research in Adults: Empirical Evidence and Clinical Implications

Chapter 14

Prepositional Processing in Spanish Speakers with Aphasia: The Role of Semantic Value and Amount of Contextual Information

BELINDA A. REYES

The vast majority of modern investigations of language processing in aphasia have been conducted with patients who are speakers of English. Thus, most information used for models of language comprehension/ production, assessment batteries, and treatment protocols has been based on data gathered from English speakers. This situation presents particular challenges for researchers and clinicians who find themselves working with non-English speakers with aphasia.

Of late, numerous investigators have begun to recognize the importance of cross-language research in aphasia (Bates *et al.*, 1987; 1988; Menn *et al.*, 1995; Paradis, 2001). It has been recognized that different languages may use different morphosyntactic features to mark various linguistic requirements. Thus, the 'same underlying deficit' may result in 'different surface manifestations' in different languages (Paradis, 2001: 5). In other words, the same aphasic syndrome may take a different form depending on the structure of the patient's premorbid language. This underscores the importance of cross-language research in order to ultimately provide proper assessment of and treatment for aphasic speakers of various languages. In an attempt to contribute to the body of cross-language data and knowledge, a research project examining Spanish speakers with aphasia was conducted. The purpose of this chapter is to describe a portion of this study designed specifically to examine the processing of prepositions by adult Spanish-speaking individuals with aphasia. Due to space limitations, this chapter discusses a portion of an earlier and larger data corpus on the use and comprehension of prepositions by Spanish-speaking aphasic individuals (Reyes, 1990). A brief review of pertinent published studies on Spanish-speaking adults with aphasia will be presented, followed by a rationale for the current investigation. Subsequently, the methodology of the current study will be outlined, findings will be described, and, finally, a discussion including clinical applications for management of Spanish-speaking aphasic patients will be presented.

Aphasia in Spanish Speakers

Although Spanish is reported to be the official language of over 20 countries (Benedet *et al.*, 1998), and the USA has been identified as the fifth largest Spanish-speaking nation in the world (behind Mexico, Spain, Colombia, and Argentina) (US Bureau of the Census, 2000), few research studies investigating language dissolution in Spanish-speaking aphasic individuals have been published (see Ardila, 2001, for a review). Regarding grammatical morphology, the area of concern in this chapter, three studies on Spanish-speaking aphasic patients have been reported. Reznik *et al.* (1995) reported an unusual case of a 55-year-old agrammatic patient with word order deficits but without major morphological errors, except for difficulty with clitic pronouns (see Anderson & Centeno, ch. 1, for related discussion on Spanish morphosyntax). Though Reznik and colleagues suggest that clitic restrictions may be interpreted using Chomsky's *Government Binding* principles, conclusions from this study are controversial. The reported case, in terms of generally intact morphosyntactic profile and right-sided lesion, did not match the typical grammatical symptomatology and left-sided etiology of agrammatism (see Ardila, 2001, for a discussion).

Benedet *et al.* (1998) investigated noun phrase morphology, verb phrase morphology, and word order in production and comprehension of active and passive sentences in agrammatic Spanish speakers from Spain. Examination of prepositions *de* 'of' (as possessive marker), *por* 'by' (signaling agency, with a passive verb), and *a* 'to' (signaling the direct object, with an active verb) comprised a small portion of this broader study of grammatical morphology. Ostrosky-Solís *et al.* (1999) examined comprehension of active versus passive sentences in patients with Broca's aphasia. Within the larger context of syntactic comprehension, comprehension of the prepositions *a* (assigning the thematic role of patient in active sentences) and *por* (marking the thematic role of agent in passive sentences) was assessed. Among the results of this study was the finding that the presence of the preposition was a significant factor in the correct assignment of thematic roles, and, thus, contributed to comprehension of active and passive sentences by the participants with Broca's aphasia.

Processing of Prepositions by Spanish-speaking Aphasic Individuals

To the author's knowledge, no study specifically designed to examine prepositional processing in Spanish-speaking aphasic adults has been documented in the literature. Examination of prepositional processing in Spanish-speaking aphasic adults merits consideration for several reasons. First, prepositions occur quite frequently in the Spanish language

(López, 1972). Secondly, prepositions serve a primary role in communication: that of relating nouns and pronouns to other words within sentences. Indeed, prepositions serve key functions in morphosyntactic structure as well as sentential meaning. Disordered language without prepositions, or some other form of marking the functions which they serve, would be quite impoverished. Thirdly, prepositional processing in Spanish aphasic speakers is worthy of investigation because prepositions have traditionally been considered to be a part of the closed-class vocabulary. It has been documented that particularly in agrammatic aphasic participants, grammatical morphemes (including inflectional word endings and closed-class words) tend to be omitted or simplified in production, and processed inadequately in comprehension (Benson & Ardila, 1996; Brookshire, 2003; Davis, 2000; Goodglass & Menn, 1985; Menn *et al.*, 1995).

Prepositions (along with determiners, conjunctions, pronouns, quantifiers, and auxiliary elements) have historically been categorized as *closed-class words or functors*. Prepositions are primarily defined in terms of their syntactic function, and are necessary in producing the syntactically correct language prerequisite for the accurate structural analysis and production of sentences (Bird *et al.*, 2002; Coslett *et al.*, 1984). On the other hand, *open-class or content words* (including nouns, verbs, adjectives) are considered to bear reference and carry the primary semantic, informational weight in communication (Bebout, 1993; Friederici, 1982; Garrett, 1980). Various investigators have documented that normal and aphasic participants do indeed respond differently to open- and closed-class words (Biassou *et al.*, 1997; Bradley *et al.*, 1980; Garrett, 1980; Nespoulous *et al.*, 1988; Weber-Fox & Neville, 2001). However, it has recently been argued that the distinction between content (open-class) and function (closed-class) words 'is not straight forwardly defined from either a syntactic or a semantic perspective,' and that 'these words do not fit into precisely circumscribed categories' (Bird *et al.*, 2002: 211).

Furthermore, agrammatism may affect different sets of free-standing functors in different patients (Caplan, 1991). Prepositions appear to present a particular dilemma in that they 'are not easily classifiable' as functors (Friederici, 1985: 136) along the sharp dichotomy between open- and closed-class items (Biassou *et al.*, 1997). Tesak and Hummer (1994: 463) point to the 'unclear status' of prepositions, while Bebout (1993: 162) suggests that prepositions are 'problematic' because, although they are always considered to be members of the closed class, they can have one meaning that is 'fully semantic' and another that is 'conventionally grammatical'. Several investigations point out that prepositions often seem to be better retained than other functors in agrammatic participants (Bird *et al.*, 2002; Friederici, 1982; 1985; Menn *et al.*, 1995). Biassou *et al.* (1997: 371) posit that prepositions constitute a 'medial category' in the

dichotomy between open-class and closed-class items, and Beyn *et al.*
(1979: 342) propose that the preposition is a 'special part of speech which
possesses not only a general grammatical meaning, but also a lexical
meaning'.

In summary, prepositions are prominent linguistic elements in the
Spanish language, and they serve important roles in communication.
Their status as closed-class items has been debated in the literature, and
no systematic investigation of these linguistic elements has been
documented in Spanish-speaking aphasic adults. Therefore, this study
was designed to investigate processing of this grammatical class of
words in aphasic Spanish speakers. The first research question asked
whether the *semantic value* of prepositions would affect their processing
in Spanish-speaking individuals with mild to moderate aphasia. It was
hypothesized that prepositions with the highest semantic value would be
the best preserved, and those with the lowest semantic load would be the
least preserved. The second research question asked whether the amount
of *linguistic contextual information* would affect prepositional processing
in Spanish-speaking individuals with mild to moderate aphasia. It was
hypothesized that tasks providing maximal linguistic contextual information would result in the best performance by the participants, whereas
tasks providing the least amount of contextual information would result
in the worst performance. It was anticipated that results of this
investigation would have clinical relevance, particularly toward the
development of possible treatment protocols and hierarchies utilizing
prepositions of varying semantic value and varying amounts of
contextual information as possible facilitating cues for aphasic patients.

Method

Participants

Twenty-four individuals, 12 control speakers and 12 aphasic speakers,
participated in this investigation. All participants were monolingual
native Spanish speakers of Mexican–American or Mexican ancestry, and
lived in south Texas along the US–Mexico border. Collected information
on language history and observations of language use were employed to
assess monolingual status in these individuals. The control group had a
negative neurological history and was matched to the experimental
aphasic group by age, sex, and educational level.

Aphasic participants consisted of eight males and four females,
ranging in age from 30 to 69 years (mean age = 57.5 years), and had an
average educational level of 8.1 years (range = 6–12 years). All aphasic
participants were right-handed, had suffered a single left cerebrovascular
accident, and had no prior neurological history or history of substance
abuse. Participants ranged from 7 to 73 months post-onset, with a mean

of 30.3 months post-onset. Aphasic participants presented with mild to moderate communication impairments, as assessed by selected subtests of a Spanish adaptation of the *Boston Diagnostic Aphasia Examination* (Goodglass & Kaplan, 1983). Eight participants were classified as nonfluent and four as fluent, based on the *Rating Scale Profile of Speech Characteristics* (Goodglass & Kaplan, 1983). All patients presented with adequate visual acuity including correction via eyeglasses where appropriate. In addition, they presented with adequate hearing acuity, demonstrating a pure tone average of 40 dB or less.

Stimuli

Forty-eight sentences containing prepositions were utilized in this investigation, 12 sentences per prepositional category. The same sentence frames were used in all four tasks in order to avoid a confounding of task type with particular stimuli. All sentences conformed to the canonical order of the constituents: subject, verb, and prepositional phrase (e.g. *el plato está en la mesa* 'the plate is on the table'). Verbs in all sentences were inflected in the present tense, and relatively high-frequency nouns and verbs were utilized (Juilland & Chang-Rodriguez, 1974).

Four categories of prepositions, varying in semantic value or content, were utilized in this experiment. The classification taxonomy was developed by the author following the criteria described below:

(1) Locative prepositions. This category consisted of prepositions that signal spatial or directional information (e.g. *el lápiz está en el cajón* 'the pencil is in the drawer'). Prepositions, such as *sobre* 'on', *entre* 'between', and *en* 'in' were used to represent locative prepositions. This prepositional category was considered to be the highest in semantic content, as the prepositions were concrete (Beyn *et al.*, 1979), had a high degree of 'imageability' (Bird *et al.*, 2002: 216; Goodglass & Menn, 1985), and they conveyed 'visual space relations' (Rivas, 1976: 23).

(2) Temporal prepositions. The second category consisted of prepositions that signal temporal information (e.g. *el tren llega a las dos* 'the train arrives at two'). Prepositions, such as *a* 'at', *desde* 'since', and *en* 'in', were used to represent temporal prepositions. This category of prepositions was also considered to be relatively high in semantic value, although conceptually it is less visual and, thus, less concrete than the locative prepositions.

(3) Case-marking prepositions. The third category consisted of prepositions that mark the following cases, as delineated by Fillmore (1977): (a) instrumental – force or object causing the action or state (e.g., *la secretaria escribe con un lápiz* 'the secretary writes with a pencil'); (b) experiencer – animate object affected by the action (e.g. *el joven le*

envía una carta a̱ la señorita 'the boy sends a letter t̲o̲ the girl'); and (c) benefactive – animate beneficiary of an action or state (e.g. *la señora cose un vestido pa̱ra la novia* 'the lady sews a dress f̲o̲r̲ the bride'). Although Fillmore notes the relational/semantic aspect of case-marking prepositions in addition to their syntactic function, upon comparison with locative and temporal prepositions, the case-marking prepositions were considered to be relatively low in semantic value.

(4) Phrasal prepositions. The fourth category consisted of prepositions that are attached to verbs (e.g. *el equipo participa e̱n el juego* 'the team participates i̱n the game'). Prepositions, such as *de* 'of', *en* 'in', and *con* 'with', were used to represent this prepositional category. All verb–preposition constructions were taken from the *Lista de Palabras que se Construyen con Preposición* (Real Academia Española, 1979). This category of prepositions was considered to possess the least amount of semantic value, as compared to the other three categories.

Procedures

Tasks for this investigation aimed to examine participants' processing of the four categories of prepositions upon being provided with various amounts of linguistic contextual information. As mentioned earlier, it was hypothesized that participants would perform best on tasks providing the most linguistic contextual information. The same sentence frames were used in all tasks, to avoid a confounding of task type with particular stimuli. The following four tasks were used, all being presented to the participants auditorily and in written form, with the exception of the repetition task, which was only presented auditorily:

(1) Repetition Task. This task consisted of single sentences each contain-ing a preposition, and being presented auditorily to the participants. Participants were required to repeat each sentence after presentation by the examiner. The repetition task was considered to provide maximal linguistic contextual information for the participants.

(2) Grammaticality Judgment Task. This task consisted of single sentences each containing a preposition. One half of the sentences included correct prepositions, while the other half contained incorrect prepositions. Participants were required to listen to each sentence (and read it silently if they so chose), and to indicate 'yes' orally or by pointing to a card if the sentence was correct or 'no' if the sentence was incorrect. This task was also considered to be relatively high in amount of linguistic contextual information provided to the participants. However, due to the fact that, in some cases, an incorrect preposition was provided and the partici-pant was required to judge the accuracy of the sentences, the

Grammaticality Judgment Task was considered to be lower in linguistic contextual cues than the Repetition Task. Although low formal education levels would make this task less natural for some participants than for others, there was no evidence that participants' responses in the current sample differed according to educational level.

(3) Multiple Choice Cloze Task. This task consisted of single sentences each containing a blank corresponding to the location of the missing preposition in the sentence. The participants were provided with three prepositions from which to choose one to complete each sentence. The three choices consisted of the correct preposition, one incorrect within-category preposition, and one incorrect across-category preposition. All three choices consisted of the same number of syllables. This task was considered to be relatively low in amount of linguistic contextual information supplied to the participants, as compared to the Repetition and Grammaticality Judgment Tasks.

(4) Spontaneous Cloze Task. This task consisted of single sentences each containing a blank corresponding to the location of the missing preposition in the sentence. Participants were required to listen to each sentence (and read it silently if they so chose), and to subsequently supply the missing preposition. This task was considered to provide the least amount of linguistic contextual information for the participants, as compared to the other three tasks.

Data analysis and results

Data analysis consisted of two basic components: statistical analysis and descriptive analysis. Due to space limitations, this discussion will focus on the former and only general comments will be made regarding the latter. Analysis of the data obtained from the normal control participants indicated that, across all 12 participants, only 4 errors occurred on 2304 stimulus items. The control group had little to no difficulty in repeating, judging the correctness of, selecting from a set of three, or spontaneously producing locative, temporal, case-marking, or phrasal prepositions. Performance of the control group suggests that the experimental tasks and stimuli used in this investigation were not complex enough to tap differences in performance as affected by semantic value of prepositions or amount of linguistic contextual information due to a ceiling effect. Since the control participants made so few errors on the experimental tasks, further discussion will focus solely on the aphasic participants' performance on the experimental tasks.

As Figure 14.1 illustrates, the error rate for stimulus items highest in semantic value (locative prepositions) was the lowest, followed by the

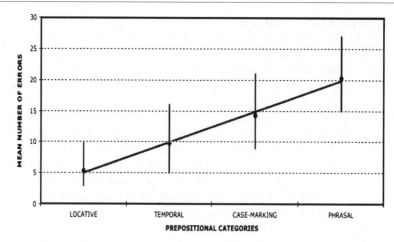

Figure 14.1 Performance of aphasic subjects on prepositional categories varying in semantic value

error rate on temporal prepositions, then case-marking prepositions, with phrasal prepositions exhibiting the highest error rate. Thus, as semantic value of the prepositions decreased, participants' error rates increased. Mean number of errors, mean error rates (expressed in terms of percentages), standard deviations, and ranges of errors for the aphasic participants on each of the four prepositional categories are shown in Table 14.1.

Again, the aphasic participants performed best on prepositions highest in semantic value, and they performed worst on prepositions with the least semantic value.

A two-factor repeated measures multivariate analysis of variance (Prepositional Category × Linguistic Context) indicated a significant main effect for Prepositional Category ($F = 89.43$; $df = 3$; $p < 0.0001$).

Table 14.1 Performance of aphasic participants on prepositional categories varying in semantic value

Prep. category	Mean no. errors	Mean error rate (%)	Standard deviation	Range of errors
Locative	5.3	11	2.3	3–10
Temporal	9.8	20.4	3.4	5–16
Case-marking	14.3	29.8	4.2	9–21
Phrasal	20.3	42.3	4.4	15–27

Post hoc analysis using profile analysis to compare the means at adjacent levels of the variable Prepositional Category revealed a significant difference at each of the adjacent levels. That is, performance on Locative prepositions was significantly different from that on Temporal prepositions ($F = 116.22$; $df = 1$, 11; $p < 0.0001$), performance on Temporal prepositions was significantly different from that on Case-marking prepositions ($F = 123.10$; $df = 1$, 11; $p < 0.0001$), and performance on Case-marking prepositions differed significantly from that on Phrasal prepositions ($F = 233.54$; $df = 1$, 11; $p < 0.0001$). As a hierarchy of semantic value of prepositional categories was proposed, given the findings of the profile analysis, it was extrapolated that performance on Locative prepositions was significantly different from performance on Case-marking and Phrasal prepositions, and performance on Temporal prepositions was significantly different from that on Phrasal prepositions. In sum, the aphasic participants included in this study demonstrated much more difficulty with prepositions low in semantic value and more success with prepositions high in semantic value.

With respect to tasks varying in amount of linguistic contextual information, four tasks were analyzed: Repetition, Grammaticality Judgment, Multiple Choice Cloze, and Spontaneous Cloze tasks.

As Figure 14.2 illustrates, the total error rate for the task highest in the amount of linguistic contextual information (Repetition Task) was the lowest, followed by the error rate on the Grammaticality Judgment Task, then the Multiple Choice Cloze Task, with the error rate on the

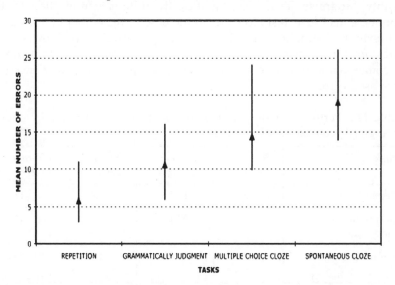

Figure 14.2 Performance of aphasic subjects on tasks varying in amount of linguistic contextual information

Spontaneous Cloze Task being the highest. Mean number of errors, mean error rates (expressed as percentages), standard deviations, and ranges of errors for the aphasic participants on each of the four tasks are shown in Table 14.2.

Again, the aphasic participants performed best on tasks high in amount of linguistic contextual information, and they performed worst on the task providing the least amount of linguistic contextual information.

A two-factor repeated measures multivariate analysis of variance (Linguistic Context x Prepositional Category) revealed a significant main effect for Linguistic Context ($F = 142.88$; $df = 3$; $p < 0.0001$). Post hoc profile analysis to compare the means at adjacent levels of the variable Linguistic Context indicated a significant difference between each of the adjacent levels. Performance on the Repetition Task was significantly different from that on the Grammaticality Judgment Task ($F = 231.16$; $df = 1$, 11; $p < 0.0001$), performance on the Grammaticality Judgment Task differed significantly from that on the Multiple Choice Cloze Task ($F = 62.79$; $df = 1$, 11; $p < 0.0001$), and performance on the Multiple Choice Cloze Task was significantly different from that on the Spontaneous Cloze Task ($F = 33.44$; $df = 1$, 11; $p < 0.0001$).

Results support a possible hierarchy in the amount of linguistic contextual information. A profile analysis indicates that performance on the Repetition Task was significantly different from that on the Multiple Choice and Spontaneous Cloze Tasks, and performance on the Grammaticality Judgment Task was significantly different from that on the Spontaneous Cloze Task. In sum, an increase in the amount of linguistic contextual information resulted in better performance (i.e. lower error rates) for the aphasic participants. Conversely, a decrease in the amount of contextual information resulted in poorer performance, evidenced by increased error rates.

Table 14.2 Performance of aphasic participants on tasks varying in amount of linguistic contextual information

Task	Mean no. errors	Mean error rate (%)	Standard deviation	Range of errors
Repetition	5.8	12.1	2.6	3– 11
Grammaticality Judgment	10.6	22.1	3.4	6– 16
Multiple Choice Cloze	14.4	30.0	4.9	10– 24
Spontaneous Cloze	19.0	39.6	4.6	14– 26

It is noted that the interaction between Prepositional Category and Linguistic Context was not significant at the chosen alpha level of 0.05 ($F = 8.62$; $df = 9$; $p < 0.0515$). However, this interaction effect closely approached significance. This may reflect the fact that differences in error rates for the four prepositional categories were smaller on the Repetition Task than they were on the subsequent three tasks, as illustrated in Figure 14.3. The primary significance of the data depicted in Figure 14.3 lies in the pattern of performance across all four tasks. That is, regardless of the task presented (i.e. Repetition, Grammaticality, Judgment, Multiple Choice Cloze, and Spontaneous Cloze), the participants performed best on locative prepositions, followed by temporal prepositions, then case-marking prepositions, and the worst performance was seen on phrasal prepositions.

Discussion and Implications

Several findings of this investigation are noteworthy. In general, the Spanish-speaking aphasic participants in the current investigation did exhibit significantly more difficulty than the normal control participants with the aspect of their morphosyntactic system consisting of prepositions. This finding is consistent with the cross-linguistic aphasia literature to date indicating a disruption to some degree of functors across Indo-European languages (Menn *et al.*, 1995). With respect to the variables addressed in this investigation, semantic value of prepositions was found to have a significant effect on participant performance:

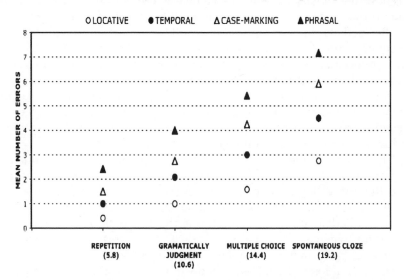

Figure 14.3 Performance of aphasic subjects on each task (mean number of errors within task shown in parentheses)

prepositions high in semantic value were better preserved than those low in semantic value. This aspect of prepositions may be at least partially responsible for the large within-class variability of error patterns on prepositions reported in the literature (Bird *et al.*, 2002; Caplan, 1991; Menn & Obler, 1990; Tesak & Hummer, 1994). Indeed, it may be the case that not only do we see 'subclasses within the closed class' itself (Bebout, 1993: 162), but we may also have subclasses with the class of prepositions, each varying with respect to semantic value. Friederici (1982: 252) has suggested that phrasal prepositions (the fourth category of prepositions in the current investigation) bear 'virtually no semantic meaning by themselves'. Again, it appears that semantic value of prepositions may be a determining factor in the preservation and disruption of these items in aphasia.

This finding has implications for the assessment and treatment of Spanish-speaking aphasic patients. With respect to cross-language research, it is not until the regularities of language dissolution are identified across different languages that the development of appropriate assessment tools in the various languages can be employed. The need is pressing for the development of *culturally and linguistically valid assessment tools* to evaluate aphasic patients in Spanish. Since prepositions constitute prominent linguistic elements in the language with important syntactic and semantic functions, it is suggested that assessment of the aphasic individual incorporate the evaluation of prepositions varying in semantic value. Inclusion of tasks designed to systematically examine prepositions of varying semantic value into our current aphasia batteries may prove to be useful in determining level of impairment, identifying subtle deficits in communication skills, differential diagnosis, and designing appropriate treatment programs. Implementation of intervention programs emphasizing comprehension and production of lexical items high in semantic value (i.e. high degree of imageability) may be warranted (Bird *et al.*, 2002). In addition, treatment protocols and hierarchies using prepositions varying in semantic value may prove useful. Furthermore, treatment tasks using prepositions high in semantic value may serve as facilitating cues for aphasic patients.

This investigation also found that amount of linguistic contextual information significantly affected participant performance: tasks providing the most linguistic contextual information resulted in the best performance, whereas tasks providing minimal linguistic contextual cues resulted in the poorest performance. It has been debated in the literature whether aphasia is a deficit of linguistic competence or linguistic performance. That is, it is questioned whether aphasia represents a loss of linguistic knowledge, or results from impaired access to/activation of linguistic rules and representations (Bates *et al.*, 1987; Friederici, 1985; McNeil *et al.*, 1991; Silkes *et al.*, 2004). Aphasic participants' performance in the current investigation on tasks providing the most linguistic contextual information suggests that underlying knowledge of prepositions (i.e. competence) in aphasia is preserved to some degree, although significant deficits in performance may be evident. Aphasic performance on tasks varying in the amount of linguistic contextual information has both clinical and theoretical relevance. It suggests that aphasic patients are able to rely on facilitating contexts when those contexts are provided for them. Incorporation of psycholinguistic principles into the development of therapeutic contexts with aphasic individuals may seek to enhance the 'underlying forms' and, in turn, facilitate their comprehension and expression (Thompson, 2001: 609). Consideration of the amount of linguistic contextual information in the construction of treatment hierarchies may also prove useful. That is, therapy may incorporate comprehension and production of prepositions in a creative manner, providing facilitation for patients by supplying more linguistic contextual information when needed. With more severely impaired patients, or in the early stages of intervention, it would seem prudent to begin with tasks providing maximal contextual cues, in order to capitalize on possible strengths and to maximize patient performance. With patient progress, tasks providing fewer contextual cues may be incorporated into the intervention program.

In conclusion, this investigation has provided preliminary information which may begin to bridge some of the gaps in our current under-standing of prepositional processing in aphasia, particularly in under-researched languages. It is hoped that this study will not only contribute to our theoretical understanding of aphasia, but that it will ultimately contribute to *cross-linguistic data* to improve clinical assessment and treatment of the aphasic patient.

References

Ardila, A. (2001) The manifestations of aphasic symptoms in Spanish. In M. Paradis (ed.) *Manifestations of Aphasia Symptoms in Different Languages* (pp. 253–263). Amsterdam: Pergamon.

Bates, E., Friederici, A.D. and Wulfeck, B. (1987) Grammatical morphology in aphasia: Evidence from three languages. *Cortex* 23, 545–574.

Bates, E., Friederici, A.D., Wulfeck, B. and Juarez, L.A. (1988) On the preservation of word order in aphasia: Cross-linguistic evidence. *Brain and Language* 33, 323–364.

Bebout, L. (1993) Processing of negative morphemes in aphasia: An example of the complexities of the closed class/open class concept. *Clinical Linguistics and Phonetics* 7, 161–172.

Benedet, M.J., Christiansen, J.A. and Goodglass, H. (1998) A cross-linguistic study of grammatical morphology in Spanish- and English-speaking agrammatic patients. *Cortex* 34, 309–336.

Benson, D.F. and Ardila, A. (1996) *Aphasia: A Clinical Perspective.* Oxford: Oxford University Press.

Beyn, E.S., Vizel, T.G. and Hatfield, F.M. (1979) Aspects of agrammatism in aphasia. *Language and Speech* 22, 327–346.
Biassou, N., Obler, L.K., Nespoulous, J.L. and Dordain, M. (1997) Dual processing of open-and-closed-class words. *Brain and Language* 57, 360–373.
Bird, H., Franklin, S. and Howard, D. (2002) 'Little words' – not really: function and content words in normal and aphasic speech. *Journal of Neurolinguistics* 15, 209–237.
Bradley, D., Garrett, M. and Zurif, E.B. (1980) Syntactic deficits in Broca's aphasia. In D. Caplan (ed.) *Biological Studies of Mental Processes* (pp. 269–286). Cambridge, NJ: MIT Press.
Brookshire, R.H. (2003) *Introduction to Neurogenic Communication Disorders.* St. Louis, MO: Mosby.
Caplan, D. (1991) Notes and discussion: Agrammatism is a theoretically coherent aphasic category. *Brain and Language* 40, 274–281.
Coslett, H.B., Rothi, L.J.G. and Heilman, K.M. (1984) Reading: Selective sparing of closed-class words in Wernicke's aphasia. *Neurology* 34, 1038–1045.
Davis, G.A. (2000) *Aphasiology: Disorders and Clinical Practice.* Boston: Allyn and Bacon.
Fillmore, C.J. (1977) The case for case reopened. In P. Cole and J.M. Sadock (eds) *Syntax and Semantics: Grammatical Relations* (pp. 59–81). New York: Academic Press.
Friederici, A.D. (1982) Syntactic and semantic processes in aphasic deficits: The availability of prepositions. *Brain and Language* 15, 249–258.
Friederici, A.D. (1985) Levels of processing of vocabulary types: Evidence from on-line comprehension in normals and agrammatics. *Cognition* 19, 133–166.
Garrett, M. (1980) Levels of processing in sentence production. In B. Butterworth (ed.) *Language Production* (pp. 177–220). New York: Academic Press.
Goodglass, H. and Kaplan, E. (1983) *The Assessment of Aphasia and Related Disorders.* Philadelphia: Lea and Febiger.
Goodglass, H. and Menn, L. (1985) Is agrammatism a unitary phenomenon? In M.L. Kean (ed.) *Agrammatism* (pp. 1–26). New York: Academic Press.
Juilland, A. and Chang-Rodriguez, E. (1974) *Frequency Dictionary of Spanish Words.* The Hague: Mouton.
López, M.L. (1972) *Problemas y Métodos en el Análisis de Preposiciones.* Madrid: Editorial Gredos.
McNeil, M.R., Odell, K. and Tseng, C.H. (1991) Toward the integration of resource allocation into a general theory of aphasia. *Clinical Aphasiology* 20, 21–39.
Menn, L. and Obler, L.K. (1990) Cross-language data and theories of agrammatism. In L. Menn and L.K. Obler (eds) *Agrammatic Aphasia* (Vol. II, pp. 1369–1389). Amsterdam: John Benjamins.
Menn, L., O'Connor, M., Obler, L.K. and Holland, A. (1995) *Non-fluent Aphasia in a Multilingual World.* Philadelphia, PA: John Benjamins.
Nespoulous, J.L., Dordain, M., Perron, C., Ska, B., Bub, D., Caplan, D., Mehler, J. and Lecours, A.R. (1988) Agrammatism in sentence production without comprehension deficits: Reduced availability of syntactic structures and/or grammatical morphemes? A case study. *Brain and Language* 33, 273–295.
Ostrosky-Solís, F., Marcos-Ortega, J., Ardila, A., Rosselli, M. and Palacios, S. (1999) Syntactic comprehension in Broca's aphasic Spanish-speakers: Null effects of word order. *Aphasiology* 13, 553–571.
Paradis, M. (2001) By the way of preface: The need for awareness of aphasia symptoms in different languages. In M. Paradis (ed.) *Manifestations of Aphasic Symptoms in Different Languages* (pp. 1–7). Amsterdam: Pergamon Press.

Real Academia Española (1979) *Gramática de la Lengua Española*. Madrid: Espasa-Calpe, S.A.

Reyes, B.A. (1990) Processing of prepositions in Spanish-speaking aphasics: Effects of semantic value and contextual information. PhD Dissertation, University of Texas at Dallas.

Reznik, M., Dubrovsky, S. and Maldonado, S. (1995). Agrammatism in Spanish: A case study. *Brain and Language* 51, 355–368.

Rivas, D.J. (1976) *Prepositions in Spanish and English: A Contrastive Study and Sample Thesaurus*. Montevideo, Uruguay: Ediciones Geminis.

Silkes, J.P., McNeil, M.R. and Dorton, M. (2004) Stimulation of aphasic naming performance in non-brain-damaged adults. *Journal of Speech, Language, and Hearing Research* 47, 610–623.

Tesak, J. and Hummer, P. (1994) A note on prepositions in agrammatism. *Brain and Language* 46, 463–468.

Thompson, C.K. (2001) Treatment of underlying forms: A linguistic specific approach for sentence production deficits in agrammatic aphasia. In R. Chapey (ed.) *Language Intervention Strategies in Aphasia and Related Neurogenic Communication Disorders* (pp. 605–625). Philadelphia, PA: Lippincott Williams and Wilkins.

US Bureau of the Census (2000) *Statistical Abstract of the United States: 2000*. Washington, D.C.: US Government Printing Office.

Weber-Fox, C. and Neville, H.J. (2001) Sensitive periods differentiate processing of open-and-closed-class words: An ERP study of bilinguals. *Journal of Speech, Language and Hearing Research* 44, 1338–1353.

Chapter 15

Cohesion in the Conversational Samples of Broca's Aphasic Individuals: Theoretical and Clinical Implications

LOURDES G. PIETROSEMOLI

Discourse analysis can provide the speech-language clinician with invaluable means to assess *functional communicative performance* in the brain-damaged population (Cherney, 1998; Lesser & Perkins, 1999; Perkins, 1995; Schiffrin *et al.*, 2001). As conversation analysis can describe how interlocutors collaborate to achieve successful discourse exchanges (Sacks *et al.*, 1974; Schegloff *et al.*, 1977), clinical observations of aphasic conversational interactions may be an important approach to evaluate current discourse status, help identify underlying cognitive and linguistic processes, and assist in treatment planning (Lesser & Milroy, 1993; Lesser & Perkins, 1999; Perkins, 1995; also see Guendouzi & Müller, 2006). In Levinson's words (1983: 284), 'conversation is clearly the prototypical kind of language usage, the form in which we are all exposed to language ... '. Conversation can be used as the basis for the study of cohesion in aphasic discourse precisely because the functional use of language seen in conversation – and not in tasks such as reading, writing, picture description, or describing procedures – has been proposed to be the ultimate target of aphasia intervention and an important skill to promote the social adaptation of the aphasic patient (Elman, 2005; Lesser, 2003; Simmons-Mackie, 2001).

Conversations selected for this study adopt the form of questions and answers. The rationale for this question–answer format goes beyond the intrinsic structure of the sociolinguistic interviews employed in the collection of linguistic data. Questions and answers naturally constitute *high-frequency structures* in the linguistic exchange of aphasics with their nonaphasic interlocutors and, as data from normal discourse analysis support, these structures are also recurrent in typical everyday speech. According to Goffman (1981: 5), 'whenever persons talk there are very likely to be questions and answers'. Moreover, talking in clinical settings is an activity in which questions and answers are typical structures between the clinician and the patient as part of assessment. Similarly, clinical personnel typically employ questions to elicit information from patients and family members. At the same time, as patients make efforts to recover important pieces of information about their interrupted life, they very often rely on question-like structures. Hamilton (1994: 81) proposes – among various reasons – an important argument for the analysis of questions and answers in Alzheimer's patients, which can also apply to aphasics: 'It is important to examine question/response routines in natural conversations with an Alzheimer's patient because the diagnosis/assessment of such a patient is based in part on the patient's responses to a tester's questions'. The analysis of questions and answers, then, is not only crucial in order to understand an important aspect of the linguistic activity in clinical populations; the analysis of the structures provided by the aphasic under the form of questions or answers can also shed some light as to the preservation of the aphasic's linguistic, cognitive, and/or social abilities.

In this chapter, I discuss an investigation and its clinical implications looking at *cohesion*, one essential property of discourse, in the conversational samples produced by three mild-to-moderate Broca's aphasic individuals and their nonaphasic interlocutors. Among the concepts developed in discourse analysis, cohesion is most suitable to incorporate in testing and intervention in aphasia (Lesser & Milroy, 1993; Liles & Coelho, 1998). Cohesion is defined as structural coherence among the sentences of a text (Halliday & Hasan, 1976). As it will be described later in the analysis section, the clear definition of boundaries between different types of cohesion makes this concept very manageable even for the nonlinguist professional.

Analysis of cohesion in discourse can successfully be employed as a reliable instrument to indicate the speakers' capacity to build pieces of a unified conversational text (e.g. Lesser & Milroy, 1993; Liles & Coelho, 1998). Yet, there are not many methods of linguistic analysis in aphasia *beyond the sentence level*. In fact, clinical analysis of discourse production is in its infancy as investigators experiment with methods for getting at the various discourse properties, such as cohesion and overall coherence (Davis, 2000). As conversation is a special type of text built between – at least – two speakers, the sentence as unit loses relevance: very often in conversation a potential sentence initiated by a speaker is completed by the interlocutor or vice versa. In this chapter, I propose the analysis of cohesion in conversation using *the turn* as the basic unit of analysis. The turn as an independent entity has been validly postulated (Coulthard, 1992; Levinson, 1983; Sacks *et al.*, 1974; Schegloff *et al.*, 1977).

The questions leading this study were the following:

(1) How does cohesion vary in conversation when one of the interlocutors is aphasic?

(2) How can we effectively incorporate the strategies followed by aphasic speakers in the process of constructing cohesive conversations into the evaluation and rehabilitation processes in aphasia?

In order to examine the above questions, conversations between three mild-to-moderate Broca-type aphasics and their nonaphasic interlocutors were analyzed following the concepts stated initially by Halliday and Hasan (1976) and applied by different authors in the analysis of unimpaired and special texts (e.g. Armstrong, 1991; Liles & Coelho, 1998; Mentis & Prutting 1987; Prutting & Kirchner 1987; Rochester & Martin 1979).

Description of the Study

This study was part of the Aphasia Research Program developed at the Universidad de Los Andes (ARPULA), Mérida, Venezuela. For the development of the ARPULA project, a corpus of neurologically based communication profiles was collected as a database for aphasiological research in the Mérida urban area (Pietrosemoli *et al.*, 1995). This corpus is expected to constitute the basis for the future development of aphasia rehabilitation programs. The data and results on the cohesion of aphasic conversationalists in comparison to their nonaphasic interlocutors discussed in this chapter are closely related to the global ARPULA project.

Participant selection

Participants were selected from a larger study (Pietrosemoli, 1998), part of the ARPULA project mentioned above. Participants included 9 monolingual Spanish-speaking patients (3 Broca's, 3 Wernicke's, and 3 anomic aphasics). The data analysis reported here focuses on the analysis of conversations produced by the three mild-to-moderate Broca's aphasic cohort, referred to here as Olga, Argen, and Cari. Aphasic participants met the following criteria: (1) completion of all neurological and linguistic evaluations required by the ARPULA protocol, including the HULA (Hospital de la Universidad de los Andes [University of The Andes Hospital]) neurological evaluation battery, CAT scan and/or MRI, sociolinguistic interview, preliminary linguistic screening, and two standardized tests, the *Token Test* (DeRenzi & Faglioni, 1978) and the *Boston Diagnostic Aphasia Examination* (BDAE) (Goodglass & Kaplan, 1983), both adapted to the Venezuelan participants, (2) evidence of no additional problems, which could mask the linguistic output, such as previous strokes, severely unintelligible speech, psychiatric problems, Alzheimer's disease, mental retardation, alcoholism or drug addiction, and (3) family and individual consent to participate in the project.

Samples of conversations with nonaphasic speakers, matched with aphasic participants according to age, gender, and socioeducational background, were employed as controls.

Procedures

The conversational pieces analyzed were extracted from a sociolinguistic interview and from conversational exchanges that took place before and after the actual therapy session. The topics were selected among the recurrent themes generated by the aphasics in the sociolinguistic interview. As aphasic productions can display a wide range of variation, in order for the speech performances to be comparable, the conversations were chosen according to the following guidelines: (1) the development and completion of at least one identifiable topic, and (2) when the topic was difficult to determine, other cues, such as prolonged pauses before or after the conversational piece or the change to a next relevant contribution, were employed as boundaries in the selection of texts. As a result, conversational pieces may vary in length. It is worth noting that this variation is also present in conversational activities of control speakers. The cohesion analysis performed on the conversational fragments is not affected by variations in length as the number of semantic links among linguistic units varies accordingly, which allowed comparisons among the different conversational fragments. Three conversations were analyzed for this chapter (Appendix A). They were transcribed following the conventions included in Appendix A. A translation in English also is provided, including an attempt to illustrate paraphasic errors.

The cohesion analysis

In Halliday and Hasan's (1976) study of cohesion, *text* is referred to as any passage, spoken or written, of whatever length, that forms a unified whole. A text is considered to be a semantic unit of language in use whose cohesion – that is, what makes it a *unified whole* – is provided by the semantic relations among its elements. The occurrence of a pair of semantically related items in a text is defined as a *tie*, and, in a given text, five different patterns of ties can be found: *reference*, *substitution*, *conjunction*, *lexical*, and *ellipsis*. This definition and classification has been employed subsequently in discourse analysis in communicatively impaired adults as a means of analyzing the cohesion of texts (e.g. Armstrong, 1991; Liles & Coelho, 1998; Mentis & Prutting, 1987; also see Prutting & Kirchner, 1987; Rochester & Martin, 1979). The analysis of cohesion in this study, then, follows the original scheme developed by Halliday and Hasan (1976). Occurrences of the five cohesive ties mentioned above were examined in the productions of each aphasic individual and his/her nonaphasic interlocutor throughout a complete conversation. Conversational samples were selected on the basis of the full development and completion of a particular topic, or other clues signaled by the interlocutor(s) concerning the initiation or completion of the conversational activity.

The indices

For every conversation, three indices were calculated in the present study (Appendix B):

(1) The *Global Conversational Cohesion Index* (GCCI) was calculated by dividing the total number of cohesive ties displayed in the conversation by the total number of conversational turns. In every conversation, however, the *opening turn* is not connected to a previous one, so the index is calculated on the basis of total of turns minus one. In Halliday and Hasan's (1976) terms, in order for a text to be cohesive, sentences must semantically relate to each other by at least one tie. The same concept applies in this study to conversations using the turn, not the sentence, as the basic unit.

(2) The *Aphasic Conversational Cohesion Index* (ACCI) was calculated by dividing the number of the aphasic speaker's cohesive ties in his/ her linguistic contributions by the total number of turns in the aphasic participant's conversation.

(3) The *Nonaphasic Conversational Cohesion Index* (NCCI) was calculated by dividing the number of ties in the nonaphasic speaker's linguistic contributions by the total number of his/her turns in conversation.

Results

According to Halliday and Hasan (1976, 1985) and Hasan (1980), every sentence in an ideal text has at least one cohesive tie that connects that specific sentence to the previous one. Correspondingly, in a conversation (considered an oral text), every turn has to be connected to the previous one by – at least – one type of tie. As shown in Table 15.1, the GCCI

Table 15.1 Cohesion indices in the conversation between Broca's aphasic and nonaphasic participants

	GCCI	*ACCI*	*NCCI*	
A				*NA*
Olga	1.5	1.6	1.4	Clinician
Argen	3.14	3.75	2.3	Clinician
Cari	1.13	1.2	1	Clinician

A, aphasic speaker; NA, nonaphasic speaker
Indices: GCCI, Global Conversational Cohesion Index; ACCI, Aphasic Conversational Cohesion Index; NCCI, Nonaphasic Conversational Cohesion Index

(total of ties per total of conversational turns) is, in every case, greater than 1, which means that every turn in the conversations analyzed is cohesively connected to the previous one through at least one type of tie. In the conversation with Argen (Appendix A: Conversation 2), the index is markedly higher than in the rest of the samples. We also observe in all three conversations that the cohesive contribution is greater in the case of the aphasic partner (ACCI: 1.6; 3.75; 1.2) than in the case of the normal speaker (NCCI: 1.4; 2.3; 1), and is also greater than the general index of the entire conversational fragment (GCCI: 1.5; 3.14; 1.13).

Some of the results on cohesive analysis in clinical populations presented in previous works seem to be at variance with these data. Several authors propose that clinical populations, in general, use fewer cohesive ties than their normal counterparts (Armstrong, 1991; Mentis & Prutting, 1987; Nicholas *et al.*, 1985; Ripich & Terrell, 1988; Ulatowska *et al.*, 1983). However, Rochester and Martin (1979) found that thought-disordered schizophrenic individuals use more cohesive ties of the lexical type than the non-thought-disordered type, and than the control normal population. Their research suggests that the greater or lesser use of cohesive ties is contingent upon linguistic genre. In their extensive study, Rochester and Martin report that all of the interlocutors – including controls – used more cohesive ties when engaged in narrative tasks than when being interviewed or in conversation. In the case of the Broca's participants' conversations in this study, it seems to be the opposite. In our sample – and this also holds true for the larger corpus in which conversations with Wernicke and Anomic aphasic speakers were included (Pietrosemoli, 1998) – Broca's speakers use more ties in conversation than in narratives. Even though we do not have sufficient data concerning the narrative abilities of all the cases under examination, we can predict that Olga and Cari, the other two Broca's participants reported here (Appendix A: Conversations 1 and 3, respectively), will have problems with cohesion when they move beyond sentence-level or turn-level. It is likely to be the case that *different strategies of cohesion vary not only with linguistic genre but also with different clinical problems, or degrees of severity within one type of problem.* In other words, thought-disordered patients could be better narrators than conversationalists, and the opposite could hold true for Broca's aphasics. Ripich and Terrell (1988), on the other hand, found no significant differences in proposi-tional form and cohesion devices in the analysis of the speech production of six unimpaired elderly and six patients with Alzheimer's disease. They concluded that the instances of disrupted cohesion found in this population were all related to missing elements in their linguistic productions.

Distribution of cohesive items

Findings of cohesive ties in this study agree with earlier findings showing a marked tendency among Broca's aphasic conversationalists to rely mainly on ellipsis or lexical ties as a means to keep conversation cohesive (Armstrong, 1991) (Table 15.2). This tendency is also supported by Milroy and Perkins (1992), who reported two severe cases of aphasia – one Broca's and one Wernicke's – in which ellipsis and lexical types are the only ties present in the first stages of the rehabilitation process. Further, Hamilton (1991) found that in the last stages of Alzheimer's disease the normal interlocutor may increase the frequency of polar questions (questions whose answer is yes/no) addressed to the Alzheimer's speaker. This fact could be interpreted as a *cooperative strategy* on the side of the normal interlocutor to privilege ellipsis – a sort of default cohesive tie – as a means of keeping cohesion in conversation. It appears then that ellipsis because of its *recycling* attributes converts itself into a linguistic mechanism that allows a person to maintain the minimal cooperation required in the conversational activity even in severe cases of syntactic loss and overall linguistic distress.

In Conversation 1 (Appendix A), the low ellipsis percentage is unexpected, considering Olga's precarious linguistic abilities. Examining her conversation, we observe that she manages to provide, in her elementary grammar, the necessary lexical items that allow her to collaborate actively in the development of conversational topics. The nonaphasic partner, on the other hand, promotes her cooperation posing wh-type questions (Conversation 1: Turns 1, 3, 9, 11, 13, and 15), instead of simpler yes/no questions, which results in a more interactive exchange. In the two cases in which yes/no questions are employed by the clinician, Olga finds a way of adding a new element to the answer,

Table 15.2 Percentage of cohesive ties in the conversational samples of both Broca's aphasic and nonaphasic participants

	Lexical (%)		Ellipsis (%)		Substitution (%)		Reference (%)		Conjunction (%)	
	A	NA	A	NA	A	NA	A	NA	A	NA
Olga	53.84	40.0	38.46	30.0	–	–	–	20.0	7.60	10.0
Argen	46.66	42.80	53.33	14.20	–	–	–	14.20	–	28.50
Cari	29.16	35.29	62.50	35.29	–	5.80	4.34	23.52	4.16	–

A, aphasic speaker; NA, nonaphasic speaker

expanding her limited capabilities as a conversational partner and raising her quota of lexical ties.

5. Clinician: *era grande?*
   was it big?
6. Olga: *grande*
   big one
7. Clinician: *era cara?*
   was it expensive?
8. Olga: *no, ocho.*
   no, eight.

Despite the severity of Olga's expression, evidenced through her linguistic parsimony (i.e. short utterances, grammatical simplicity, and phonological paraphasias; e.g. Turns 4, 8), her conversation sample presents itself as strikingly efficient and smooth; the only interruptions being her attempts at self-repairs (Turns 4, 10). Such smooth pattern in the conversation could be explained on the basis of the shared knowledge existing, in this particular case, between the therapist and the patient, a common feature sometimes developed during long-term rehabilitation programs (also see Guendouzi & Müller, 2006, for similar patterns in other communication contexts with neurologically impaired speakers).

In Conversation 2, there is a slightly higher proportion of lexical ties in the aphasic person's speech relative to the unimpaired speaker (Table 15.2: 46.66% versus 42.80%). Following Milroy and Perkins (1992), this can be interpreted as though the aphasic interlocutor is in charge of the topical unity. This holds true for this particular example. In this conversational sample, and due to the phonologically induced aphasic error (e.g. Turn 4: *contusión–construcción* 'construction'), both interlocutors find themselves at a *dead end* (Conversation 2: Turns 4–7). The aphasic speaker acknowledges his responsibility in correcting this situation by way of explaining the meaning of the unknown word. His production of semantically related words (Turn 8: *fablical edificio* 'to construct building') or repetitions (*contusión* appears five times in eight turns: Turns 4, 6, 8) unbalances the distribution of lexical ties.

In Conversation 3, the aphasic interlocutor presents a more serious expressive problem, but this difficulty does not lead to a real misunderstanding. In this conversational sample, in which two nonaphasic interlocutors (i.e. the clinician and the patient's sister) participate, the nonaphasic participants essentially take an active role to keep a smooth topic flow in the conversation, based on the aphasic speaker's responses, hence circumventing potential miscommunication problems. The aphasic speaker, however, also participates using her expressive resources. She shows no doubts as to the timing and syntactic/semantic adequacy of her next contribution in conversation. In this manner, the aphasic speaker contributes by repairing the nonaphasic participants' turn as soon as she perceives the speaker's difficulty in finding the precise word:

> 20 Clinician: *ajá ... mira, y cuál es tu santo, tu santo (pausa) ... ?*
> uhu, say, and which one is your saint, your saint (pause)?
> 21 Cari: *preferido.*
> favorite.

Discussion

Broca's aphasia has been commonly associated with effort, slowness, and difficulties in oral expression. In the samples examined, the efficiency in the turn-taking process and the adequacy of responses in conversation seem to compensate for the expressive impairment. The absence of pauses between turns is especially notable. This readiness in the turn-taking activity in conversation has been described by Coulthard (1992) as a central characteristic of normal conversationalists, and as requiring a high degree of skill and sophistication on the side of interlocutors. The evidence gathered in the conversations analyzed suggests that underlying processing operations involved in the expressive output of Broca's aphasics does not impinge upon the system controlling conversation. As clearly supported by analysis of the third conversational sample, even in situations of severe linguistic stress, Broca's speakers can *participate meaningfully* in conversation using their limited resources and by being aware of the *timing and syntactic/semantic adequacy* of their contributions.

Returning to the research questions posed at the beginning of this chapter, findings suggest that conversational structure and strategies in our mild-to-moderate Broca's aphasic group seemed to be well preserved, as evidenced by the cohesive indices. Regarding cohesion indices, the figures displayed in Table 15.2 are to some extent unexpected. Our intuition tells us that a discourse characterized as *telegraphic and agrammatic* (impoverished grammatical structure), as generally observed in Broca's aphasia, must be noncohesive to some extent. Yet, a lack of cohesion has been reported in the narratives of thought-disordered patients by Rochester and Martin (1979). In the development of a conversation, however, other resources that assemble the conversational text may appear. Repetitions and/or synonyms (lexical cohesion) or recycling of own, or the other participant's interventions (ellipsis) may contribute to provide the wholeness desired in a conversational exchange in precarious linguistic situations. In the conversational samples described here, the aphasic and nonaphasic interlocutors engaged in similar repetitions thus providing the required cohesive elements, and, at the same time, actively cooperating in the construction of a cohesive piece of conversation. Additionally, it is likely that different strategies of cohesion are not only at variance with linguistic genre but also with different clinical problems, or degrees of severity within one type of problem.

This study supports earlier research (Davis, 1986; Davis *et al.*, 1985; Holland, 1991; Lesser & Milroy, 1993; Pulvermuller & Roth, 1991). Essentially, this investigation emphasizes the fact that mild-to-moderate Broca's aphasic patients, in spite of their expressive restrictions, still behave as social individuals who can sustain a conversational exchange, and who still can function as *information providers*. These findings have important clinical implications. Particularly, the tendency for the Broca's aphasic speakers in this study to exhibit well preserved conversational structure and strategies may be valuable for rehabilitation purposes and for *post-stroke social adaptation*. Hence, in addition to addressing specific linguistic skills in treatment (i.e. naming, sentence production, and so forth), conversational activities can be incorporated into the therapy protocol and the patient's daily routines. Using this approach, clinicians and relatives jointly work in creating conversational contexts (e.g. topics and activities) well known to the patient. Awareness of the conversational scenario provides a facilitating context that relieves aphasic speakers from any difficulties with information retrieval and shifts their efforts to conversational devices that would keep a smooth flow in the interaction. This approach is consistent with intervention programs with the elderly based on the most optimal linguistic and physical contexts to enhance communication (e.g. Harris, 1997) and aphasia treatment methods emphasizing collaborative interactional routines between the patient and unimpaired speakers (Elman, 2005; Lesser, 2003; Simmons-Mackie, 2001; also see Guendouzi & Müller, 2006). In this manner, intervention would incorporate meaningful life contexts that encourage the patient to participate in more social and meaningful communicative activities beyond stimulus-response treatment tasks (Elman, 2005).

References

Armstrong, E.M. (1991) The potential of cohesion analysis in the analysis and treatment of aphasic discourse. *Clinical Linguistics and Phonetics* 5, 39–52.

Cherney, L.R. (1998) Pragmatics in discourse. In L.R. Cherney, B.B. Shadden and C.C. Coelho (eds) *Analyzing Discourse in Communicatively Impaired Adults* (pp. 1–7). Gaithersburg, MD: Aspen.

Coulthard, M. (1992) *An Introduction to Discourse Analysis*. London: Longman.

Davis, G.A. (1986) Pragmatics and treatment. In R. Chapey (ed.) *Language Intervention Strategies in Adult Aphasia* (pp. 121–142). Baltimore: Williams and Wilkins.

Davis, G.A. (2000) *Aphasiology: Disorders and Clinical Practice*. Boston, MA: Allyn and Bacon.

Davis, G.A., Wilcox, M.J. and Leonard, L. (1985) *Adult Aphasia Rehabilitation: Applied Pragmatics*. Windsor: NFER-Nelson.

DeRenzi, F. and Faglioni, P. (1978) Normative data and the screening power of a shortened version of the Token Test. *Cortex* 14, 41–49.

Elman, R. (2005) Social and life participation approaches to aphasia intervention. In L.L. LaPointe (ed.) *Aphasia and Related Neurogenic Language Disorders* (pp. 39–50). New York: Thieme.

Goffman, E. (1981) *Forms of Talk*. Philadelphia: University of Pennsylvania Press.

Goodglass, H. and Kaplan, E. (1983) *The Assessment of Aphasia and Related Disorders*. Philadelphia: Lea and Febiger.

Guendouzi, J.A. and Müller, N. (2006) *Approaches to Discourse in Dementia*. Mahwah, NJ: Lawrence Erlbaum.

Halliday, M. and Hasan, R. (1976) *Cohesion in English*. London: Longman.

Halliday, M. and Hasan, R. (1985) *Language, Context and Text: Aspects of Language in a Social-Semiotic Perspective*. Oxford: Oxford University Press.

Hamilton, H. (1991) *Inappropriateness of Response: A Longitudinal Study of the Conversation of one Elderly Female Alzheimer's Patient*. Washington, DC: Georgetown University.

Hamilton, H. (1994) *Conversations with an Alzheimer's Patient*. Cambridge, UK: Cambridge University Press.

Harris, J.L. (1997) Reminiscence: A culturally and developmentally appropriate language intervention for older adults. *American Journal of Speech-Language Pathology* 6, 19–25.

Hasan, R. (1980) What's going on: A dynamic view of context in language. In J.E. Copeland and P.W. Davis (eds) *The Seventh LACUS Forum* (pp. 47–57). Columbia, SC: Hornbeam Press.

Holland, A. (1991) Pragmatic aspects of intervention in aphasia. *Journal of Neurolinguistics* 6, 197–211.

Lesser, R. (2003) Conversation analysis and aphasia therapy. In I. Papathanasiou and R. De Bleser (eds) *The Sciences of Aphasia: From Therapy to Theory* (pp. 173–185). Amsterdam: Pergamon.

Lesser, R. and Milroy L. (1993) *Linguistics and Aphasia. Psycholinguistic and Pragmatic Aspects of Intervention*. London: Longman.

Lesser, R. and Perkins, L. (1999) *Cognitive Neuropsychology and Conversation Analysis as Guidelines for Aphasia Therapy: An Introductory Case-based Workbook*. Portland, OR: Taylor and Francis.

Levinson, S.C. (1983) *Pragmatics*. Cambridge: Cambridge University Press.

Liles, B.Z. and Coelho, C.A. (1998) Cohesion analysis. In L.R. Cherney, B.B. Shadden and C.C. Coelho (eds) *Analyzing Discourse in Communicatively Impaired Adults* (pp. 65–82). Gaithersburg, MD: Aspen.

Mentis, M. and Prutting, C.A. (1987) Cohesion in the discourse of normal and head-injured adults. *Journal of Speech and Hearing Research* 30, 88–98.

Milroy, L. and Perkins, L. (1992) Repair strategies in aphasic discourse: Toward a collaborative model. *Clinical Linguistics and Phonetics* 6, 27–40.

Nicholas, M., Obler, L.K., Albert, M. and Helm-Estabrooks, N. (1985) Empty speech in Alzheimer disease and fluent aphasia. *Journal of Speech and Hearing Research* 28, 405–410.

Perkins, L. (1995) Applying conversational analysis to aphasia: Clinical implications and analytic issues. *European Journal of Disorders of Communication* 30, 372–83.

Pietrosemoli, L. (1998) Cohesion and coherence in aphasic conversational discourse. Ph.D. thesis, Georgetown University.

Pietrosemoli, L., Vera, M. and González, S. (1995) Corpus para el estudio de la afasia. Unpublished manuscript, Universidad de Los Andes, Mérida, Venezuela.

Prutting, C.A. and Kirchner, D.M. (1987) A clinical appraisal of pragmatic aspects of language. *Journal of Speech and Hearing Disorders* 52, 105–19.

Pulvermuller, F. and Roth, V.M. (1991) Communicative aphasia treatment as a further development of PACE therapy. *Aphasiology* 5, 39–50.

Ripich, D. and Terrell, B. (1988) Patterns of discourse cohesion and coherence in Alzheimer's disease. *Journal of Speech and Hearing Disorders* 53, 8–15.

Rochester, S. and Martin, J.R. (1979) *Crazy Talk*. New York: Plenum Press.

Sacks, H., Schegloff, E. and Jefferson, G. (1974) A simplest systematics for the organization of turn-taking for conversation. *Language* 50, 696–735.

Schegloff, E., Jefferson, G. and Sacks, H. (1977) The preference for self-correction in the organization of repair in conversation. *Language* 53, 360–382.

Schiffrin, D., Tannen, D. and Hamilton, H. (eds) (2001) *The Handbook of Discourse Analysis*. Malden, MA: Blackwell Publishers.

Simmons-Mackie, N. (2001) Social approaches to aphasia intervention. In R. Chapey (ed.) *Language Intervention Strategies in Aphasia and Related Neurogenic Communication Disorders* (pp. 246–268). Baltimore, MD: Lippincott Williams and Wilkins.

Ulatowska, H.K., Doyel, A.W., Stern, R.F. and Haynes, S.M. (1983) Production of procedural discourse in aphasia. *Brain and Language* 18, 315–341.

Appendix A: Three samples of the conversations between the clinician and the Broca's aphasic participants

Conversation 1: 'The weekend'

1. Clinician: *qué hizo el fin de semana … el sábado, qué hizo?*
   what did you do during the weekend … Saturday, what did you do?

2. Olga: *sábado … bajal … combral fruta y … todo a compral.*
   Saturday … go down … buy fruit and … everything buy.

3. Clinician: *qué fruta compró?*
   what fruit did you buy?

4. Olga: **kesoña, lesocha, esoya, nelosia**
   (phonological paraphasias. Possible target *lechosa* 'papaya').

5. Clinician: *era grande?*
   was it big?

6. Olga: *grande*
   big one

7. Clinician: *era cara?*
   was it expensive?

8. Olga: *no, ocho.*
   no, eight.

9. Clinician: *qué mas compró?*
   what else did you buy?

10. Olga: *todo compral: **parro, bárrago** ... compré ... no acuerda*
               everything buy (phonological paraphasias; possible target
               pargo 'Porgy') I bought ... not remember
11. Clinician: *cómo lo prepararon?*
               how did you (plural) prepare it?
12. Olga: *freito, hija*
               fried (paraphasia), darling.
13. Clinician: *y usted, que hizo?*
               and you (singular), what did you do?
14. Olga: *ayudar.*
               to help.
15. Clinician: *con qué lo prepararon?*
               what did you prepare it with?
16. Olga: *arroz.*
               rice

Conversation 2: 'My previous job'

1. Clinician: *qué hacía usted antes de enfermarse?*
              what did you do before your illness?
2. Argen: *era promero*
              [I] was plumber
3. Clinician: *y ... trabajaba a domicilio, o en algún sitio?*
              and ... did you work independently or in a specific
              place?
4. Argen: *no, ninguno, por negocio, eh:: como. como. vamos a decir eh::
              habitacionar, ve? este:: en **contusión**.*
              no, neither one, for profit, eh:: how. how. let's say eh:: to
              inhabit, you see? eh:: in contution (construction)
5. Clinician: *qué es eso?*
              what is that?
6. Argen: *bueno ... habitacionar, en **contusión**, o sea. cómo es que se
              llama? la: bueno ... yo tabajo en **contusión**, ve?*
              well ... to inhabit, in contusion, that means. how do you
              call it? the: well ... I work in contusion, you see?
7. Clinician: *pero, qué es la **contusión**, es un término de plomería?*
              but, what is 'contution', a plumbing term?
8. Argen: *ajá, bueno, todo la. la. cómo es qué es? ... la **contusión** es
              fablical edificio, entiende?*
              uhu, okay, all the. the. how is it? ... contution is to
              fablicate buildings, you see?

Conversation 3: 'My favorite saint'

1. Clinician: *tú eres religiosa?*
       are you a religious person?
2. Cari: *y es ... religiosa*
       and is ... religious
3. Clinician: *qué religión?*
       what religion?
4. Cari: *le católica*
       the catholic
5. Clinician: *católica?*
       Catholic?
6. Cari: *si*
       yes
7. Clinician: *practicante?*
       (are you a) practicing (Catholic)?
8. Cari: *si*
       yes
9. Clinician: *así, todos los domingos?*
       like that, every Sunday?
10. Cari: *no: no: ... **teo comingo** no.*
       no: no: ... on Cunday no.
       [all participants laugh]
11. Clinician: *no.*
       no.
12. Cari: *no: ... yo bue- eh- eh- **mi ii sie moenti**..*
       no: ... I we- eh- eh- me and sie moenti. (paraphasia)
13. Hermana: *ella va cuando puede.*
       Sister: she goes whenever she can
14. Cari: *cuando puedo ... eh pone la ...*
       when I can ... eh puts the ...
15. Hermana: *una velita al ... al San Judas ...*
       Sister: a candle to the ... to Saint Judas ...
16. Clinician: *ajá, velita.*
       uhu, candle.
17. Cari: *si, velita un ... un ...*
       yes, candle a ... a ...
18. Clinician: *lo haces*
       you do that
19. Cari: *esa ... tamente.*
       Exact ... ly.
20. Clinician: *ajá ... mira, y cuál es tu santo, tu santo ...*
       uh ... say, and which one is your saint, your saint ...

21. Cari: *preferido.*
             favorite.
22. Clinician: *cuál es?*
                 which one?
23. Cari: *si, San Judas Tadeo.*
            yes, Saint Judas Tadeus.
24. Clinician: *porqué? qué ... cuéntame de San Judas, quién era él?*
                 why is that? what ... tell me about Saint Judas, who was
                 he?
25. Cari: *hombre caramba!*
            On boy!

Key to transcription conventions
.   falling intonation at the end of declarative sentence
?   rising intonation
,   continuing intonation
...   noticeable pause
:   lengthened syllable
boldface used to highlight paraphasias

Appendix B: Example of the calculation of analysis and cohesion indices based on Conversation 2

Turn	Speaker	Number of ties	Type and sequence of ties
1	NA	0	
2	A	1	1 Ellipsis
3	NA	4	1 Conjunction 1 Lexical 1 Conjunction 1 Ellipsis
4	A	4	4 Ellipsis
5	NA	1	1 Reference
6	A	5	2 Lexical 1 Ellipsis 2 Lexical
7	NA	2	2 Lexical
8	A	5	1 Ellipsis 3 Lexical 1 Ellipsis

A, aphasic speaker; NA, nonaphasic speaker

Calculation of indices:

Number of turns: 8-1 = 7. In every conversation, the opening turn is not connected to a previous one, so the index is calculated on the basis of the total number of turns minus one.

Number of turns by aphasic speaker: 4

Number of turns by nonaphasic speaker: 3

Total of ties in conversation = 22

Global Conversational Cohesion Index: 22/7 = 3.14 (Total ties/Total turns)

Aphasic Conversational Cohesion Index: 15/4 = 3.75 (Ties per speaker/turns per speaker)

Nonaphasic Conversational Cohesion Index: 7/3 = 2.3 (Ties per speaker/turns per speaker)

Chapter 16

Language Switching in the Context of Spanish–English Bilingual Aphasia

ANA INÉS ANSALDO and KARINE MARCOTTE

Bilingual individuals frequently switch between languages and mix elements of the two languages they speak. In fact, the ability to switch and mix between languages is a trademark of proficient bilinguals (see Centeno, ch. 3, this volume). The study of language switching (LS) and language mixing (LM) in non-brain-damaged and brain-damaged populations has been the focus of interest in a wide variety of disciplines. One of the reasons for this interest, particularly in linguistics, speech-language pathology, and psychology, is that the study of LM and LS provides information regarding the possible ways two or more languages are represented and processed in the mind of bilingual speakers.

Brain damage can impair the mechanisms that allow the appropriate use of LM and LS. Curiously, it is rare that appropriate language choice breaks down in aphasia that is due to frank lesions; rather, one sometimes sees problems with language selection in the aphasia resulting from Alzheimer's dementia (Obler *et al.*, 1995). Nonetheless, there are circumstances in which non-Alzheimer's aphasic bilinguals may show inappropriate mixing of languages, such as during episodes of *anomia* (word-finding limitations) in which the aphasic bilingual may use the wrong language when searching for the target lexical item (Obler *et al.*, 1995). Given that more than half of the world is multilingual (Fabbro, 2001), bilingual and polyglot aphasia can be considered frequent conditions. Hence, studying impaired LS profiles constitutes an important aspect in bilingual aphasiology.

The purpose of this chapter is to discuss LM and LS in the context of aphasia and its intervention. The first part of the chapter will discuss the general principles of normal LM and LS to provide a theoretical framework for the description of LM and LS following aphasia. An overview of clinical case reports on pathological LM and LS will follow. In addition, we will discuss the case of EL, a Spanish–English bilingual man who presented impaired LM and LS secondary to aphasia. Finally, the assessment and therapy designed to overcome pathological LM and LS will be described.

Language Mixing and Language Switching: Two Distinct Phenomena

Although they are sometimes used interchangeably, LM and LS actually correspond to different expressive behaviors. There is a general agreement that LM consists of the importation of linguistic units from one language into a sentence or a sequence of sentences (e.g. narrative discourse or conversation) produced in another language (Fabbro, 2001). In LM, phonemes, morphemes, words, modifiers, and clauses from one language (e.g. L2) are imported into a sentence or discourse uttered in a different language (e.g. L1). In other words, LM is intrasentential, and may occur at the phonological, morphological, lexical, or syntactic level (see Centeno, ch. 3, in this volume for further discussion).

Language mixing needs to be distinguished from borrowing. In borrowing, the imported lexical item is assimilated into the phonological and morphological processes of the matrix language, which gives the sentence its structural properties (e.g. I threw the *basura* into the basket, where *basura* 'rubbish' is the borrowed item, and English is the matrix language). Nouns are more easily borrowed than verbs, followed by derivational morphological material and inflectional material, with syntactic structures the least likely to be borrowed (Romaine, 1989). According to Fabbro (1999), LM respects a series of rules: (1) the subject (if it is a pronoun) and predicate (verb) of a sentence belong to the same language; (2) prepositions and function words are rarely expressed in a language other than the matrix language; and (3) function words are generally produced in the mother tongue. Phonology can also be borrowed; more specifically, the embedded item may be pronounced in accordance with the phonotactic rules dictating permissible phoneme combinations of the matrix language.

In contrast to LM, LS is the alternation between languages across clause boundaries, and at points where juxtaposition of the two languages does not violate a syntactic rule in either one. Some authors (e.g. Poplack, 1979) consider that LS occurs only at points where the surface structures of both languages map onto each other. Sridhar (1978) argues that the internal structure of the guest language (*embedded language*) need not conform to that of the host language (*matrix language*), as long as the placement of the host sentence obeys the rules of the host language. This concept is known as the *dual structure principle* (Sridhar, 1978), and has been systematically verified among bilingual populations (e.g. *Quiero agua por favor; I am thirsty.* 'I want water please; I'm thirsty').

Language switching is constrained by both linguistic and pragmatic factors. The former concern the formal and functional constraints imposed by the structural features of either language as well as lexical availability and the speaker's proficiency in L1 and L2, whereas pragmatic factors relate to the contextual demands of the communicative event. For example, bilinguals may use LS to specify the addressee of a message, to relate to a particular topic, to convey a meaning above and beyond the explicit message, or to express a social role. Compliance with these linguistic and pragmatic constraints is, in turn, modulated by the requirements of effective and economical communication. In this regard, LS demands the on-line actualization of cognitive abilities that relate to *planning and strategy*.

A Model of Language-Switching Control in Bilinguals

Control of LS is a major issue for bilinguals (Green, 1986). This communicative ability relates to pragmatic aspects of communication, and reflects bilingual proficiency, as mentioned earlier. In order to account for normal and pathological LS, different approaches can be used. Among them, the *lesion approach* examines the impact of brain damage on LS, whereas the *cognitive approach* describes LS in terms of *processing devices* representing computational operations or requirements. More recently, the *neurocognitive approach* states how the processing devices map onto the corresponding *neuroanatomical networks* (Green, 2005).

Green (1986) proposed a cognitive model of LS control in bilinguals. According to this model, the outputs from the bilingual lexicosemantic system are controlled by two types of devices: those representing the linguistic units, at the semantic, syntactical, phonological, and morphological levels (i.e. bilingual lexicosemantic system), and those involved in the control of the output. In non-brain-damaged bilinguals, this subtle balance depends upon proficiency in either language and is modulated by pragmatic factors. According to Green's model (1986; 1998a,b), the schemas for word production in L1 and L2 are in permanent competition (Figure 16.1). Consequently, naming in L1 requires the activation of the target word in L1 (English: *apple*), together with the inhibition of its

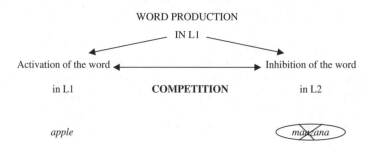

Figure 16.1 A simplified model of language switching in bilinguals (based on Green, 1986)

equivalent in L2 (Spanish: *manzana*). Moreover, during LS, the previously activated schema has to be inhibited (L1), whereas the formerly inhibited schema (L2) needs to be activated. Those competitive costs in LS may be asymmetrical, depending upon the level of proficiency in both languages. Accordingly, the more proficient language is inhibited less easily than the less proficient one.

Following brain damage, the control of the bilingual system may be affected, as a result of a *reduction in the cognitive resources* available. Particularly, a lesion involving frontal and subcortical circuits that allow for the control of the bilingual system may lead to impairment in a variety of language tasks (Price *et al.*, 1999). In this regard, the inhibition and control model proposed by Green (1986; 1998a,b) constitutes a suitable framework to examine the cognitive mechanisms underlying LM and LS and accounts for both normal and impaired LM and LS in bilingual populations.

Neuroimaging Studies of Language Switching

The search for a language switch has proceeded not only by means of behavioral studies, but also through the examination of neuroanatomical structures related to LS. Using neuroimaging techniques, researchers have examined brain activations associated with the alternation between languages in a wide variety of tasks. Studies with positron emission tomography (PET), evoked related potentials (ERP), and functional magnetic resonance imaging (fMRI) have provided mixed evidence about the cost of LS and how it affects performance in healthy bilingual adults. A number of factors, such as age (Hernández & Kohnert, 1999), task demands (Price *et al.*, 1999), and sociolinguistic factors (Fabbro, 2001; Muñoz *et al.*, 1999), may have an impact on the bilingual's ability to switch between languages.

The impact of age on the capacity to switch between languages has been explored (e.g. Hernández & Kohnert, 1999; Hernández *et al.*, 2001). Using a wide variety of experimental tasks (e.g. cued picture naming with mixed and blocked conditions, lexical decision, repetition and translation), LS was compared in different populations: 65-year-old and older bilinguals and college-age bilinguals (Hernández & Kohnert, 1999) and across 5–20-year-old participants (Hernández *et al.*, 2001). Results of these series of studies revealed that LS processing costs of interference are high in young children, remain stable between the ages of 18 and 50, and decrease after age 65, concurrently with the *rise and fall theory* of the frontal lobes (Cerella & Hale, 1994). According to this theory, rate of information processing changes during the lifespan: it rises during infancy, remains stable at the adult-age and decreases after 50 years old, particularly with regards to executive functions and working memory.

Moreover, and specifically with regard to the neural basis of LS abilities during naming, Hernández *et al.* (2001) reported an increased activation in the dorsolateral prefrontal cortex in both cerebral hemispheres in young English–Spanish bilinguals. Interestingly, this region has been found to be active in nonverbal task switching (Meyer *et al.*, 1997), which suggests that LS is not a language-specific ability, but depends upon *general executive functioning*.

Another factor that has been shown to modulate LS costs is task demands. Price *et al.* (1999) found different activation patterns during LS, depending on the type of experimental task used. Specifically, using an oral translation task during silent reading, the authors found an increased activation in the neural regions associated with articulation: the insula, the cerebellum, and the supplementary motor area. They argued that this increased activation resulted from the fact that oral translation during silent reading specifically requires the inhibition of the articulatory output activated by the orthographic information from the written stimuli. Conversely, covert LS in L2 during silent reading in L1 resulted in an increased activation in Broca's area, and in the supramarginal gyrus, bilaterally. Price *et al.* (1999) interpreted these findings as evidence that switching modulates word processing at the phonological level.

Yet, in none of the above cases did Price *et al.* (1999) find increased activation of the dorsolateral prefrontal cortex, as reported by Hernández and Kohnert (1999). Hernández *et al.* (2001) argue that the apparent discrepancy between their results (Hernández & Kohnert, 1999) and those reported by Price *et al.* (1999) stems from: (1) the different load on executive function demands with either task (i.e. a naming task in the Hernández *et al.* (2001) study, and a translation task in the Price *et al.* (1999) study); (2) the different types of instructions used, and (3) the different timing parameters in the two fMRI studies.

In summary, the evidence from neuroimaging studies of LS in normal bilinguals suggests that switching depends upon a non-language-specific ability related to executive functions. The neural structures that show increased activation during switching vary depending on the tasks performed: switching languages within a naming task is associated with an increased activation in the dorsolateral prefrontal cortex in both cerebral hemispheres (Hernández *et al.*, 2001), whereas increased activation associated with translation varies depending on the type of information to be inhibited during the task (Price *et al.*, 1999). The fact that switching costs have been shown to be related to age (Hernández *et al.*, 2001) and task demands (Price *et al.*, 1999) is in line with the *executive function hypothesis*, given that the processing load on the executive function increases with age (Hasher & Zacks, 1988; Zacks & Hasher, 1997), and is also known to vary depending upon task demands (Hernández *et al.*, 2001). Executive function impairment can result from brain damage, as well. Thus, lesions involving the frontal-subcortical circuits (e.g. pallidum, corona radiata, or centrum semiovale) lead to executive dysfunction (Vataja *et al.*, 2003). Accordingly, bilingual aphasia resulting from lesions in these regions should impair LS.

The next section presents a case report of a bilingual speaker with aphasia resulting from a subcortical lesion, who presented pathological LM and LS. The participant was assessed with a series of tests requiring both lexical access and abilities, and his performance was analyzed within the framework of the *inhibitory control model* (Green, 1998b). The results of the assessment guided the choice of intervention strategies, which resulted in an improvement in the patient's communication abilities.

Case Report

Participant description

EL, a 56-year-old Spanish–English bilingual man, suffered a left subcortical perisylvian embolic lesion in the internal capsule (Ruíz & Ansaldo, 1990). The patient presented with transcortical motor aphasia characterized by word-retrieval deficits, agrammatism, and LM (see the section on clinical assessment, below, for further details). EL had no previous history of neurological disease. He was right-handed and Spanish was his native language.

EL had learned English during childhood. He completed his primary and secondary school in a bilingual school in Buenos Aires, Argentina. He later moved to the USA for his college education, and returned to Argentina after completing his degree. He considered himself to be bilingual, and was equally at ease in Spanish and English, according to his and his relatives' reports. However, his family reported that EL's communication style before the stroke did not include LM or LS. He used Spanish both at work and at home, although he would read books and newspapers, and watch films in English. At the time of the stroke, EL had only been speaking Spanish in his daily routines for more than ten years.

Clinical assessment

Language assessment with the original English version and a Spanish adaptation of the *Western Aphasia Battery* (Kertesz, 1982) was conducted by two monolingual speech-language pathologists (SLPs) in separate sessions, one month after the stroke. The assessment revealed a transcortical motor aphasia in both languages, although scores were slightly better in Spanish than in English. The aphasia profile in both languages was characterized by functional oral language comprehension, agrammatic oral expression, and severe anomia. Further, EL would frequently mix languages within a single utterance, and could not avoid using LM and LS, even when he was speaking to a monolingual partner.

Two months after the stroke, EL showed some recovery. The pattern of recovery was consistent with *parallel deficits* (Paradis, 2004); thus, Spanish and English recovered at the same time and to the same extent. Spanish remained the stronger language. At the sentence level, EL would produce a larger number of syntactically correct sentences, but would still substitute or omit grammatical words on spontaneous speech. Anomia was characterized by a difficulty in accessing the phonological information corresponding to the target word in either language. Hence, EL could easily access the semantic information corresponding to the target word, but had difficulty retrieving the sequence of sounds that corresponded to the spoken form of the same target. When attempting to name items, he would, thus, exhibit a great deal of effort and produce phonemic paraphasias. Additionally, EL presented mild apraxia of speech, and, in turn, showed a deficit in programming the sequence of movements corresponding to the phonemic or syllabic structure of the target lexical item.

The most striking features in EL's oral expression – and the focus of this chapter – were *pathological LM and LS* in the context of conversation and picture description. Hence, two months after the stroke EL's oral expression still was characterized by LM phenomena. He would frequently produce English words in the context of a sentence in Spanish, even when he knew that his communication partner was a monolingual Spanish speaker; a behavior that seemed strategically compensatory as EL appeared to be relying on his most available expressive resources. The following examples (1–5) include utterances produced during conversation and picture description tasks with a monolingual Spanish-speaking SLP. In the transcription, ellipses stand for pauses and italicized words stand for English. The possible target follows the example, and is given in both Spanish and English.

1. El niño ... se cayó y ... rompió la ... mb ... be ... *fishbowl.*
   El niño se cayó y rompió la pecera 'The boy fell down and broke the fishbowl.'
2. No vine porque estaba m ... a ... b ... a *ill*, con un eh ... eh *headache.*
   No vine porque estaba enfermo, con dolor de cabeza 'I did not come because I was ill, with a headache.'
3. ... y la *mother* le dijo *come here*, m'hijito.
   ... y la madre dijo: Venga aqui, m'hijito '... and the mother said: come here my boy.'
4. No quiero ... *speakear*[1] Inglés.
   No quiero hablar Inglés 'I don't want to speak English.'
5. Iba corriendo y se *fall*ió.[2]
   Iba corriendo y se cayó 'He was running and he fell down.'

Borrowings from L2 occurred at the word level (Examples 1, 2, and 3), regardless of the grammatical class of the item (nouns, verbs, adjectives, prepositions), or at the morphemic level, by replacing the root of the verb and combining it with a Spanish grammatical morpheme corresponding to the infinitive form of the verb (Examples 4 and 5). Moreover, from additional samples, alternative LS was observed within the context of conversational and narrative discourse (e.g. *Yo estaba en la Universidad estudiando . . . a . . . ba . . . at Berkley University for four years in . . . ach ar . . . arquitectura, and I got married there* 'I was at the University studying . . . at Berkley University for four years in . . . arch . . . architec-architecture, and I got married there').

Interestingly, EL was aware of his LM and LS productions but could not avoid them, even when asked to speak Spanish only. Thus, EL would switch to English while conversing in the waiting room with monolingual Spanish-speaking patients, even when they told him they did not speak English. Attempts to control involuntary LM and LS would result in an exacerbation of anomia and anomia-related signs (i.e. a larger number of gaps, silences as well as groping behaviors). EL underwent additional experimental testing in order to further describe his expressive behaviors, and provide the basis for further model-based intervention.

Experimental assessment

Tasks

EL was assessed on confrontation naming of nouns and verbs, repetition, and translation of the same items from Spanish to English, and from English to Spanish. He also was tested on a picture description task and on story retelling. Stimuli for naming, repetition, and translation were taken from the *Boston Naming Test* (Kaplan *et al.*, 1983) (for nouns and for verbs); for picture description and story retelling, we developed two six-picture stories. The pictures corresponded to the sequence of events in either story. Performance in either language was examined by a monolingual examiner, except for the translation task, which was performed by a bilingual examiner. Spanish was assessed first. There was a three-day interval between assessments in either language, translation being examined at the end of each series of tasks.

The next section presents a summary of the results of the experimental assessment, followed by a description of EL's performance within a model of language-switching control (Green, 1986; 1998a,b).

Results

We calculated the percentage of correct responses, number of LM utterances, and response times for correct answers with the confrontation naming, repetition, and translation tasks, in either language. With the picture description and narrative discourse tasks, we calculated the number of LS utterances.

Oral Picture Naming and Word Repetition Tasks. EL's performance on the repetition tasks was 100% correct in both Spanish and English. With oral picture naming, the pattern was different: specifically in Spanish, nouns were named more easily and faster than verbs, whereas in English, naming verbs was faster and led to fewer errors than for nouns (Figure 16.2).

Overall, these results show a different pattern for naming tasks in each language. Thus, while there was a slight difference between Spanish and English in terms of access to the verb category, the noun category was definitely more impaired in English than in Spanish. This indicates that preserved access to a grammatical category in L1 does not necessarily facilitate access to the same category in L2.

Translation. The results show that translation was better than naming when it corresponded to the less available word category in the given language (Figure 16.3). More specifically, translating nouns into English resulted in a higher score (65%) than naming nouns in English (47.5%). In the same way, translating verbs into Spanish resulted in a higher score (72.5%) than naming verbs in Spanish (60%). In other words, translation would benefit from lexical availability in the other language. Consequently, there was a task effect in both languages, given that the translation task was easier to perform than the naming task.

Picture Description Task. LM and LS were observed with L1 (Spanish) and L2 (English), and across tasks. EL could not help switching even when he was explicitly asked to respond in a specific language, although he was aware of the fact that the examiner was monolingual. Furthermore, switching was generally preceded by a latency, and increased with fatigue.

EL's performance on the picture description task was better in Spanish than in English. More specifically, his discourse in Spanish was fluent,

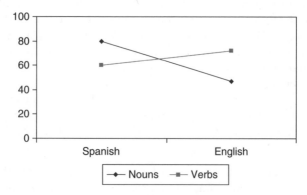

Figure 16.2 Percentage of correct responses on the confrontation naming task

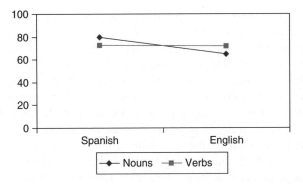

Figure 16.3 Percentage of correct responses in the translation task

with hardly any agrammatic errors, with a few latencies; two borrowings and six LS occurrences were observed. The following utterances (Examples 6 and 7) show LM and LS during picture description in Spanish:

6. Toma el omnibus co ... emp ... *outside* empieza a llover fuerte.
   LM: *He takes the bus ... Outside it is beginning to rain heavily.*

7. Se ponen a correr tras de ... *to the bus stop and they see* otra vez nubes, *clouds.*
   LS: *They start running behind ... to the bus stop and they see again clouds, clouds.*

Picture description in English was agrammatic and less fluent than in Spanish. Anomia was very frequent, and was generally followed by LM and LS. Specifically, we observed six borrowings and eight LS occurrences. The following examples (8–10) illustrate LM and LS during the picture description task in English:

8. The storm is very strong, and ... go ... *van al omnibus y empieza a llover. Después bajan y* they play outside, running and jumping, and suddenly ... *de nuevo hay nubes en el cielo* ... the sky is cloudy.
   LS: *The storm is very strong and ... go ... they go to the bus, and it starts to rain. After that, they get off and they play outside, running and jumping and suddenly ... again there are clouds in the sky ... the sky is cloudy.*

9. They are running behind the ... ba ... *van corriendo el autobus y se apuran porque llueve* ... mucho ... it is raining a lot.
   LS: *They are running behind the ... they are running the bus and they hurry up because it is raining ... a lot ... it is raining a lot.*

10. They are going to school ... or going back ... *a casa* ... I don't really know.
    LM: *They are going to school ... or going back ... home I don't really know.*

Story Retelling Task. Story retelling was better in Spanish than in English, which was probably due to better preserved lexical availability in Spanish (see the results for the naming tasks above). As in the picture description task, LS was more frequent in English than in Spanish, probably because word retrieval in English was more impaired than in Spanish (see results of naming tasks). In other words, difficulty accessing a word in one language would contribute to switching to the other language. EL pointed out that LS was involuntary, as he could not avoid switching even within a monolingual conversational context. Moreover, LS would sometimes be followed by translation back to the previous language. This is evident in Examples 8 and 9, where, in the context of a picture description task in English, EL switches to Spanish, and then translates back to English (Example 8: *de nuevo hay nubes en el cielo* ... the sky is cloudy; Example 9: *llueve ... mucho ... it is raining a lot.*)

Analysis of EL's Performance within a Model of Language-switching Control in Bilinguals

EL's word-finding impairment was observed in the presence of preserved comprehension and occurred very unsystematically. The same word was available at one point and not retrieved some minutes later. Errors were latencies, anomia, phonological substitutions, and phonological approximations of the target. Conversely, EL did not make any semantic substitutions of the target (i.e. semantic paraphasias). This type of word finding problem is generally observed in cases of impairment in the access to phonological information, and is known as *phonological anomia* (Ellis *et al.*, 1994). The word finding problem seemed to interact with difficulties in controlling each language. Thus, EL had difficulties not only in accessing the phonological form of the target word in language A but he was also impaired in suppressing its equivalent in language B. Though appearing to be used as a strategy to overcome anomia, LM and LS seemed to occur involuntarily, even with monolingual communication partners.

Green's (1986) model of control and LS in bilinguals provides a theoretical frame to analyze EL's language impairment. According to this model, EL's communication impairment concerned two levels: the *lexical level* (i.e. anomia), and the L1–L2 *control level* (i.e. involuntary mixing and switching). Thus, EL's language impairment concerned both the devices representing the linguistic units (i.e. phonological information required for the production of nouns and verbs), and those involving language control (e.g. inhibitory resources to prevent involuntary switching to English within a Spanish utterance, or the opposite). For EL, a word retrieval impairment combined with a lack of inhibitory resources determined switching alternatively from one language to the other.

According to Green (1986), in the bilingual language system (Figure 16.4), word output in either language is modulated by (1) the flow of activation and (2) a sufficient amount of inhibitory resources to suppress the language that is not spoken. Moreover, as bilinguals can speak one or the other language, translate into either language, and switch between them, Green proposed a device, *a specifier*, that defines the mode of functioning of the system, if a person is to act in one or the other of these ways.

Selection of L1 is partially a matter of increasing activation in L1, but also requires suppressing the activation of L2. The output in L2 can be suppressed externally (external suppression, represented by an inhibitory link at the stage of L2 phonological assembly), or within the system itself (internal suppression, represented by a loop). Thus, when L1 is spontaneously used, L2 is externally suppressed at the *phonological assembly* level. During LS, there is no need for external suppression, as the output is free, according to which words or syntactic structures reach threshold first. Finally, translation into L1 requires internal suppression, as the speaker has to avoid repeating the word or phrase in L2.

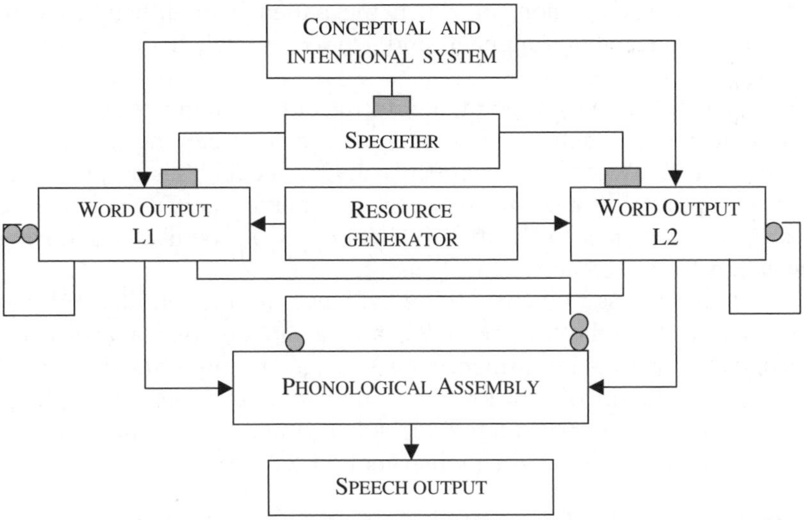

→ flow of activation, ▬ control instructions, ●● adequate inhibitory resources, ● inadequate inhibitory resources

Figure 16.4 A state of the system in the inhibitory control model during alternate language switching, as proposed by Green (1986)

Brain damage seemed to have resulted in insufficient activation flow and inhibitory resources within EL's bilingual system. This imbalance alternatively favored one or the other language. For example, let us suppose that, at a certain point in time, activation flow favors L1 and external suppression of L2 is achieved. EL will, therefore, speak in L1 and L2 will be suppressed. However, consuming resources at a faster rate than they are produced will lead to insufficient activation of L1 items, and lack of inhibitory resources to suppress L2 items; hence, switching to L2 will occur. Figure 16.4 depicts a state of the system in which switching to L2 occurs due to a lack of inhibitory resources. If the rate of *resource generation* continues to be insufficient to replenish resources as they are consumed, L2 will in turn cease to dominate, and the system will flip back to the previous state.

From a neuroanatomical perspective, the fact that EL presented a left subcortical perisylvian lesion is well in line with this pattern of performance. Studies using fMRI with bilinguals have shown that left subcortical lesions impair language control in dual-language users (Abutalebi *et al.*, 2000), and impaired access to lexical representations, such access probably being under the control of frontal-basal-ganglia circuits (Abutalebi *et al.*, 2000). Further, our findings are consistent with Agliotti *et al.* (1996), who reported a case of bilingual aphasia, secondary to a left subcortical lesion, in which the patient had difficulties with maintaining the native language and tended to switch to the second language.

From a behavioral standpoint, the results of EL's language assessment showed that translation was better preserved than naming (see Figure 16.2 and 16.3). According to Green's (1986) model, this implies that internal suppression mechanisms were functioning better that external ones. Moreover, it is likely that availability of L2 equivalents during translation facilitated access to L1 items.

In summary, based on converging evidence from lesion data (Abutalebi *et al.*, 2000; Agliotti *et al.*, 1996) and a model-based analysis (i.e. Green, 1986) of EL's performance, EL's language impairment resulted from a combination of word-retrieval deficits and a lack of language control, as a consequence of left-sided subcortical damage. This rationale provided the basis for language intervention with EL.

A Model-based Intervention Approach for Pathological Language Switching in Bilingual Aphasia

Based on the above analysis, a therapy strategy that could make use of better preserved language abilities (i.e. translation from English to Spanish) to enhance impaired skills (i.e. LS control and word access in L1) was developed. Therapy was provided in Spanish only, as this was the language used by the patient in his everyday life. The patient received one 60-min speech-therapy session per week, over 4 months, with a bilingual Spanish–English SLP. Word finding difficulties and pathological switching were approached simultaneously.

For word finding difficulties, a *Semantic Feature Analysis* (SFA) (Boyle & Coelho, 1995) was applied. SFA stimulates and reinforces the reciprocal links between semantically related words within the semantic network (e.g. chair, couch). In this way, SFA boosts the semantic representations and contributes to the access to word forms. As EL presented phonological anomia, with difficulties in the access to word forms and preserved semantic information, SFA was considered to be a suitable approach to improve his word finding difficulties.

With regards to LM and LS, an approach that we called *Switch-back through Translation* (SBT) was developed. The choice of this approach was made because of EL's better preserved ability to translate in comparison to naming (see behavioral results above), particularly when translating into Spanish (see Figure 16.3). According to Green's model (1986), the fact that translation was better preserved than naming means that EL could make use of *intentional and internal mechanisms* much better than he could do with regards to external suppression ones (see Figure 16.4). Thus, when speaking in L1 spontaneously, L2 is externally suppressed (i.e. inhibitory link to the output of L2) whereas, when translating from L2 to L1, the output of L2 is internally suppressed (i.e. inhibitory loop). Accordingly, by using SBT, the aim was not to inhibit pathological switching but to *transform it into translation*. For this purpose, immediately after the occurrence of pathological LM or LS to English, the SLP cued EL with the Spanish expression *que quiere decir ...* 'which means ... ', using an interrogative accent, as a supplementary prosodic cue. This would cue EL to proceed to translation and, consequently, to return to L1, the language of use in the ongoing conversation.

Initially, the SLP's role was directive, as she directed EL to switch back to Spanish by means of the cue phrase every time pathological LS or LM occurred. Gradually, the SLP replaced the cue phrase by a cue gesture, a movement of the hand indicating that EL should switch back to Spanish. With time elapsed, the SLP's cues were faded out, and EL produced the cue gesture himself. EL gradually achieved on-line translation of English utterances to Spanish hence switching back to the language of discourse. This strategy, combined with anomia therapy, which was carried out in parallel, resulted in an improvement in naming and conversational discourse abilities. Overall, intervention allowed for a *compensatory strategy* in which LM and LS use improved EL's functional communication.

Concluding Remarks

LM and LS are frequent phenomena among bilinguals. As discussed above, these complex and fascinating communication abilities depend on the degree of proficiency in each language and contextual requirements of the communication event. Indeed, smooth LM and LS use call for both efficient language abilities and control resources to achieve optimal communication. Brain damage may have an impact on the balance of this complex system, hence resulting in disordered deployment of LM and LS.

We presented the case of a bilingual individual, EL, who suffered from aphasia, and could no longer control switching between languages. A simultaneous impairment in both control and lexical access caused pathological LM of English words in the context of conversation with monolingual Spanish speakers; the global pattern of language impairment resulting from left subcortical damage. Results from language assessment and a model-based analysis of EL's performance allowed the development of an individualized intervention for pathological LM and LS. Combined with SFA therapy for word-retrieval deficits, this approach led to an overall improvement of functional communication.

These results support the use of theory-based intervention in cases of impaired LM and LS use in aphasic bilinguals. This conceptual approach to therapy highlights plausible theoretical grounds that may optimize communication abilities in bilingual speakers with aphasia, thus allowing SLPs to target the possible impaired processes underlying the observed deficit. Hence, the connections between disrupted linguistic and cognitive mechanisms and their neural substrates exploited by this approach may provide important explanatory grounds in clinical communication. As recently proposed by Green (2005), a neurocognitive approach to linguistic deficits characterizes the language impairment at a cognitive level by specifying possible mappings of cognitive operations onto neuroanatomical networks, hence establishing possible relationships between neurological damage and the observed communication behaviors. Regarding bilingual speakers, our results and clinical observations, although previous to Green's (2005) proposal, support that the integration of clinical data and cognitive analysis of the patient's performance may provide a suitable rationale for aphasia intervention with bilinguals.

Advances in neuroimaging techniques will contribute to enrichment of neurocognitive interpretations of language processing in both monolingual and bilingual contexts. However, in terms of dual-language users, as clearly stated by Paradis (2004), if neuroimaging is to advance our understanding, neuroimaging studies will need to be framed within neurolinguistically informed theories of bilingualism that provide the rationale for the hypotheses to be tested, the tasks that are better suited to assess those hypotheses, and the interpretive approaches applied to the resulting data.

Notes

1. *Speakear* is formed by 'speak', which means *hablar* in Spanish, and the morpheme *-ear*, which corresponds to the first-conjugation verb class in Spanish.
2. *Falliõ* is formed by 'fall', which means *caer* in Spanish, and the morpheme *-iõ*, which corresponds to the simple past tense in Spanish.

References

Abutalebi, J., Miozzo, A. and Cappa, S.F. (2000) Do subcortical structures control language selection in bilinguals? Evidence from pathological language mixing. *Neurocase* 6, 101–106.

Agliotti, S., Beltramello, A., Girardi, F. and Fabbro, F. (1996) Neurolinguistic follow-up study of an unusual pattern of recovery from bilingual subcortical aphasia. *Brain* 119, 1551–1564.

Boyle, M. and Coelho, C.A. (1995) Application of semantic feature analysis as a treatment for aphasic dysnomia. *American Journal of Speech-Language Pathology* 4, 94–98.

Cerella, J. and Hale, S. (1994) The rise and fall in information processing rates over the life-span. *Acta Psychologica* 86, 109–197.

Ellis, A.W., Franklin, S. and Crerar, A. (1994) Cognitive neuropsychology and the remediation of disorders of spoken language. In M.J Riddoch and G.W. Humphreys (eds) *Cognitive Neuropsychology and Cognitive Remediation* (pp. 207–227). London: Lawrence Erlbaum.

Fabbro, F. (1999) *The Neurolinguistics of Bilingualism: An Introduction*. East Sussex, UK: Psychology Press.

Fabbro, F. (2001) The bilingual brain: Cerebral representation of languages. *Brain and Language* 79, 211–222.

Green, D.W. (1986) Control, activation, and resource: A framework and a model for the control of speech in bilinguals. *Brain and Language* 27, 210–223.

Green, D.W. (1998a) Mental control of the bilingual lexico-semantic system. *Bilingualism* 1, 67–81.

Green, D.W. (1998b) Schemas, tags and inhibition. Reply to commentators. *Bilingualism* 1, 100–104.

Green, D.W. (2005) The neurocognition of recovery patterns in bilingual aphasics. In J.F. Kroll and A.M.B. de Groot (eds) *Handbook of Bilingualism: Psycholinguistic Approaches* (pp. 516–530). New York: Oxford University Press.

Hasher, L. and Zacks, R.T. (1988) Working memory, comprehension, and aging: A review and a new view. In G.H. Bower (ed.) *The Psychology of Learning and Motivation* (pp. 193–225). New York: Academic Press.

Hernández, A.E. and Kohnert, K. (1999) Aging and language switching in bilinguals. *Aging, Neuropsychology, and Cognition* 6, 69–83.

Hernández, A.E., Dapretto, M., Mazziotta, J. and Bookheimer, S. (2001) Language switching and language representation in Spanish–English bilinguals: An fMRI study. *Neuroimage* 14, 510–520.

Kaplan, E., Goodglass, H. and Weintraub, S. (1983) *Boston Naming Test*. Philadelphia: Lea and Febiger.

Kertesz, A. (1982) *Western Aphasia Battery.* San Antonio: Psychological Corporation.

Meyer, D.E., Evans, J.F., Lauber, E.J., Rubinstein, J., Gmeindi, L., Junck, L. and Koeppe, R.A. (1997) Activation of brain mechanisms for executive mental processes in cognitive task switching. Poster presented at the meeting of the Cognitive Neuroscience Society, Boston, MA.

Muñoz, M.L., Marquardt, T.P. and Copeland, G. (1999) A comparison of the code-switching patterns of aphasic and neurologically normal bilingual speakers of English and Spanish. *Brain and Language* 66, 249–274.

Obler, L.K., Centeno, J. and Eng, N. (1995) Bilingual and polyglot aphasia. In L. Menn, M. O'Connor, L.K. Obler and A. Holland (eds) *Non-fluent Aphasia in a Multilingual World* (pp. 132–143). Amsterdam: John Benjamins.

Paradis, M. (2004) *A Neurolinguistic Theory of Bilingualism.* Amsterdam: John Benjamins.

Poplack, S. (1979) Sobre la elisión y la ambigüedad en el español puertorriqueño: El caso de la (n) verbal. *Boletín de la Academia Puertorriqueña de la Lengua Española* 7, 129–143.

Price C.J., Green D.W. and Von Studnitz, R. (1999) A functional imaging study of translation and language switching. *Brain* 122, 2221–2235.

Romaine, S. (1989) *Bilingualism.* Oxford: Basil Blackwell.

Ruíz, A. and Ansaldo, A.I. (1990) Specific anomia for one language: A cause for language mixing. *Journal of Clinical and Experimental Neuropsychology* 12, 373–426.

Sridhar, S.N. (1978) On the functions of code-mixing in Kannada. *International Journal of Sociology of Language* 16, 109–117.

Vataja, R., Pohjasvaara, T., Mäntylä, R., Ylikoski, R., Leppävuori, A., Leskelä, M., Kalska, H., Hietanen, M., Aronen, H.J., Salonen O., Kaste, M. and Erkinjuntti, T. (2003) MRI correlates of executive dysfunction in patients with ischaemic stroke. *European Journal of Neurology* 10, 625–631.

Zacks, R. and Hasher, L. (1997) Cognitive gerontology and attentional inhibition: A reply to Burke and McDowd. *Journal of Gerontology: Psychological Sciences* 52B, 274–283.

Chapter 17
Description and Detection of Acquired Dyslexia and Dysgraphia in Spanish

I. CAROLINA IRIBARREN

Developmental dyslexia has been defined as difficulty in learning to read in spite of adequate intelligence, instruction, and sociocultural environment. Acquired dyslexia, on the other hand, refers to reading loss or deterioration due to brain injury. The corresponding deficits in writing are called dysgraphia. Psycholinguistic studies concerning the breakdown patterns of reading and writing disorders point towards the existence of different subtypes of dyslexia and dysgraphia. Following the works of Marshall and Newcombe (1966, 1973) and Beauvois and Dérouesné (1979), at least three types of central dyslexias have been identified: *deep dyslexia*, *surface dyslexia*, and *phonological dyslexia*. These syndromes stand for the description of reading difficulties ranging from problems accessing the pronunciation of a word from its graphic representation to problems of accessing the meaning of a word from its written form. Corresponding breakdown patterns have been described for writing (Beauvois & Dérouesné, 1981; Bub & Kertesz, 1982; Hatfield, 1985; Shallice, 1981; also see Ijalba & Obler, ch. 18; Weekes, ch. 7, this volume).

Based on observations of this pathological behavior, *dual-route models* of reading and writing with different degrees of complexity and specificity have been proposed by several authors (Lecours, 1996; Monsell *et al.*, 1992; Morton & Patterson, 1987). These models permit explanation of the differential behavior of patients that show understanding of written words but are incapable of reading them aloud correctly, or patients that can read aloud correctly a list of words but show confusion in understanding the meaning of the same words. According to these models, readers and writers have at least two possible activation systems at their disposal that they can use according to their needs, task demands, skills, and quality of the input. This activation can be directed through two main routes: a *lexical route* leading to the direct access to meaning or graphic representation from the whole visual or acoustic image of the word, and a *sublexical route*, which requires the segmentation of the word into its corresponding grapheme–phoneme

231

units with their posterior assemblage. In other words, the word can be processed as a whole (as a lexical unit) or as units smaller than the word (a sublexical unit).

However, a common criticism about these types of models and explanations is that they have been developed mainly for reading and writing in English and French, with their particular orthographies and do not consider other kind of orthographies (Ardila, 1991; Ardila *et al.*, 1989) or writing systems (Karanth, 2003). Accordingly, differential dyslexic and dysgraphic patterns, as well as access to the different routes when reading and writing, are fostered by the fact that the English and French orthographies are *deep* – that is, the grapheme–phoneme correspondence in these languages is not regular – and this necessarily requires the development of both routes in the first place. At the same time, *superficial* orthographies, presumably like that of Spanish – that is, orthographies where the grapheme–phoneme correspondence is regular – or completely deep orthographies, like that of Chinese, do not require that readers or writers develop both routes, and, hence, differential dyslexic and dysgraphic patterns should not be observed or are not pertinent.

The orthographic structure of a language plays an important role in its acquisition, practice, and breakdown patterns. In this chapter, the aim is to show that, in the description and diagnosis of acquired dyslexia and dysgraphia in Spanish, the orthographic structure of the language must indeed be taken into account. Yet, two factors warrant attention in Spanish. First, the conception of Spanish orthography has to be interpreted in alternative ways, and, second, the cognitive operations developed by readers and writers of Spanish are the same as that of readers and writers of other languages. That is, as it will be argued in this chapter, the reading and writing models proposed for other languages are universal, and, hence, although certain orthographies may favor one or the other route, normal readers *even for nonalphabetic writing systems* develop both options and, in turn, the same breakdown patterns described for other orthographies can be observed in Spanish speakers. In a sense, as discussed later in this chapter, we can refer to a certain *universality of reading and writing processes*. In this chapter, it is claimed that the problem of the description and detection of acquired dyslexias and dysgraphias in Spanish is related more to the assumptions and methodologies in evaluating the reading and writing deficits of patients than to the orthographic structure of the language *per se*. Understanding the different factors that interact in normal and pathological reading and writing in different languages would lead to better research and clinical practices.

The Orthographic Structure of Spanish

The Orthographic Depth Hypothesis (ODH)

The standard argument of the ODH claims that, among orthographies, there are differences with respect to the unit of graphemic representation and that these are the result of morphological and graphological characteristics of each language. In turn, such graphemic differences have consequences on the strategies used by readers and writers when accessing the meaning or pronunciation of a written word (Katz & Frost, 1992). It is assumed that superficial orthographies (also called *transparent* or *regular*) support a word recognition process mediated by the phonology of the language while, in contrast, deep orthographies (also referred to as *opaque* or *irregular*) force the reader to resort somehow to his/her morphological and lexical knowledge to recognize the written word globally. A number of authors refer to Spanish orthography as transparent (Coulmas, 1990; Sampson, 1989), as it operates on a level close to the phonetic surface structure that reflects phonemic distinctions of the language.

However, most experimental studies carried out with different languages to examine the ODH have given conflicting and unpredicted results (Katz & Frost, 1992). For instance, comparisons of lexical and priming effects in Farsi, Spanish, Dutch, Italian, and Serbo-Croatian revealed that the psychological operations carried out by readers of these languages have many more things in common with that of readers of opaque orthographies than previously thought (Besner & Smith, 1992). In contrast to the ODH, these findings support that there is nothing in any orthography that can prevent a healthy brain from developing the associations between the semantic and orthographic patterns when the grapheme–phoneme correspondence is regular.

Spanish orthography

Comparatively, Spanish orthography is far more regular than that of English and French. Rules of grapheme–phoneme correspondence to read Spanish are almost one-to-one. There are very few exceptions: letters, such as < c >, < x >, < y >, and < r >, can take different phonological values depending on specific contexts, and some letters are not pronounced, such as < h > and other letters in digraphs like the < u > in < qu > or < gu >. In lexical borrowings, some letters may take different phonological values than those proper of Spanish (e.g. *ballet* read as /ba'le/ and not as /ba'ʎe/ or *home run* read as /hom'ron/ and not as /ome'run/) (Iribarren, 2005). Sampson (1989) points out that among modern European languages, Spanish is the only one that scrupulously marks the stress pattern of the words with a diacritic accent mark. The accent mark is used when the stress falls in a syllable that does not correspond to the unmarked stress pattern of Spanish. Except in the case of verbs, this information must be provided in the lexicon (Harris, 1983). Because the use of phonological segmentation is not always a reliable strategy to mark the stress of a word properly, this type of information must be learned by the reader and must become part of the information of his/her mental lexicon in order to read and write a word correctly.

On the other hand, the rules of phoneme–grapheme correspondence for writing are not so straightforward and require a good *orthographic memory*. Particularly confusing are the writing of the phonemes /b/, /x/, and /s/, which can be written as < b > or < v >, < j > or < g >, and < s >, < c >, or < z > respectively, depending on the lexical or morphological context. These phonemes are found in highly frequent words. Also, the writing of the letter < h > is problematic, as it does not possess any phonological value (Justicia *et al.*, 1999; Valle Arroyo, 1984). But these are not the only phonemes with more than one graphemic representation (see Iribarren, 2005). The marking of the diacritic accent is also a source of difficulty for writing Spanish (Gutiérrez *et al.*, 2001).

Since 1726, the orthographic rules of Spanish have been dictated by the Spanish Royal Academy (Real Academia Española, RAE) which has ensured the preservation of a common *grapholect* among Spanish-speaking countries and communities in the world. Considering the great dialectal variations and some historic phonological changes, the RAE opted for an intermediate policy to determine the adoption of orthographic rules. Visual morphological identity is maintained by the choice of some graphemes over other phonologically equivalent ones (e.g. < b > and < v >). Yet, it is not quite true that we write as we speak (Iribarren, 2005). The same graphemes can be read according to the dialect of the reader and, in order to read and write adequately, the correct orthographic rules as well as lexical and morphological information must be learned (see Anderson & Centeno, ch. 1, this volume for further discussion on Spanish dialects). Neither a simple phonological transcription nor a pronunciation by segmental units alone will give satisfactory results. These facts have consequences for the acquisition, practice, and breakdown patterns of reading and writing Spanish.

Dyslexias in Spanish

Surface dyslexia

The central symptom of surface dyslexia is the production of *regularization errors*; that is, the patient will give an irregularly spelled word an incorrect but phonologically possible reading (e.g. the word *bough* read as /boʊf/) (also see Weekes, ch. 7, in this volume). Usually comprehension depends on oral production; therefore, if the word is pronounced incorrectly, the patient will misunderstand it. The confusion caused by reading heterographic homophonic words (e.g. *piece–peace*, *nose–knows*) is another of the symptoms associated with surface dyslexia. Legal nonwords (a string of letters that resemble a real word but do not belong to the lexicon of the language) are read correctly and usually lexical effects (e.g. frequency, word category, imageability, and word length) are not observed. This behavior is interpreted as reading by the sublexical route due to impairment of the lexical route (Patterson *et al.*, 1985).

The diagnosis of this syndrome in Spanish can be problematic due to the highly regular grapheme-to-phoneme correspondence. However, with the proper design of testing methods adapted to the orthographic characteristics of Spanish, a case of surface dyslexia has been documented (Iribarren *et al.*, 1996). Based on the highly lexicalized stress pattern of words, a test was constructed to test production of regularization errors. The reading of heterographic homophonic words was examined as well as the reading aloud of different word categories. Patient IT was a 67-year-old, right-handed, monolingual Spanish-speaking, retired medical doctor who suffered a CVA in the left hemisphere. At the time of examination his speech was fluent but anomic. IT was able to correctly read 148 real words controlled for grammatical category, frequency, length, and imageability. He read 20 legal nonwords without mistakes. He was also shown a list of 30 words, controlled for frequency, syllable stress place, and length, with graphic stress markings erased. IT made 12 stress pattern regularization mistakes. For example, the target word *corazon* (without accent) was read incorrectly as **corázon* /ko'rason/ instead of *corazón* /kora'son/ 'heart'; *aqui* (without accent) was read as **áqui* /'aki/ instead of *aquí* /a'ki/ 'here'. From a pair of homophonic words, IT was asked to underline the correct word for a given sentence read aloud to him. In a first trial he answered only 46% correctly; in a second trial, six months later, he was able to get 65% of the responses correct. In a multiple choice reading comprehension test ($n = 20$), IT gave 95% correct responses, but in order to answer he vocalized the choices to himself several times. IT was diagnosed as a surface dyslexic. The high regularity of the Spanish orthography permitted him to read most kinds of words aloud without mistakes. However, his regularization mistakes with lexical accented words and confusion with homophonous words permitted us to diagnose his reading problem.

In order to detect surface dyslexia in Spanish, given the characteristics of the orthographic system, it is necessary to design tests to check understanding of written words and see whether the patient produces regularization mistakes. Discrimination of heterographic homophonous words and reading of words with erased accent might be two useful tasks for this purpose.

Deep dyslexia

In general, the reading skills of deep dyslexics are very poor for all kinds of words. However, the central symptom of deep dyslexia is that the patient has the tendency to make a type of error called *semantic paralexias*; that is, they substitute the target word with a synonym or a circumlocution (e.g. instead of reading *motor* the patient reads *car* or *in the garage*) (also see Weekes, ch. 7, this volume). Morphological errors are very common (e.g. *direct* instead of *direction*). They commit visual errors (e.g. *sword* instead of *word*). Word category effects are observed (frequency, length, grammatical category, and imageability), hence affecting reading of certain kinds of words more than others. The reading of nonwords poses a great problem to these patients, and, sometimes, they substitute them with visually similar real words; thus making *lexicalization errors* (e.g. the nonword *fonce* read as *force*) (Barry & Richardson, 1988; Coltheart, 1987; Coltheart *et al.*, 1987). The type of mistakes, that is, the dominance of semantic confusions and substitutions, the effect that different classes of words have on the reading performance of these patients, the inability to read legal non-words, and less than adequate general reading abilities can be considered as the typical symptoms of deep dyslexia. The explanation of this syndrome is controversial. However, there seems to be certain agreement that, to some extent, these patients tend to rely more on their somehow preserved lexical strategy and that their sublexical reading strategy is seriously compromised (e.g. Coltheart *et al.*, 1987; Lecours, 1996).

Ruíz *et al.* (1994) published the first two cases of deep dyslexia in Spanish. For example, patient ON read *terraza* 'terrace' instead of *balcón* 'balcony', *francés* 'French' instead of *italiano* 'Italian', and *pasar* 'to pass' instead of *seguir* 'proceed'. Patient MG read *pibe* 'kid' (in the Argentinean Spanish dialect) in place of *niño* 'child', *Ernesto* for *Oswaldo*, and *ser* 'to be' instead of *existir* 'to exist'. Both patients made morphological errors when reading. For example, ON read *violines* 'violins' instead of *violinista* 'violinist', and MG read *está* 'he/she is' for *estaba* 'he/she was'. Neither patient was able to read phonologically legitimate nonwords. Ferreres and Miravalles (1995) present another case of deep dyslexia in Spanish. This patient shows word category effects and 56% of his mistakes were semantic substitutions. For example, he read *cultura* 'culture' for *estatua* 'statue', *fuerza* 'force' for *gimnasia* 'gymnastics', and *chequera* 'checkbook' for *banco* 'bank'. He was unable to read nonwords. In another case reported by Iribarren (1996), a monolingual Spanish-speaking patient, when reading words aloud, showed word class, length, and frequency effects. He was unable to read nonwords, and he produced numerous circumlocutions when reading words (e.g. *representación* 'representation' read as *otro por mí* 'some one else in my place', and *humanidad* 'humankind' read as *todo el mundo* 'everybody'). In a test of discrimination of homophonous words in context, he chose the correct response for

19 out of 20 sentences. He read 24 of 30 words with erased accents correctly, and his mistakes consisted of visual confusions and not regularization errors.

Based on the above findings, the origin and interpretation of symptoms in deep dyslexia have several explanations (e.g. Cuetos, 2002); however, we considered it interesting that, in Spanish, with a quite regular orthography, we can observe this syndrome. This fact seems to indicate that Spanish readers develop all strategies, sublexical and lexical, and that, in Spanish-speaking individuals, these routes of reading can be impaired differentially as in readers of any other language.

Phonological dyslexia

The central symptom of phonological dyslexia is the contrast observed in the adequate reading of words with a marked deficiency in the reading of nonwords. There is also a certain degree of visual confusion when reading words and nonwords. These patients tend to read much better than deep dyslexics, but when they encounter new words or are presented with nonwords, their reading deteriorates considerably. Word category effects may or may not affect their reading, and they make almost no semantic paralexias; they make mostly visual or derivational errors (Beauvois & Dérouesné, 1979; Beauvois *et al.*, 1980; Funnell, 1983).

Cuetos *et al.* (1996) described a case of phonological dyslexia in Spanish, comparable to what has been described for users of opaque orthographies, where a clear dissociation in the reading of words versus nonwords was observed. Iribarren *et al.* (1999) reported two more cases of phonological dyslexia in monolingual Spanish-speaking patients. Both patients, TR and CP, showed word category effects when reading words; they read short words better than long words, but imageability had no significant effect on their reading. Regular as well as irregular words (words with erased accent) were read about equally well. For both patients, most deficits consisted of morphological or visual errors, as for example, giving the wrong inflection or derivation (e.g. *olvidar* 'to forget' for *olviden* 'that they forgot'; *pereza* 'laziness' for *perezoso* 'lazy'). Both patients had great difficulty reading nonwords: TR read only 4 out of 20 nonwords, and CP was unable to read any nonwords correctly. On the other hand, both patients performed quite well in a vocabulary comprehension test (90% for TR and 100% for CP of correct responses) and a paragraph comprehension test (100% of correct responses for both cases). A homophonic reading discrimination task was done very accurately by both patients. As in the cases described for opaque orthographies, these patients showed a marked contrast between the readings of words versus nonwords.

These data suggest that reading via a lexical route is also an option in Spanish. Thus, if we were to adopt the stance that, because Spanish orthography is regular, we would need to develop a sublexical strategy of reading, which brings another perspective to the interpretation of the preceding data. Reading legal nonwords demands the use of a sublexical route, and these patients cannot read this kind of word. On the other hand, they read legal words quite adequately. A most likely explanation is that they might be using a sort of global lexical matching strategy. In order to give an appropriate diagnosis in this case, the development of tests that check for the reading of different types of nonwords must be employed.

Dysgraphias in Spanish

Patterns of writing impairments equivalent to those of reading have been found for opaque orthographies: surface dysgraphia (Beauvois & Dérouesné, 1981), deep dysgraphia (Bub & Kertesz, 1982), and phonological dysgraphia (Shallice, 1981). As explained earlier, the rules of phoneme–grapheme correspondence in Spanish writing are less direct than those for reading. As these rules depend on morphological and lexical knowledge, they might cause the need for the writer to develop a visual lexicon in order to write correctly and, consequently, this should be reflected in writing breakdown patterns as well.

Iribarren *et al.* (2001) described two cases, IT and AM, of differential writing impairments in monolingual Spanish-speaking patients. Both patients had good handwriting and were able to write their names fluently and correctly. In copying real words, both patients performed relatively well; however, when asked to copy nonwords, IT made two legal phonological substitutions, and AM refused to perform the test. For a dictation test, 160 words were selected, controlling for regularity of spelling, grammatical category, length, frequency of occurrence, and imageability. AM performed with a high level of accuracy, making only two mistakes, which could be attributed to her level of education. On the other hand, from the 80 regularly spelled words, IT made 7 errors, and from the 80 irregularly spelled words, he committed 31 mistakes. Ninety percent of his mistakes were phonologically plausible substitutions (e.g. *excases* instead of *escasez* 'shortage', *cullo* instead of *cuyo* 'whose', and *haguafiestas* instead of *aguafiestas* 'spoilsports'), and he made 10% of other letter substitutions producing neologisms (e.g. *melleza* instead of *belleza* 'beauty'). Out of 20 legal nonwords, IT was able to write 17 (85%), but AM did not succeed with any of the nonwords and showed great frustration with this task. In writing 10 homophonous words in context to dictation, IT made four mistakes, all of them phonological substitutions, and AM wrote nine words correctly. AM's only mistake was a semantic substitution: she wrote *uno* 'one' instead of *As* 'Ace'. IT was diagnosed as a surface dysgraphic. AM, on the other hand, was diagnosed as a phonological dysgraphic.

Although acquired dysgraphias are less well studied than other language deficits, probably because patients either have physical impediments that prevent them from writing or they get very frustrated very easily, the appropriate tests for writing different kinds of words and nonwords should be developed and used with patients. The classification of patients' mistakes should also be used as a guide to make the proper diagnosis. In Spanish, the dictation of words with regular and irregular spellings as well as the dictation of nonwords is crucial to determine the possible source of the writing difficulty in the patient.

Conclusions

Dyslexic and dysgraphic syndromes are far more complex than what has been presented here. Usually, *pure* cases can be observed but are not common in any language. However, there are clear tendencies in which patients favor either a sublexical strategy or a lexical strategy, and show difficulties with the opposite strategy of reading and writing. The precise source of the problem is not so well understood for any language either. This requires further research.

With respect to the observations of these syndromes in Spanish-speaking patients, two possible explanations may be offered. The first one is related to the orthographic structure of Spanish. It has been assumed that Spanish orthography is transparent because its unit of graphemic representation is alphabetic; that is, each character stands for either a vowel or a consonant. However, the consistent use of groups of graphemes related to morphological or lexical units allows them to function as pleremic units. Therefore, using the taxonomy proposed by Hass (1983), functionally, written Spanish uses cenemic as well as pleremic units. Cenemic units do not have meaning in themselves but are used to differentiate meanings; on the other hand, pleremic units have meaning (Hass, 1983). The consistent use of written units bigger than the syllable serves the reader/writer as indicators of semantic and syntactic associations between words (Iribarren, 2005). Catach (1996) makes a distinction between the linguistic description of a graphemic unit used in a language and its functional definition.

The second possible explanation for the observation of similar reading and writing breakdown patterns as those found in other orthographies is related to the capacity of all human beings for developing their cognitive potentials equally when confronted by similar cognitive tasks. There is nothing in the Spanish orthography that will prevent a reader from developing the same strategies used by readers of other languages. Studies performed with healthy Spanish-speaking readers of different ages and degrees of schooling support the use of sublexical as well as lexical strategies for reading and writing (see Iribarren, 2005). Reading and writing in Spanish is not substantially different from reading and writing in any other language (Besner & Smith, 1992). Hence, the data and arguments presented here support the *universality of reading and writing processes*. Further discussion of this notion is beyond the scope of this chapter. The reader is advised to refer to additional works for further cross-linguistic support to this claim (e.g. Coulmas, 1990; Hass, 1983; Lecours, 1996).

It is undeniable that the orthographic structure of each language plays an important role in the acquisition, practice, and breakdown patterns of reading and writing. Yet, a better understanding of an orthography and its pertinent processing demands in reading and writing should be taken into consideration to arrive at an appropriate determination of a patient's problem. Accurate diagnosis will crucially depend on the understanding of the complexity of the reading and writing processes as well as the design of the appropriate testing methods suitable to the patient's language. For Spanish-speaking patients, it would be crucial to test their reading and writing using different word categories, heterographic homophonic pairs of words, nonwords, and irregular words (e.g. words with erased graphic accent). Once the proper diagnosis has been made, therapy can be directed more effectively towards the development of facilitating intervention contexts and stimuli that would, in turn, help patients to overcome their particular difficulties and to develop necessary compensatory strategies.

References

Ardila, A. (1991) Errors resembling semantic paralexias in Spanish-speaking patients. *Brain and Language* 41, 437–445.

Ardila, A., Roselli, M. and Pinzón, O. (1989) Alexia and agraphia in Spanish speakers: CAT scan correlations and interlinguistic analysis. In A. Ardila and F. Ostrosky-Solís (eds) *Brain Organization of Language and Cognition* (pp.147–230). New York: Plenum Press.

Barry, C. and Richardson, T. (1988) Accounts of oral reading in deep dyslexia. In H. Whitaker (ed.) *Phonological Processes and Brain Mechanisms* (pp. 118–171). New York: Springer-Verlag.

Beauvois, M.F. and Dérouesné, J. (1979) Phonological alexias: Three dissociations. *Journal of Neurology, Neurosurgery, and Psychiatry* 42, 1115–1124.

Beauvois, M.F. and Dérouesné, J. (1981) Lexical or orthographic agraphia? *Brain* 104, 21–49.

Beauvois, M.F., Dérouesné, J. and Saillant, B. (1980) Syndromes neuropsychologiques et psychologie cognitive: Aphasie tactile, alexie phonologique et agraphie lexicale. *Cahiers de Psychologie* 23, 211–245.

Besner, D. and Smith, M.C. (1992) Basic processes in reading: Is the Orthographic Depth Hypothesis sinking? In R. Frost and L. Katz (eds) *Orthography, Morphology, and Meaning* (pp. 45–66). Amsterdam: Elsevier.

Bub, D. and Kertesz, A. (1982) Deep agraphia. *Brain and Language* 17, 146–165.

Catach, N. (1996) La escritura como plurisistema o teoría de L prima. In N. Catach (ed.) *Hacia una Teoría de la Escritura* (pp. 310–331) Barcelona: Gedisa.

Coltheart, M. (1987) Deep dyslexia: A review of the syndrome. In Coltheart, K. Patterson and J.C. Marshall (eds) *Deep Dyslexia* (2nd edn, pp. 22–47). London: Routledge and Kegan Paul.

Coltheart, M., Patterson, K. and Marshall, J.C. (1987) Deep dyslexia since 1980. In M. Coltheart, K. Patterson and J.C. Marshall (eds) *Deep Dyslexia* (2nd edn, pp. 407–451). London: Routledge and Kegan Paul.

Coulmas, F. (1990) *The Writing Systems of the World*. Oxford: Basil Blackwell.

Cuetos, F. (2002) Sistemas de lectura en ortografías transparentes: Evolución de la dislexia profunda en español. *Cognitiva* 14, 133–149.

Cuetos, F., Valle, F. and Suárez, P. (1996) A case of phonological dyslexia in Spanish. *Cognitive Neuropsychology* 13, 1–24.

Ferreres, A.R. and Miravalles, G. (1995) The production of semantic paralexias in a Spanish-speaking patient. *Brain and Language* 49, 153–172.

Funnell, E. (1983) Phonological processes in reading: Evidence from a deep and shallow orthographies. *Journal of Experimental Psychology: Learning, Memory, and Cognition* 20, 116–129.

Gutiérrez, N., Palma, A. and Benavides, I. (2001) Lexical stress and reading: A study with children. *Electronic Journal of Research in Educational Psychology* 2, 143–160.

Harris, J.W. (1983) *Syllable Structure and Stress in Spanish: A Nonlinear Analysis, Linguistic Inquiry – Monograph 8*. Cambridge, MA: The MIT Press.

Hass, W. (1983) Determining the level of a script. In F. Coulmas and K. Ehlich (eds) *Writing in Focus* (pp. 15–29). Berlin: Mouton.

Hatfield, F. (1985) Visual and phonological factors in acquired dysgraphia. *Neuropsychologia* 23, 13–29.

Iribarren, I.C. (1996) Un Posible Caso de Dislexia Profunda en Español, Unpublished manuscript.

Iribarren, I.C. (2005) *Ortografía Española: Bases Históricas, Lingüísticas y Cognitivas*. Caracas: Los Libros de EL Nacional. Universidad Simón Bolívar.

Iribarren, I.C., Jarema, G. and Lecours, A.R. (1996) The assessment of surface dyslexia in a regular orthography. *Brain and Cognition* 32, 196–198.

Iribarren, I.C., Jarema, G. and Lecours, A.R. (1999) Lexical reading in Spanish: Two cases of phonological dyslexia. *Applied Psycholinguistics* 20, 407–428.

Iribarren, I.C., Jarema, G. and Lecours, A.R. (2001) Two different dysgraphic syndromes in a regular orthography, Spanish. *Brain and Language* 77, 166–175.

Justicia, F., Defior, S., Pelegrina, S. and Martos, F. (1999) The sources of error in Spanish writing. *Journal of Research in Reading* 22, 198–202.

Karanth, P. (2003) *Cross-linguistic Study of Acquired Reading Disorders: Implications for Reading Models, Disorders, Acquisition, and Teaching*. New York: Kluwer.

Katz, L. and Frost, R. (1992) The reading process is different for different orthographies: The orthographic depth hypothesis. In R. Frost and L. Katz (eds) *Orthography, Morphology, and Meaning* (pp. 67–84). Amsterdam: Elsevier.

Lecours, A.R. (1996) *L'ecriture: Histoire, Théorie et Maladies*. Isberges: Ortho.

Marshall, J.C. and Newcombe, F. (1966) Syntactic and semantic errors in paralexias. *Neuropsychologia* 4, 169–176.

Marshall, J.C. and Newcombe, F. (1973) Patterns of paralexias: A psycholinguistic approach. *Journal of Psycholinguistic Research* 2, 175–199.

Monsell, S., Patterson, K., Graham, A., Hughes, C. and Milroy, R. (1992) Lexical and sub-lexical translation of spelling to sound: Strategic anticipation of lexical status. *Journal of Experimental Psychology: Learning, Memory, and Cognition* 18, 452–467.

Morton, J. and Patterson, K. (1987) A new attempt at an interpretation or an attempt at a new interpretation. In M. Coltheart, K. Patterson and J.C. Marshall (eds) *Deep Dyslexia* (2nd edn, pp. 91–118). London: Routledge and Kegan Paul.

Patterson, K., Marshall, J.C. and Coltheart, M. (1985) *Surface Dyslexia: Neuropsychological and Cognitive Studies of Phonological Reading*. London: Lawrence Erlbaum.

Ruíz, A., Ansaldo, A.I. and Lecours, A.R. (1994) Two cases of deep dyslexia in unilingual hispanophone aphasics. *Brain and Language* 46, 245–256.

Sampson, G. (1989) *Writing Systems: A Linguistic Introduction*. Stanford, CA: Stanford University Press.

Shallice, T. (1981) Phonological agraphia and the lexical route in writing. *Brain* 104, 413–429.

Valle Arroyo, F. (1984) The importance of grapheme-to-phoneme conversion rules in beginning readers. In R.N. Malatesha and H. Whitaker (eds) *Dyslexia: A Global Issue* (pp. 511–516). The Hague: Martinu.

Chapter 18

Cross-linguistic Aspects of Dyslexia in Spanish–English Bilinguals

ELIZABETH IJALBA and LORAINE K. OBLER

This chapter aims to describe the particular problems in reading that may be evident in Spanish–English bilinguals and in those Spanish speakers who are in the process of learning English as a second language. The speech-language pathologist (SLP) who works in the schools is well aware of the large numbers of bilingual students referred to special education and to speech-language therapy because of reading failure. The English as a Second Language (ESL) teacher who works with high-school and college students learning English as a foreign language (FL) is also aware of the problems in reading and language learning that a select group of these students display. Why is it that reading deficits and problems with language learning may go together? Why is it that some Spanish speakers who are English Language Learners (ELLs) have particular difficulty in reading English but may nevertheless read relatively well in their native Spanish orthography?

We can even argue that reading in English is a task that may be particularly difficult for Spanish readers who first learned to read in the highly consistent orthography of their native language. In order to lay the groundwork for our understanding of the particular difficulties faced by Spanish speakers learning to read English, a detailed exploration of the *neurocognitive basis* of reading and reading disorders is indicated. Though we focus here on Spanish and English alphabetic orthographies (i.e. reading is based on grapheme-to-phoneme correspondences), similar principles may be applicable to readers of other alphabetic scripts, such as Italian, French, and other European languages. This chapter complements other discussions in this volume addressing ethnographic influences in literacy acquisition in bilingual readers (Kayser & Centeno, ch. 2), and reading and writing impairments in Spanish users (Iribarren, ch. 17; Ostrosky-Solís *et al.*, ch. 19; Weekes, ch. 7).

The Neurocognitive Basis for Word Reading

Reading can be described as deriving meaning from print. Whereas skilled readers can access semantic, syntactic, and phonological forms from print, cognitive models of reading attempt to delimit these processes by focusing on word recognition (see Ellis, 1998). As detailed in the discussions by Iribarren (ch. 17) and Weekes (ch. 7) earlier, in dual-route models of reading (Coltheart *et al.*, 2001), new or unfamiliar words and nonwords (word-like structures) can be decoded and sounded-out by grapheme (printed letter)-to-phoneme (sound) conversion through a *sublexical route*. Familiar words that have often been encountered in print are recognized without the need for decoding and irregularly spelled words must also be recognized to be read. Both familiar and irregularly spelled words are accessed via a *lexical route*, which allows immediate access to their meaning. Whereas both routes are known to play important roles in reading acquisition, the lexical route (word recognition) is the primary mechanism that proficient readers use. The sublexical route (decoding) plays a greater role at beginning reading stages and remains as an alternative route used by proficient readers when orthographically mediated lexical access fails (see Iribarren, ch. 17, this volume for further description on dual-route models of reading).

Our knowledge of how reading is processed comes in great measure from cases of *acquired dyslexia* (impaired reading after brain damage in someone who was able to read premorbidly) and also from cases of *developmental dyslexia* (difficulty learning to read despite normal intelligence and educational opportunities). The early interpretations of developmental dyslexia centered on visual deficits as exemplified by the term *congenital word blindness* (Hinshelwood, 1917; Pringle-Morgan, 1896). However, more recent interpretations attribute dyslexia to a verbal deficit, particularly in phonological processing (Shankweiler *et al.*, 1979; Snowling, 2001; Vellutino, 1979), which prevents readers from building word-recognition strategies and establishing an orthographic lexicon.

An alternative interpretation of reading deficits is proposed by Wolf and Bowers (1999) in the *double-deficit hypothesis*. Based on experimental data and cross-linguistic research, these authors identify two main deficit categories that may occur independently in impaired readers. The *phonological-deficit readers* experience phonological processing problems. Their main difficulty is in establishing the phonological representation of words and in learning sound-to-letter correspondences. The *naming-speed deficit readers* experience naming-speed problems for visually presented symbols. They have difficulty automatizing the reading of familiar words and must, therefore, rely on decoding. The *combined-deficit type* constitutes the most impaired readers. They experience difficulty in both phonological processing and in naming speed. In this double-deficit form, impaired readers have few compensatory strategies available and remediation is more difficult.

The multicomponential aspects of reading have generated difficulty in reaching a uniform interpretation of disordered reading. Coltheart *et al.* (2001) caution against a unitary characterization of dyslexia by pointing out that in order for reading development to proceed smoothly, several reading subsystems must operate and interact (e.g. a letter-recognition system, a word recognition system, a letter-to-sound rules system, etc.). Jackson and Coltheart (2001) recommend that, in order to effectively diagnose reading difficulties, it is essential to differentiate between proximal causes of a reading disorder (i.e. what system is altered) from distal causes (i.e. why a system is altered). When following this format, we may find, in answering what is wrong (i.e. what subsystem is altered), that a child may have difficulty with the establishment of grapheme-to-phoneme associations or mappings between letters and letter-strings to phonology. When we ask why, it may be that the child comes to the task with poorly specified phonological representations. However, for another child with the same proximal cause (e.g. difficulty establishing grapheme-to-phoneme associations), the distal cause may, for example, be instruction that eschewed the teaching of phonics. A detailed breakdown from word analysis to word recognition in alphabetic orthographies is provided in Table 18.1.

Influence of Orthography on Reading

Across the languages of the world a number of different writing systems have developed, from those that represent all phonemes (e.g. Spanish) to those that represent only some (e.g. Arabic) to those that use symbols representing syllables (e.g. Japanese) to those whose symbols represent whole morphemes or words (e.g. Chinese). In addition, in any of these systems, current writing can transparently reflect current speech forms, or more opaquely represent historically earlier speech forms, thus appearing inconsistent.

A main difference in how readers derive meaning from print in an inconsistent orthography (e.g. English) when compared with a more consistent one (e.g. Spanish) is that, in addition to decoding, the reader must learn to recognize irregularly spelled words. For instance, Foorman *et al.* (1997) estimate that approximately 13% of words in English are unpredictable from the way they are spelled and must be memorized to be effectively recognized and read. Hanna *et al.* (1966) point out that pronunciation in English can be predicted from the way that words are spelled in only approximately 50% of the lexicon. The phonology–orthography demands that are placed on English readers are, thus, much greater than those for readers of consistent orthographies like that of Spanish, who must learn univocal (consistent) sound-to-letter correspondences (cf. Iribarren in this publication – there are exceptions).

The way in which first-language reading strategies influence the learning of another language was revealed in a study by Ijalba and Obler (2002). In that study, we compared two groups of monoscriptal readers, Spanish readers and English readers, on the learning of two versions of a

Table 18.1 In order to read, a reader must possess basic knowledge about the language, including sufficient vocabulary and syntax. The following skills are necessary for achieving word recognition in alphabetic orthographies:

- Letter identification and ability to form grapheme–phoneme associations.
- Online processing of grapheme–phoneme associations, which includes decoding (breaking down the word into its corresponding sound units or phonemes), combining phonemes, and recoding the printed word to say it aloud.
- Recoding requires accurate phonological representations (a reader must be able to access how a word sounds from the mental lexicon).
- Practice in decoding–recoding rapidly evolves in the formation of orthographic representations (the reader develops an orthographic lexicon that is intimately associated with the phonological representation of words).
- Phonological awareness and orthographic awareness are intimately related and advance in unison, facilitating each other during the reading progress.
- Orthographic representations facilitate phonological access.
- Phonological representations facilitate orthographic access.
- There is a direct link between the orthography of a word and its meaning (sight vocabulary). Efficient readers access meaning directly from word recognition. Reading becomes fast or automatized, allowing the reader to read silently for meaning and to process larger amounts of text.
- There is an indirect link between the letter components in a word and its meaning: letters within a word must be recognized, converted to phonemes and recombined in order for meaning to be accessed via 'sounding out' the word. Beginning readers heavily rely on sublexical processing as they build an orthographic lexicon. Efficient readers also 'slow down' and use sublexical processing to read new or unfamiliar words.
- Either a sublexical or a lexical processing reading strategy may be favored at different points in development, e.g. a lexical or 'holistic' strategy is used by pre-readers to recognize logos and names; sublexical processing is used by beginning readers to focus on elements within words during decoding; lexical processing is used by efficient readers to focus on word recognition (sight words) as reading speed improves.
- Online processing at the word level is influenced by short-term memory, particularly for sublexical processing that requires holding grapheme–phoneme conversions in memory as they are being recombined to obtain the final word form. Short-term verbal memory also plays an important role in online text processing as the reader strings words together to form sentences and sentences into paragraphs.

---

novel writing system. In one version, the orthography of this novel writing system was consistent and maintained univocal grapheme-to-phoneme correspondence. In the second version, the orthography was rendered less consistent by allowing multiple grapheme-to-phoneme correspondences for the vowels, such that each syllabic unit could have two possible pronunciations. The task of the reader was to learn the multiple grapheme-to-phoneme correspondences and to memorize only one pronunciation for each target word in the orthographically less consistent version.

Findings from this study revealed that everyone learned the orthographically consistent version of the novel writing system with greater ease than the orthographically less consistent version. However, the Spanish readers learned the orthographically consistent version with greater ease than the English readers and a trend in the opposite direction was also noted, that is, English readers outperformed the Spanish readers in learning the orthographically less consistent version of this novel writing system.

One may infer that when readers are faced with the task of learning a new orthography, they tend to apply or transfer the most reliable and/or predominant strategies used in their native language orthography. Research findings concur in showing that language transfer across many levels (from phonological awareness to semantic and syntactic aspects) is implicated in second language acquisition (August *et al.*, 2002; Bialystok, 2001; Bialystok & Hakuta, 1994; also see Kayser & Centeno, ch. 2, this volume). August and Hakuta (1998) point out that it takes longer to learn a language that is typologically very different from the native language than one that is relatively similar, a conclusion consistent with the findings by Ijalba and Obler (2002) vis-à-vis orthographic systems.

Learning a second language and its writing system are challenging enough tasks that require the learner to apply only those most effective reading strategies from the native language, a decoding or sublexical strategy for Spanish readers, and both sublexical and lexical strategies by English readers. Problems would arise, however, the more that the first-language orthography and the second-language orthography differ.

An important focus of research on the relationship between orthography and reading is whether dual-route processing is present in languages with varying degrees of orthographic transparency or consistency. Valle-Arroyo (1996) analyzed the use of sublexical and lexical processing on lexical decision tasks with 2nd-, 3rd-, and 5th-grade elementary students in Spain. He found that the 3rd- and the 5th-grade students made more mistakes than the 2nd graders in the reading aloud of nonwords created by altering one letter in real words such as *escuella* derived from *escuela* 'school'. Whereas the reaction times were faster for the older readers, particularly the 5th graders, their reading accuracy decreased when compared to their younger peers. The older readers tended to *lexicalize* or read as real words the altered target words. Valle-Arroyo interpreted these findings as showing a shift from decoding to the automatization of reading processes and an increased use of the lexical-route (word recognition) as readers become faster and more efficient.

Results congruent with those of Valle-Arroyo (1996) that point to the increased use of lexical reading strategies by older readers in Spanish are evident in a study by Calvo and Carrillo (2000). Performance on reading tasks by poor readers from 4th, 5th, and 6th grades in Spain showed that older students (5th and 6th grade) read nonwords faster but with less accuracy than younger students (4th grade). However, the older students also identified correct words from pseudohomophones (i.e. *vaso/baso*) better than their younger peers, suggesting they had acquired a better orthographic lexicon. On a more detailed analysis of their data, the authors noted that phonological processing problems were evident in relation to the speed of reading nonwords. That is, whereas the older students could read nonwords faster than the younger students, the older students made more lexicalization mistakes than their younger peers, which was indicative of their efforts in attempting to use lexical strategies that were, for this task, incompletely grounded in deficient sublexical processing.

A conceptualization of reading that departs from the influence of the orthography and centers on the experience of the learner is that proposed by Share (1995). He posits that, in learning to read, children *self-teach* by learning the associations between letters and phonemes, which in turn allows them to decode and derive the meaning of written words. As children progressively apply this procedure and are successful, the words they repeatedly encounter become incorporated into an ortho-graphic lexicon and are used in the future for lexical reading. In this model, both regularly and irregularly spelled words become part of the orthographic lexicon. Thus, the use of the lexical route in reading depends more on experience than on spelling regularity. The increased use of lexical processing evident in the studies by Valle-Arroyo (1996) and Calvo and Carrillo (2000) would, thus, result from the increased reading practice schooling brings. In the case of adult Hispanic ELLs, this model would also predict increased use of sublexical processing rather than lexical processing in the reading of English for two reasons. First, this would result because prior experience in L1 (Spanish) would tend to support decoding strategies. Second, it would occur because most words in L2 (English) would be unfamiliar and predispose the reader toward decoding rather than toward sight-word reading. In contrast, English readers, who must rely on lexical processing in their L1, would tend to apply sight-word reading when learning a foreign language.

In summary, orthographic differences in writing systems influence reading processes and the strategies used in learning to read, consistent with Iribarren (ch. 17) in this volume. Highly consistent, transparent, writing systems facilitate sublexical processing, whereas less consistent orthographies require more use of lexical processing for the reading of irregularly spelled words. Even with these underlying differences, dual-route processing in highly consistent alphabetic writing systems, such as the one used for Spanish, indicates increased use of sublexical processing by less experienced readers and increased use of lexical processing by more experienced readers.

Biliterates with Dissociations in Impaired Reading

More conclusive evidence in support of dual-route processing in reading can be found in the few but highly revealing clinical cases reported that show a dissociation between the sublexical and lexical routes (decoding and word recognition). Given the varying demands that writing systems impose on readers, it comes as no surprise that some bilingual readers may experience more reading problems in one language than in the other language, particularly when there are differences in orthographic consistency between the two scripts.

A clinical case showing a dissociation in the reading and spelling of English and Spanish was reported by Meara *et al.* (1985). The authors described the case of FE, a 29-year-old bilingual (Spanish–English) college student from Colombia, residing in England for 14 years and attending college there. FE spoke fluent English, however he had severe reading and spelling problems in English, but only mild (mostly spelling) problems in Spanish. FE made twice as many errors reading irregularly spelled words when compared with regularly spelled words in English. He also made spelling errors on more than 50% of the words in a spelling test and most of these errors were phonological in nature, e.g. *serch* for *search*, *coff* for *cough*. FE also had great difficulty identifying target words from homophone pairs, e.g. *beach* and *beech*. When tested in Spanish, FE showed few reading errors for both words and nonwords. However, spelling errors were present in words in which there was not a direct mapping between graphemes and phonemes (a few consonant letters in Spanish have more than one phoneme equivalent, e.g. < c > may be /s/ and /k/; also see Iribarren, ch. 17, this volume for additional examples). The authors concluded that FE relied too heavily on a phonological strategy without use of a lexical route, typical of surface dyslexia (difficulty establishing word recognition). FE showed essentially the same symptoms in English and in Spanish, but his overall performance reflected the regularity of the Spanish orthography and the reading deficit could, therefore, pass undetected in the writing system of his native language.

A proposal that attempts to bridge orthographic consistency from alphabetic to ideographic writing systems has been suggested by Wydell and Butterworth (1999). The authors report the case of AS, a bilingual (Japanese–English) adolescent who experienced severe difficulties reading in English but near normal reading in Kana and Kanji, the syllabic and whole-word scripts, respectively, used for writing Japanese. In order to account for the dissociation that AS revealed in his ability to read Japanese (both Kana and Kanji) and English, the authors proposed the hypothesis of *transparency and granularity*, which posits that irrespective of the granule or unit size (i.e. phoneme, syllable, or character), phonological dyslexia (difficulty in establishing grapheme-to-phoneme correspondences essential for decoding) cannot be present as long as there is a one-to-one correspondence between the unit and sound. This hypothesis predicts that the occurrence rate of developmental dyslexia, particularly phonologically based dyslexia, should be low in transparent or consistent orthographies and also unlikely in orthographies with large granules of print-to-sound mapping (such as Kanji or Chinese). The case of AS, who was an early Japanese–English bilingual, and schooled in the three types of script, provided clinical evidence in support of this hypothesis.

Several cases of developmental dyslexia are reported in biliterate speakers of Hindi–English and Kannada–English (Karanth, 1992, 2003). Both Hindi and Kannada use syllabic scripts that are highly transparent. Increased difficulty reading and writing English over that for either Kannada or Hindi was evident in all cases. Errors in reading English words reflected poor use of orthographic strategies (e.g. *fond* for *found*, *does* for *did*), while spelling errors reflected phonological recoding and confirmed difficulties recalling orthographic forms (e.g. *laf* for *laugh*, *tabel* for *table*). Most of the errors in the reading and writing of Hindi and Kannada were visual in nature and far fewer than the number of errors noted in English.

To summarize, case studies of biscriptal readers that show a dissociation in reading one writing system better than the other provide clear evidence of dual-route processing in reading. Dyslexia can go unnoticed in the more consistent writing systems that facilitate one-to-one grapheme-to-phoneme mappings because sublexical processing is supported by the orthography. Difficulty in reading only becomes more obvious in less consistent orthographies that require increased use of those lexical processes involved in word recognition. Spanish readers with dyslexia may rely heavily on sublexical processing when reading Spanish, a strategy that may be neither efficient nor sufficient to support reading in English.

Diagnostic Tasks Used to Identify Reading Deficits across Orthographies

Most of the literature on reading impairment originates from research conducted on English readers. Indeed, Ziegler *et al.* (2003) point out that two thirds of all publications on developmental dyslexia since 1998 are on English-speaking individuals, which raises the question as to whether results from these studies can be generalized to orthographies that are different from English. This question acquires more relevance when considering the data reviewed above indicating that the manifestation of reading disorder varies across orthographies (see also Bowers & Wolf, 1993; Jiménez González & Hernández Valle, 2000; Landerl *et al.*, 1997; Paulesu *et al.*, 2001; Rodrigo López & Jiménez González, 1999; Tressoldi *et al.*, 2001; Wimmer *et al.*, 2000; Wimmer & Mayringer, 2002; Wolf *et al.*, 2000). Let us focus, then, on those papers that treat languages like German, whose orthographic transparency is similar to that of Spanish.

In a study comparing English and German dyslexic readers (9–13 years), Ziegler *et al.* (2003) used three psycholinguistic measures relevant in understanding underlying reading processes. The lexicality effect (difference between word and nonword reading) was selected to investigate phonological decoding deficits across the orthographies. The length effect was chosen to quantify serial processes in word and nonword decoding and the large units' effect (complex syllables) was selected to identify sensitivity to body neighborhood effects (words that share the same orthographic rime [that is, the part of the syllable including the vowel and the subsequent consonant], e.g. *street, meet, feet*). Results showed that reading speed and slow, serial phonological decoding deficits were of similar size across the two orthographies. For instance, both groups of dyslexic readers showed significant effects for length (number of letters) in the reading of words and nonwords (processing costs per letter were up to 11 times greater than in normal readers). The English readers, however, made more decoding errors than the German readers and they relied more on larger orthographic units than the German dyslexics, reflecting the facilitatory effects of the German orthography, which is highly consistent.

The measures that best discriminated between dyslexic readers and normal readers in a consistent orthography were studied by Landerl (2001) in a large sample of German 3rd graders. Dyslexic readers were first selected from a group by using measures of timed-reading comprehension that indirectly measured reading speed. Those who performed lowest were then individually assessed with a standardized battery, which included tests of word and nonword reading, spelling, reading speed, phoneme deletion, nonword repetition, rapid automatized naming, and visual-processing speed (processing of letter-like characters). Findings from this study revealed that, on measures of word and nonword reading, dyslexics read accurately but slowly, and there were no differences between the two tasks, showing the effectiveness of sublexical processing. What this study failed to do was to compare the reading of nonwords between 3rd graders and older readers, as was done in the Valle-Arroyo (1996) study, which showed increased mistakes in nonword reading as older students relied more heavily on lexical processing.

Landerl *et al.* (1997) assessed reading speed by using a sentence-reading test in which participants silently read simple sentences and indicated if the content of each sentence was right or wrong (the number of sentences understood was divided by the time in minutes taken to read, reflecting the reading speed measure). The performance of the dyslexic readers was within the 4th percentile when compared to the normal control group. In the phoneme-deletion task, participants were asked to say a word without the first phoneme (i.e. *(b)rief*). Dyslexic readers committed twice as many errors as the normal readers in this task. The spelling measure consisted of single words dictated and dyslexic readers performed significantly lower when compared to the normal controls. Dyslexics also showed phonetic spellings, suggesting difficulty recalling orthographic forms. The visual processing task consisted of two tasks assessing visual processing speed. The child was required to cross out a letter-like character within a word-like sequence of seven characters. Dyslexic readers performed significantly worse than normal readers on this task, indicating the presence of visual-processing deficits in addition to phonological processing problems in their reading. Finally, the rapid automatized naming task consisted of rapidly naming five items randomly repeated. The task contained pictures of animals and single digits. Rapid naming was found to be the most discriminative in differentiating between the dyslexic and normal readers. In conclusion, German dyslexic readers had extremely slow reading speed. The children also had severe delays in spelling (reflecting the complex syllabic structure of German). The most prominent cognitive deficits were reduced rapid-naming speed, followed by deficits in phonological awareness. In the clinical practice of the first author of this chapter, similar deficits observed in Spanish readers with dyslexia (excepting the severity of spelling deficits because Spanish has a simple syllabic structure) highlight that reading speed, rapid naming, and phonological awareness are key aspects of reading that may show dyslexia.

In other studies aimed at identifying dyslexia in bilinguals of different ages, phonological awareness, decoding, word recognition, and fluency are found to be among the most effective measures. The use of grapheme-to-phoneme correspondence rules necessary for decoding and important in building word recognition not only differentiate good from poor readers in L1 but also apply to reading in L2. Geva *et al.* (2000) found a strong correlation between reading speed and accuracy in L1 and L2 for young readers from various language backgrounds. Sparks *et al.* (1998) found that decoding and word identification measures differentiated good from poor readers in foreign language learners. Lindsey *et al.* (2003) found that phonological awareness in L1 (Spanish) was predictive of word-identification skills in L2 (English) among first-grade Spanish-speaking English learners. Other L1 variables that showed high correlation with L2 reading were word knowledge (picture vocabulary), memory for sentences, and rapid object naming, which was the most significant task even when tested one year later. Findings in young readers, such as in this study, are consistent with findings in the adult foreign-language literature and even with research that shows dyslexia to be a lifelong disorder.

In summary, the tasks used in many of the studies reviewed are generally aimed at uncovering underlying reading processes that may explain how we are able to derive meaning from print. In line with the claim that there are some universal strategies in reading and writing (see Iribarren, ch. 17, this volume), cognitive and language-specific processes interact in common ways across orthographies to reflect subtle and, sometimes, more obvious differences when part of the overall reading system does not function efficiently. The basic processes of establishing grapheme-to-phoneme mappings (sublexical processing) and achieving word recognition (lexical processing) are typically assessed through the decoding of nonwords, reading of regularly spelled words, exception words (irregular), and spelling tasks among others. The influence of phonemic awareness and orthographic knowledge is also highly correlated with the encoding and recoding processes that allow reading and writing. Word frequency, lexicality, and orthographic neighbors have an effect on reading performance, across consistent and less consistent orthographies. The effects of fluency, automaticity, and word recognition are correlated with readers' performance on rapid-naming tasks across orthographies. Furthermore, the value of psycholinguistic tasks able to predict reading problems in L2 by measuring skills in the more proficient language is also particularly important in education. The studies reviewed in this chapter indicate that the most reliable measures that can predict reading problems in L2 by testing in L1 include phonological awareness, rapid naming, decoding, and fluency or reading proficiency.

Conclusions

This chapter was aimed at exploring the particular problems that many Spanish readers encounter when reading in English. These problems were explored within the context of neurocognitive cross-linguistic reading research. Understanding these core deficits that make reading in English difficult is particularly important when working with bilingual populations whose native languages, like Spanish, may have more consistent orthographies than English. Undetected reading problems in the native language may only surface when the reader is faced with the task of learning to read in an inconsistent orthography such as English. The role of diagnosing and planning appropriate remediation for these problems is incumbent upon SLPs who work with Spanish speakers and Spanish-speaking English-language learners, as well as speakers of other languages faced with similar challenges.

References

August, D., Calderón, M. and Carlo, M. (2002) Transfer of skills from Spanish to English: A study of young learners. In *Report for Practitioners, Parents, and Policy Makers*. Washington, DC: Center for Applied Linguistics.

August, D. and Hakuta, H. (1998) *Educating Language-minority Children*. Washington, DC: National Academy Press.

Bialystok, E. (2001) *Bilingualism in Development: Language, Literacy, and Cognition*. Cambridge: Cambridge University Press.

Bialystok, E. and Hakuta, K. (1994) *In Other Words: The Psychology and Science of Second Language Acquisition*. New York: Basic Books.

Bowers, P.G. and Wolf, M. (1993) Theoretical links among naming speed, precise timing mechanisms and orthographic skill in dyslexia. *Reading and Writing* 5, 69–85.

Calvo, A. and Carrillo, M. (2000) Dificultades de aprendizaje de la lectura: Hay diferentes tipos de malos lectores? PhD. thesis, Universidad de Murcia, Spain.

Coltheart, M., Rastle, K., Perry, C., Langdon, R. and Ziegler, J. (2001) DRC: A dual route cascaded model of visual word recognition and reading aloud. *Psychological Review* 108, 204–256.

Ellis, A.W. (1998) *Reading, Writing and Dyslexia: A Cognitive Analysis*. Hove, UK: Psychology Press.

Foorman, B.R., Francis, D.J., Shaywitz, S.E., Shaywitz, B.A. and Fletcher, J.M. (1997) The case for early reading intervention. In B. Blachman (ed.) *Foundations of Reading Acquisition and Dyslexia: Implications for Early Intervention* (pp. 243–264). Mahwah, NJ: Lawrence Erlbaum.

Geva, E., Yaghoub-Zadeh, Z. and Schuster, B. (2000) Understanding individual differences in word recognition skills of ESL children. *Annals of Dyslexia* 50, 123–154.

Hanna, P.R., Hanna, J.S., Hodges, R.E. and Rudorf, E.H. (1966) *Phoneme–grapheme Correspondences as Cues to Spelling Improvement*. Washington, DC: US Government Printing Office.

Hinshelwood, J. (1917) *Congenital Word-blindness*. London: Lewis.

Ijalba, E. and Obler, L.K. (2002) *Grapheme–phoneme Correspondence Learning in Spanish and English Speakers*. Paper presented at the conference of the Multilingual International Dyslexia Association, Washington, D.C.

Jackson, N.E. and Coltheart, M. (2001) *Routes to Reading Success and Failure: Toward and Integrated Cognitive Psychology of Atypical Reading*. New York: Psychology Press.

Jiménez González, J.E. and Hernández-Valle, I. (2000) Word identification and reading disorders in the Spanish language. *Journal of Learning Disabilities* 33, 40–60.

Karanth, P. (1992) Developmental dyslexia in bilingual-biliterates. *Reading and Writing* 4, 297–306.

Karanth, P. (2003) *Cross-linguistic Study of Acquired Reading Disorders: Implications for Reading Models, Disorders, Acquisition, and Teaching*. New York: Kluwer.

Landerl, K. (2001) Word recognition deficits in German: More evidence from a representative sample. *Dyslexia* 7, 183–196.

Landerl, K., Wimmer, H. and Frith, U. (1997) The impact of orthographic consistency on dyslexia: A German–English comparison. *Cognition* 63, 315–334.

Lindsey, K.A., Manis, F.R. and Bailey, C. (2003) Prediction of first-grade reading in Spanish-speaking English-language learners. *Journal of Educational Psychology* 95, 482–494.

Meara, P., Coltheart, M. and Masterson, J. (1985) Hidden reading problems in ESL learners. *The TESL Canada Journal/Revue TESL du Canada* 3, 29–36.

Paulesu, E., Demonet, J.F., Fazio, F., McCrory, E., Chanoine, V., Brunswick, N., Cappa, S.F., Cossu, G., Habib, M., Frith, C.D. and Frith, U. (2001) Dyslexia: Cultural diversity and biological unity. *Science* 291, 2165–2167.

Pringle-Morgan, W. (1896) A case of congenital word blindness. *British Medical Journal* 2, 1378.

Rodrigo López, M. and Jiménez González, J.E. (1999) An analysis of the word naming errors of normal readers and reading disabled children in Spanish. *Journal of Research in Reading* 22, 180–197.

Shankweiler, D., Liberman, I.Y., Mark, L.S., Fowler, C.A. and Fischer, F.W. (1979) The speech code and learning to read. *Journal of Experimental Psychology: Human Learning and Memory* 5, 531–545.

Share, D.L. (1995) Phonological recoding and self-teaching: Sine qua non of reading acquisition. *Cognition* 55, 151–218.

Snowling, M.J. (2001) *Dyslexia*. Oxford: Blackwell.

Sparks, R., Artzer, M., Ganschow, L., Siebenhar, D., Plageman, M. and Patton, J. (1998) Differences in native-language skills, foreign-language aptitude, and foreign language grades among high-, average-, and low-proficiency foreign-language learners: Two studies. *Language Testing* 15, 181–216.

Tressoldi, P.E., Stella, G. and Fagella, M. (2001) The development of reading speed in Italians with dyslexia: A longitudinal study. *Journal of Learning Disabilities* 33, 414–417.

Valle-Arroyo, F. (1996) Dual-route models in Spanish: Developmental and psychological data. In Carreiras, M., García-Albea, J.E. and Sebastian-Gallés, N. (eds) *Language Processing in Spanish* (pp. 89–118). Mahwah: Lawrence Erlbaum.

Vellutino, F.R. (1979) *Dyslexia: Research and Theory.* Cambridge, MA: MIT Press.

Wimmer, H. and Mayringer, H. (2002) Dysfluent reading in the absence of spelling difficulties: A specific disability in regular orthographies. *Journal of Educational Psychology* 94, 272–277.

Wimmer, H., Mayringer, H. and Landerl, K. (2000) The double-deficit hypothesis and difficulties in learning to read a regular orthography. *Journal of Educational Psychology* 92, 668–680.

Wolf, M. and Bowers, P.G. (1999) The double deficit hypothesis for the developmental dyslexias. *Journal of Educational Psychology* 91, 415–438.

Wolf, M., Bowers, P.G. and Biddle, K. (2000) Naming-speed processes, timing, and reading: A conceptual review. *Journal of Learning Disabilities* 33, 387–407.

Wydell, T.N. and Butterworth, B.I. (1999) A case study of an English–Japanese bilingual with monolingual dyslexia. *Cognition* 70, 273–305.

Ziegler, J., Conrad, P., Ma-Wyatt, A., Ladner, D. and Schulte-Korne, G. (2003) Developmental dyslexia in different languages: Language-specific or universal? *Journal of Experimental Child Psychology* 86, 169–194.

Chapter 19

Neuropsychological Profile of Adult Illiterates and the Development and Application of a Neuropsychological Program for Learning to Read

FEGGY OSTROSKY-SOLÍS, AZUCENA LOZANO, MAURA J. RAMÍREZ and ALFREDO ARDILA

The ability to read and write is important for an individual's success and survival in the contemporary world. About 9.5% of Mexicans over 15 years are illiterate, and 18.6% of the adult population have not finished elementary school (Instituto Nacional para la Educación de los Adultos [INEA], 2001). The INEA has developed education programs for the illiterate adult population in Mexico. Despite all the efforts, failure in learning to read is found in a significant percentage of the INEA participants. Approximately, only 28.6% succeed in learning to read (INEA, 2001). The rest (over 60%) either do not complete the program or simply fail in learning to read. It can be assumed that different variables can account for this high percentage of failure, ranging from personal factors to the teaching methods. Understanding the variables that affect success in learning to read represents a very important question in overcoming illiteracy not only in Mexico, but also in other countries (see Kayser & Centeno, ch. 2, this volume for related discussion on bilingual readers).

Reading represents a major cognitive tool (Vygotsky, 1962) and it is not surprising that a significantly decreased neuropsychological test performance has been documented in illiterate individuals (Ardila et al., 1989, 2000; Goldblum & Matute, 1986; Lecours et al., 1987; Manly et al., 1999; Matute et al., 2000; Ostrosky et al., 1998, 2004; Reis & Castro-Caldas, 1997; Rosselli, 1993; Rosselli et al., 1990). Lower scores are observed in most cognitive domains, especially naming, phonological verbal fluency, verbal memory, and conceptual functions.

Departing from the previous considerations, we developed an *evidence-based intervention program*. The study, which provided the empirical evidence, included the following stages (1) the identification of the cognitive profile of adult individuals who attended the literacy program at INEA, (2) the development of a neuropsychological learning-to-read method based on the identified neuropsychological profile of adult illiterates, and (3) the evaluation of the efficiency of the reading program. In this chapter, we will describe this study and its clinical implications in literacy assessment and intervention in monolingual Spanish speakers.

Assessing the Cognitive Profile of Illiterate Individuals

Method

In order to accomplish the first objective, that is, the identification of the cognitive profile of adult individuals, a 238-participant sample (72 men, 166 women) in the INEA literacy program, named *Palabra Generadora*, was selected in four different Mexican states (Mexico City, Jalisco, Zacatecas, and Colima). The larger proportion of women in the sample arises out of the circumstance that many more women than men attended the program.

The major purpose of the *Palabra Generadora* program is to provide basic reading strategies. It usually takes eight months, six devoted to the development of basic reading and writing skills, and two to the study of the elementary reading books used in Mexican schools.

Table 19.1 shows the general characteristics of the sample. Previous schooling time and time at INEA were recorded. This information was taken directly from the INEA files.

Materials

The *NEUROPSI* neuropsychological test battery (Ostrosky *et al.*, 1997, 1999) was used to evaluate cognitive functioning. In addition, based on the notion that phonological awareness (phonological synthesis and analysis skills) and lexical access (measured by naming speed) are correlated with success in single word decoding (Shaywitz, 1996; Stanovich & Siegel, 1994), we developed specific tests to assess these skills: a phonological processing and awareness test; a naming test and a

Table 19.1 General characteristics of the illiterate group

n	*Age*		*Gender*		*Handedness*			*Previous schooling (months)*		*Time at INEA (months)*	
	χ	*sd*	*M*	*F*	*RH*	*LH*	*AD*	χ	*sd*	χ	*sd*
238	44.1	17.4	72	166	230	6	2	18.3	25.9	5.5	6.8

χ, mean; *sd*, standard deviation; M, male; F, female; RH, right handed; LH, left handed; AD, ambidextrous

reading test of words and pseudowords. Specific descriptions of these materials follow.

Neuropsychological Test Battery

The *NEUROPSI*, a brief neuropsychological test battery developed and standardized in Mexico (Ostrosky *et al.*, 1997, 1999), was employed. In total, 26 different scores are obtained. Maximum total score is 130. Administration time is 25–30 min. The *NEUROPSI* distinguishes four levels of performance in each age and education range: normal (within one standard deviation), mildly abnormal (between one and two standard deviations), moderately abnormal (between two and three standard deviations), and severely abnormal (over three standard deviations with regard to the means scores in that age and education group). Subjects in this study were compared with the norms corresponding to their schooling (illiterates or 1–4 years of formal education). For further details on tests and scores included in this battery, see Ostrosky *et al.* (1997, 1999).

Phonological Processing and Awareness

Phoneme-Blending Test. The individual phonemes in a word were presented to the subject to put together into a word (e.g. the following question was stated in Spanish: *What word is formed with the sounds* /s/, /a/, *and* /l/? The subject had to answer *sal* 'salt'; maximum score = 12).

Phoneme-Deletion Test. A word was read, and the subject was asked how it would sound if a sound were omitted (e.g. the following statement was made in Spanish: *If in the word* /gol/ *the sound* /l/ *were deleted, how would it sound?* The correct answer was *go*; maximum score = 12).

Phoneme-Segmentation Test. The subject was asked how many and which sounds were included in a word (e.g. the following question was stated in Spanish: *Which sounds are included in the word* /mesa/? The correct answer was: four sounds /m/, /e/, /s/, and /a/; maximum score = 12).

Naming Test

Eighteen drawings (Snodgrass & Vanderwart, 1980), previously standardized according to middle and high frequency of occurrence nouns in Spanish, were used. Correct answers and naming time were scored (maximum score = 18).

Reading of Words and Pseudowords (Matute et al., in press)

Reading of Words. A card containing eight words (three to eight letters) was used. Correct reading and time were scored (maximum score = 8).

Reading of Pseudowords. A card containing eight pseudowords (three to eight letters) was used. Correct reading and time were scored (maximum score = 8).

The score obtained in the NEUROPSI Reading task was used as an indicator of reading understanding.

Procedures and statistical analyses

Testing was conducted in a single session, lasting about 60 min. The participants were divided into three groups according to their performance in the *NEUROPSI*: normal, moderately abnormal, and severely abnormal neuropsychological performance. ANOVAs were performed and a Tukey post hoc analysis was used to compare groups. Bonferroni corrections were performed and a statistical level of significance was set at $p < 0.05$. Finally, to analyze the contribution of phonological and naming skills to adequate word decoding and reading comprehension, a multiple linear regression analysis was performed. The regression model used oral reading comprehension (from the *NEUROPSI*), oral reading of words, and oral reading of pseudowords scores as dependent variables and the *NEUROPSI* subtest scores as independent variables.

Results

NEUROPSI scores (Table 19.2) for the literacy groups showed that 201 participants (84.5%) scored in the normal range (68–94 points), 25 participants (about 11%) had scores corresponding to a moderately abnormal range (54–67), and 12 participants (5%) scored as severely abnormal (41 or below). When comparing the three groups, statistically significant differences were observed in 19 scores between the normal and moderately abnormal and severe groups: orientation in person, digits backward, visual detection, 20 minus 3, naming, repetition, similarities, calculus, left and right hand position, alternate movements, opposite reactions, copy and recall of a figure, and verbal memory (free recall and cueing). Intrusions in encoding and recalling of words significantly increased in the moderately abnormal and severe groups.

Regarding phonological processing, that is, tasks including naming and reading subtests administered to the literacy program group ($n = 238$) (Table 19.3), naming ability decreased in the severe group, as suggested by the results for correct words produced and time taken to produce those words. Word reading ability was also inferior in those individuals with abnormal *NEUROPSI* scores. Reading of pseudowords, however, was similarly low in the three groups. Regarding instruction time, individuals from the moderately abnormal and severe groups showed longer previous schooling time as well as time spent in the INEA program than the normal group (Table 19.4).

Table 19.2 Illiterate group. Means, standard deviations, and differences among the three subgroups for NEUROPSI subtests ($n = 238$)

Subtest	Normal (n = 201)		Moderately abnormal (n = 25)		Severely abnormal (n = 12)		F	Level of significance	Differences among groups
	χ	sd	χ	sd	χ	sd			
Orientation									
Time	2.44	0.84	2.04	1.17	1.83	0.93	4.38	0.00	
Place	1.88	0.35	1.88	0.33	1.75	0.45	0.74	0.48	
Person	1.00	0.00	0.76	0.44	0.67	0.49	32.4	0.00	N vs. M, S
Attention									
Digits backwards	2.19	1.28	1.68	1.41	0.92	1.44	6.74	0.001	N vs. S
Visual detection	10.18	4.20	8.28	4.46	5.58	5.07	8.19	0.00	N vs. S
20 minus 3	2.84	1.99	1.50	1.89	1.17	1.70	8.49	0.00	N vs. M, S
Encoding									
Verbal memory (VM)	4.17	0.88	3.88	0.83	3.67	0.78	2.96	0.05	
VM: intrusions	0.71	1.22	0.92	1.12	1.75	1.76	4.13	0.01	N vs. S
Copy of a figure	8.46	2.16	7.18	3.17	4.79	3.19	16.27	0.00	N vs. M, S

(Continued)

Table 19.2 (*Continued*)

Language									
Naming	7.58	0.63	7.20	0.65	6.58	0.79	16.51	0.00	N vs. M, S
Repetition	3.85	0.36	3.72	0.46	3.25	1.14	10.86	0.00	N, M vs. S
Comprehension	4.24	1.18	3.72	1.06	3.58	1.37	3.79	0.02	
Semantic fluency	13.34	4.04	11.36	4.19	11.08	4.37	4.07	0.01	
Letter fluency	3.30	3.23	2.12	2.72	2.17	3.33	2.09	0.12	
Reading	0.94	2.49	0.24	0.59	0.50	1.00	1.16	0.31	
Writing; dictation	0.12	0.32	0.08	0.27	0.17	0.39	0.30	0.73	
Writing; copy	0.18	0.39	0.12	0.33	0.00	0.00	1.59	0.21	
Conceptual functions									
Similarities	2.98	1.72	1.96	1.62	2.33	2.33	4.32	0.01	N vs. M
Calculus	1.20	1.06	0.84	0.99	0.33	0.49	4.95	0.00	N vs. S
Sequences	0.22	0.42	0.04	0.20	0.00	0.00	3.92	0.02	
Motor functions									
Left hand position	0.69	0.76	0.32	0.62	0.33	0.65	3.83	0.02	N vs. M
Right hand position	0.83	0.77	0.32	0.56	0.33	0.49	7.34	0.00	N vs. M

(*Continued*)

Table 19.2 (*Continued*)

Subtest	Normal (n = 201)		Moderately abnormal (n = 25)		Severely abnormal (n = 12)		F	Level of significance	Differences among groups
	χ	sd	χ	sd	χ	sd			
Alternate movements	0.89	0.71	0.28	0.46	0.67	0.78	9.04	0.00	N vs. M
Opposite reactions	1.39	0.62	1.04	0.73	1.17	0.72	3.74	0.02	N vs. M
Recall									
VM	2.69	2.12	1.56	1.85	1.50	1.68	4.78	0.00	N vs. M
VM: intrusions	0.71	1.22	0.84	1.70	1.67	1.62	3.04	0.04	N vs. S
Cueing	3.16	1.18	2.04	1.59	1.0	1.21	12.11	0.00	N vs. M, S
Recognition	5.46	1.12	5.24	1.50	4.82	1.78	1.73	0.17	
Recognition: intrusions	1.02	1.73	2.24	3.11	2.82	3.09	7.82	0.00	N vs. M, S
Recall of a figure	6.86	2.62	5.20	2.40	3.95	3.38	10.41	0.00	N vs. M, S

χ, mean; N, normal; M, moderately abnormal; S, severely abnormal

Table 19.3 Illiterate group. Means, standard deviations and differences among the three subgroups in the phonological processing, naming and reading subtests ($n = 238$)

Subtest	Normal (n = 201)		Moderately abnormal (n = 25)		Severely abnormal (n = 12)		F	Level of significance	Differences among groups
	χ	sd	χ	sd	χ	sd			
Phonological processing									
Phoneme blending	2.29	3.52	0.90	2.17	1.00	2.09	2.14	0.11	
Phoneme deletion	4.50	4.42	2.70	3.56	3.18	4.35	1.91	0.14	
Phoneme segmentation	2.75	4.36	1.25	3.39	1.27	3.28	1.64	0.19	
Naming Test									
Correct	17.11	1.43	16.35	2.13	15.91	1.76	5.12	0.006	N vs. S
Time	41.9	29.9	43.4	25.3	67.8	35.9	3.56	0.030	N vs. S
Reading									
Words	5.09	3.17	3.10	3.59	3.45	3.05	4.66	0.01	N vs. M, S
Pseudowords	3.86	2.86	2.81	3.23	2.36	2.42	2.48	0.08	

χ, mean; N, normal; M, moderately abnormal; S, severely abnormal

Table 19.4 Illiterate group. Time at INEA and previous schooling. Means, standard deviations, and level of significance are presented

	Normal (n = 201)		Moderately abnormal (n = 25)		Severely abnormal (n = 12)		F	Level of significance	Differences among groups
	χ	sd	χ	sd	χ	sd			
Time at INEA	4.98	6.33	9.96	9.42	7.38	7.44	5.02	0.007	N vs. M, S
Previous schooling	14.50	21.25	30.27	33.91	42.45	39.19	9.12	0.000	N vs. M, S

χ, mean; N, normal; M, moderately abnormal; S, severely abnormal

Finally, multiple linear regression analyses were carried out for reading comprehension and adequate decoding skills, as measured by reading of single words and reading pseudowords (Table 19.5). Six variables were

Table 19.5 Illiterate group. Linear regression analysis for reading comprehension and adequate decoding skills

Variables	*Adjusted* **R** *square*	F	p
Reading comprehension			
NEUROPSI	0.278	50.999	0.000
Semantic fluency	0.308	29.864	0.000
Sequences	0.343	23.655	0.000
Orientation: time	0.372	20.225	0.000
Visual detection	0.391	17.712	0.000
Oral reading time	0.414	16.323	0.000
Reading of words			
NEUROPSI	0.300	102.664	0.000
Letter fluency	0.411	83.602	0.000
Orientation: time	0.451	66.011	0.000
Phoneme blending	0.486	57.130	0.000
Copy of a figure	0.514	51.098	0.000
Delayed Verbal Memory	0.516	53.902	0.000
Reading of pseudowords			
Phoneme segmentation	0.566	162.768	0.000
Letter fluency	0.678	131.793	0.000
NEUROPSI	0.734	114.811	0.000
Phoneme blending	0.757	97.483	0.000
Calculus	0.766	82.401	0.000
Delayed Verbal Memory	0.774	71.904	0.000
Naming	0.782	64.431	0.000

significant predictors of reading comprehension: *NEUROPSI* total score, visual detection, semantic fluency, sequences, orientation to time, and total reading time. For reading of single words, six variables were significant predictors: *NEUROPSI* total score, letter fluency, delayed verbal memory, phoneme blending, copy of a figure, and orientation to time; finally, the variables that best predicted the reading of pseudowords were: letter fluency, calculus, delayed verbal memory, phoneme segmentation, *NEU-ROPSI* total score, phoneme blending, naming, and calculus. Altogether, the seven variables accounted for 74% of the variance.

COGNIALFA: A Neuropsychologically Based Program for Teaching to Read

It was hypothesized that a teaching-to-read program directed to reinforce specific neuropsychological abilities having an impact on literacy acquisition could facilitate the learning-to-read process. Based on the above findings on the neuropsychological profile of adult illiterates and related research (Ardila *et al.*, 2000; Morais *et al.*, 1979), the abilities that should be most stimulated and reinforced include verbal memory, visuoperceptual abilities, and phonological processing. Furthermore, a successful teaching-to-read program should at best use personal and concrete information dealing directly with the learner's personal background and interests (Ardila *et al.*, 2000; also see Kayser & Centeno, ch. 2, this volume for pertinent discussion).

A teaching-to-read method called COGNIALFA was developed. It consisted of an instructor's manual and a reading book for the student. The instructor's manual included 55 exercises grouped in 12 lessons. Each lesson took about 3–4 hours, and each exercise took about one hour. The method can be accomplished in about four months, working three times weekly.

This teaching method attempts to emphasize those abilities in which illiterates frequently get low scores in common neuropsychological tests. These abilities are reinforced throughout the learning-to-read process, not in separate training sessions. The method includes the following types of exercises: (1) phonological awareness (phoneme discrimination, phonological similarity, decomposition of words into sounds and letters, grouping of words with common phonemes, and crossword puzzles), (2) attention and concentration (letter cancellation, discrimination of letters), (3) visual and verbal memory (encoding and retrieval), (4) language (acquisition of vocabulary, semantic associations, and text comprehension), and (5) executive functions (proverb interpretation, ordering of sentences and stories).

Method

Twenty illiterate individuals, the total enrollment at the INEA in Zacatecas, participated in the program. The sample was divided into two groups according to each teaching method, COGNIALFA and the *Palabra Generadora* (Table 19.6). The COGNIALFA group consisted of 9 individuals (7 men, 2 women; mean age: 32.33, SD 13.36), whereas the *Palabra Generadora* group included 11 participants (6 men, 5 women; mean age: 41.09, SD 15.46). All the participants had a normal performance in daily-life activities.

The tests applied to the sample were included in the *NEUROPSI* battery (Ostrosky *et al.*, 1997, 1999) as well as additional tasks including phoneme blending, phoneme deletion, phoneme segmentation, and naming and reading of words and pseudowords. They were individually administered to all participants before and after the learning-to-read programs in order to evaluate the efficiency of each teaching method.

Results

NEUROPSI scores before and after completing each learning-to-read training program were compared. In general, an increase in the scores is observed with both methods. However, improvement is stronger in the COGNIALFA group (Table 19.7).

An improvement was observed in 25 out of 36 subtests in the COGNIALFA group. Yet, a significant difference was only observed in reading comprehension, similarities, sequences, phoneme blending, phoneme segmentation, and time of naming. Similarly, 15 out of 36 subtests showed improvement, but only naming, hand position, and phoneme blending reached significant differences in the *Palabra Generadora* group.

Discussion and Conclusions

This study has shown that individuals with a lower performance in a neuropsychological test battery have learning difficulties or are slower learners than people presenting higher scores. Time at school was negatively associated with *NEUROPSI* scores. Obviously, the learning-disabled and slow learners spend a longer time learning to read and write. Having the *neuropsychological profile* could help them in avoiding frustration while spending many years trying to learn how to read and write before adequate diagnosis is made. Lower scores in the abnormal groups were observed, especially in motor, memory, and conceptual subtests. In the memory subtests, a significantly increased frequency of intrusions was observed.

Lower neuropsychological test performance has been additionally associated with difficulties in phonological processing. Our findings agree with other studies on illiterate adults showing that Portuguese-speaking

Table 19.6 General characteristics of the total sample participating in the COGNIALFA and Palabra Generadora learning-to-read programs

	n	NEUROPSI			Age		Gender		Handedness		Time at INEA (months)		Previous schooling (months)	
		N	M	S	χ	sd	M	F	RH	LH	χ	sd	χ	sd
Total sample	20	13	6	1	37.1	15.1	13	7	20	0	2.6	1.7	30.3	37.3
COGNIALFA	9	4	4	1	32.3	13.3	7	2	9	0	3.5	1.9	28.6	26.8
Palabra Generadora	11	9	2	0	41.0	15.4	6	5	11	0	1.9	1.3	31.6	29.0

N, normal; M, moderately abnormal; S, severely abnormal; χ, mean; M, male; F, female; RH, right handed; LH, left handed

Table 19.7 Means and standard deviations for the neuropsychological battery subtests before and after completing the COGNIALFA ($n = 9$) and Palabra Generadora programs ($n = 11$)

Subtest	COGNIALFA		Palabra Generadora	
	Pre-test x (sd)	Post-test x (sd)	Pre-test x (sd)	Post-test x (sd)
Orientation				
Time	1.67 (1.00)	1.89 (1.45)	2.36 (0.92)	2.27 (1.01)
Place	1.67 (0.71)	1.89 (0.33)	1.91 (0.30)	2.00 (0.00)
Person	0.89 (0.33)	1.00 (0.00)	0.91 (0.30)	0.91 (0.30)
Attention				
Digits backwards	1.95 (1.03)	1.89 (0.78)	2.00 (1.18)	2.36 (0.67)
Visual detection: correct	12.44 (3.13)	12.33 (3.81)	11.82 (4.60)	12.45 (2.73)
20 minus 3	2.22 (1.92)	2.33 (1.73)	2.36 (2.11)	3.09 (1.92)
Coding				
Verbal memory: correct	3.78 (0.67)	4.22 (0.67)	4.45 (0.52)	4.82 (0.75)
Copy of a figure	8.38 (2.92)	7.88 (2.48)	9.09 (1.90)	9.00 (2.52)
Language				
Naming	7.44 (1.01)	7.11 (1.27)	7.36 (0.67)	7.73 (0.47)*
Repetition	3.67 (0.50)	3.78 (0.67)	3.91 (0.30)	3.91 (0.30)

(Continued)

Table 19.7 (*Continued*)

Subtest	COGNIALFA		Palabra Generadora	
	Pre-test x (sd)	*Post-test x (sd)*	*Pre-test x (sd)*	*Post-test x (sd)*
Comprehension	3.67 (1.32)	4.44 (1.59)	5.18 (0.98)	4.45 (1.04)
Semantic fluency	10.89 (2.20)	11.33 (4.18)	15.27 (4.67)	13.09 (3.08)
Phonological fluency	2.44 (2.70)	4.67 (6.78)	2.82 (4.05)	2.45 (3.17)
Reading	0.87 (1.25)	1.89 (1.45)	0.73 (1.27)	1.00 (1.18)
Reading time	182.5 (88.4)	208.6 (97.7)	140 (95.26)	269.6 (233.1)
Conceptual functions				
Similarities	1.67 (1.50)	3.89 (2.03)*	3.82 (1.66)	2.73 (1.68)
Calculation abilities	0.56 (0.73)	1.22 (1.48)	1.27 (1.35)	1.36 (1.21)
Sequences	0.22 (0.44)	0.67 (0.50)*	0.36 (0.50)	0.36 (0.50)
Motor functions				
Hand position	1.89 (1.27)	2.67 (1.73)	0.64 (1.29)	2.09 (1.58)*
Alternating movements	1.00 (0.71)	1.22 (0.67)	0.91 (0.54)	1.36 (0.50)
Opposite reactions	1.33 (0.50)	1.56 (0.73)	1.64 (0.50)	1.27 (0.47)

(*Continued*)

Table 19.7 (*Continued*)

Recall			
Recall of a figure	6.72 (3.02)	7.50 (1.88)	8.04 (1.87)	8.09 (2.51)
Words: correct	2.89 (1.83)	3.67 (1.58)	3.27 (1.62)	3.27 (2.24)
Cueing	2.56 (1.94)	3.11 (2.03)	3.55 (0.93)	3.64 (2.11)
Recognition: correct	5.67 (0.71)	5.78 (0.44)	5.91 (0.30)	5.18 (1.60)
NEUROPSI	74.88 (13.40)	81.61 (14.66)	83.81 (12.12)	85.54 (13.73)
Other tests				
Phonemic blending	5.50 (3.82)	8.56 (3.91)*	6.56 (3.43)	8.55 (3.17)*
Phonemic deletion	0.29 (0.76)	4.22 (5.43)	1.44 (2.96)	2.36 (3.91)
Phonemic segmentation	2.63 (3.54)	6.56 (5.64)*	2.67 (4.77)	3.36 (4.46)
Naming	17.00 (2.00)	17.11 (1.62)	17.64 (0.67)	17.64 (0.50)
Naming time	55.55 (17.93)	29.25 (8.68)*	38.81 (18.53)	37.90 (25.76)
Reading of words	4.86 (3.48)	4.67 (3.64)	4.89 (3.30)	4.64 (3.04)
Reading of words time	61.33 (45.52)	64.50 (66.84)	51.12 (25.65)	64.77 (42.66)
Reading of pseudowords	3.43 (3.05)	4.44 (3.54)	4.00 (3.12)	3.27 (3.13)
Reading of pseudowords time	61.83 (26.27)	69.12 (71.07)	69.25 (37.02)	90.88 (67.07)

*Statistically significant differences $p > 0.05$ between pre-test and post-test

χ, mean

illiterates can perform very poorly in phoneme deletion (e.g. take away the first sound of *porto*: *orto*) and short-term verbal recall tasks (Morais *et al.*, 1979). Of course, enhanced performance in phoneme awareness tasks may also be a consequence of learning to read, as the relationship seems to be reciprocal (Swank & Larrivee, 1998). Further, difficulties in phonological awareness have been thought to be secondary to verbal short-term memory among English readers (Pennington *et al.*, 1991). Thus, phonological awareness and short-term verbal memory may be associated.

Several studies have additionally revealed that single-word-decoding problems in poor readers of different ages, including children, adolescents, and adults, can be primarily associated with problems segmenting words and syllables into phonemes (Pratt & Brady, 1998; Shaywitz, 1996; Stanovich & Siegel, 1994). Results of our stepwise regression analysis support the assumption that *high scores in neuropsychological tests and phonological processing tasks* represent important predictors of decoding skills. Recall that, when reading words and pseudowords, several variables emerged as significant predicting factors including phoneme segmentation, letter fluency, phoneme blending, delayed verbal memory, naming (time), and total NEUROPSI score.

These data support the notion that, in order to become a proficient decoder, individuals have to learn the rules for relating sound structures to print. They also have to become aware and remember that words have internal structures, based on the sounds represented by the alphabet. Some of these skills involved separating words into constituent phonemes (phoneme segmentation) while others involved putting phonemes together into words (phoneme blending). Particularly, the association between phonological awareness and the total NEUROPSI scores deserves special consideration because it may suggest that phonological processing represents a predictor of a verbal cognitive level. Phonological awareness, as a matter of fact, is a *metalinguistic (metacognitive) ability*, which may be informative about language awareness and ability to use language (see Swank & Larrivee, 1998). Indeed, though multiple interacting factors have been identified in the process of learning to read (see Catts & Kamhi, 2005, for review), our findings are in line with the compelling evidence supporting that phonemic awareness is an important psycholinguistic component in reading development (see Swank & Larrivee, 1998; Torgesen *et al.*, 2005; also see Kayser & Centeno, ch. 2, this volume).

Regarding the high reading comprehension scores, several factors, including semantic fluency, measures of attention as well as accuracy and fluency (as reflected in total reading time), were significant predictors of adequate reading comprehension. These findings reflect the *multivariate complexity* of poor reading comprehension.

It may be conjectured that, even though illiteracy may be associated with a diversity of factors, two major variables can be distinguished. First, on one hand, socioeconomic factors play a fundamental role in illiteracy in Mexico and, undoubtedly, in any country (also see Kayser & Centeno, ch. 2, this volume for related discussion). Most illiterate people never had the opportunity to attend school and to learn to read. They can function appropriately in their routine environment with minimal or no literacy demands. Yet, they can learn to read and write if the opportunity is provided. According to our results, this illiterate subgroup may represent about 80– 90% of illiterates in Mexico. Second, illiteracy, on the other hand, is also associated with learning disabilities, and increased frequency of neurological abnormalities. Interestingly, in our sample, the abnormal groups (according to the *NEUROPSI* scores) had significantly lower scores in all the motor ability subtests, suggesting subtle neurological abnormalities. By the same token, intrusions in the memory subtests were significantly increased, particularly in the moderate and severe groups. Intrusions in memory tests are usually regarded as abnormal, pointing to some inability to separate memory traces, and frequently found in confused and disoriented individuals (Ostrosky *et al.*, 1997).

Regarding the findings of the learning-to-read methods, the COGNI-ALFA group obtained better post-test scores than the *Palabra Generadora* cohort. Such differences may arise because the COGNIALFA method focuses on the knowledge of a system of visual symbols and a system of equivalence between graphemes and phonemes. That is, the COGNIALFA directs the learner's attention to a sequential string of graphemes and the spatial organization and phonological equivalence of those symbols. It also emphasizes the abilities required in oral and written comprehension, such as phonological discrimination, verbal memory, and morphological and lexical associations. In contrast, the *Palabra Generadora* method emphasizes practice in coding and decoding of isolated phonemes. Furthermore, the COGNIALFA method included more participants with an altered profile, as measured by the *NEUROPSI*, than the other group.

Some caution should be stated with regard to our current results. Previous time spent at school (and probable socioeconomic levels and possibly unreported medical conditions) cannot be ruled out as confounders in poor performance. Some other uncontrolled variables, such as familiarity with the testing situation, attitude toward testing, cultural values, etc., may have also impacted the observed results. Indeed, test-taking strategies may be culturally determined, hence having an impact on research results (see Centeno & Gingerich, ch. 8, this volume).

All in all, some important implications emerge from our study with special relevance to those professionals who diagnose and treat reading-disabled or illiterate individuals. Our results point out that it is possible to identify the cognitive profile of adult individuals with normal and abnormal learning and literacy abilities through a brief *neuropsychological evaluation*. Specific learning-to-read programs can be developed for such individuals focusing on phonological awareness, memory strategies, and some executive function abilities; that is, those abilities required to learn to read successfully, and found to be insufficient in learning-disabled persons. Further, our findings support the assumption that *direct training and reinforcement* of those abilities in which illiterates significantly underperform will result in a significant improvement in neuropsychological test scores. Recall that improvement was observed in various cognitive domains, but especially in phonemic abilities, determining similarities, naming, and reading comprehension. Hence, knowledge of brain–behavior correlations can help us to better understand the possible cognitive–verbal interactions important in learning and instruction, and plan suitable remedial programs. Our findings and implications, based on monolingual Spanish-speaking illiterates, may provide useful theoretical and clinical grounds to investigators and practitioners working with other illiterate populations.

Acknowledgements

This research was partially supported by a grant given to Dr. Feggy Ostrosky-Solís, Laboratory of Psychophysiology and Neuropsychology, National University of Mexico, by the Consejo Nacional de Ciencia y Tecnología (CONACYT-38570-H) and the Programa de Apoyo a Proyectos de Investigación e Innovación Tecnológica (PAPIIT IN -308500.)

References

Ardila, A., Ostrosky-Solís, F. and Mendoza, V. (2000) Learning to read is much more than learning to read: A neuropsychologically-based learning to read method. *Journal of the International Neuropsychological Society* 6, 789–801.
Ardila, A., Rosselli, M. and Rosas, P. (1989) Neuropsychological assessment in illiterates: Visuospatial and memory abilities. *Brain and Cognition* 11, 147–166.
Catts, H.W. and Kamhi, A.G. (2005) Causes of reading disabilities. In H.W. Catts and A.G. Kamhi (eds) *Language and Reading Disabilities* (2nd edn, pp. 94–126). Boston, MA: Pearson.
Goldblum, M.C. and Matute, E. (1986) Are illiterate people deep dyslexics? *Journal of Neurolinguistics* 2, 103–114.
Instituto Nacional de Educación para los Adultos (2001) *Dirección de Planeación y Evaluación*. México: Instituto Nacional de Educación para los Adultos.
Lecours, R.L., Mehler, J., Parente, M.A., Caldeira, A., Cary, L., Castro, M.J., Dehaout, F., Delgado, R., Gurd, J., Karmann, D., Jakubovitz, R., Osorio, Z., Cabral, L.S. and Junqueira, M. (1987) Illiteracy and brain damage I: Aphasia testing in culturally contrasted populations (control subjects). *Neuropsychologia* 25, 231–245.
Manly, J.J., Jacobs, D.M., Sano, M., Bell, K., Merchant, C.A., Small, S.A. and Stern, Y. (1999) Effect of literacy on neuropsychological test performance in

non-demented, education-matched elders. *Journal of the International Neuropsychological Society* 5, 191– 202.

Matute, E., Leal, F., Zarabozo, D., Robles, A. and Cedillo, C. (2000) Does literacy have an effect on stick construction tasks? *Journal of the International Neuropsychological Society* 6, 668– 672.

Matute, E., Rosselli, M., Ardila, A. and Ostrosky, F. (in press) *Examen Neuropsicológico Infantil*. Guadalajara: Universidad de Guadalajara.

Morais, J., Cary, L., Alegría, J. and Bertelson, P. (1979) Does awareness of speech as a sequence of phones arise spontaneously? *Cognition* 7, 323– 331.

Ostrosky, F., Ardila, A. and Rosselli, M. (1997) *NEUROPSI: Una Batería Neuropsicológica Breve*. Mexico, D.F: Laboratorios Bayer.

Ostrosky, F., Ardila, A. and Rosselli, M. (1999) NEUROPSI: A brief neuropsychological test battery in Spanish. *Journal of the International Neuropsychological Society* 5, 413– 433.

Ostrosky, F., Ardila, A., Rosselli, M., López-Arango, G. and Uriel-Mendoza, V. (1998) Neuropsychological test performance in illiterates. *Archives of Clinical Neuropsychology* 13, 645– 660.

Ostrosky-Solís, F., Ramírez, M., Lozano, A., Picasso, H. and Velez, A. (2004) Culture or education: Neuropsychological test performance of a Maya indigenous population. *International Journal of Psychology* 39, 36– 46.

Pennington, B., Van Orden, G., Kirson, D. and Haith, M. (1991) What is causal relation between verbal STM problems and dyslexia? In S.A. Brady and D.P. Shankweiler (eds) *Phonological Processes in Literacy: A Tribute to Isabelle Y. Liberman* (pp. 173– 186). Hillsdale, NJ: Lawrence Erlbaum.

Pratt, A.C. and Brady, S. (1998) Relation of phonological awareness to reading disability in children and adults. *Journal of Educational Psychology* 80, 19– 323.

Reis, A. and Castro-Caldas, A. (1997) Illiteracy: A cause for biased cognitive development. *Journal of the International Neuropsychological Society* 5, 444– 450.

Rosselli, M. (1993) Neuropsychology of illiteracy. *Behavioral Neurology* 6, 107– 112.

Rosselli, M., Ardila, A. and Rosas, P. (1990) Neuropsychological assessment in illiterates II: Language and praxic abilities. *Brain and Cognition* 12, 281– 296.

Shaywitz, S.E. (1996) Dyslexia. *Scientific American* 7, 98– 104.

Snodgrass, J. and Vanderwart, M. (1980) A standardized set of 260 pictures: Norms for name agreement, image agreement, familiarity and visual complexity. *Journal of Experimental Psychology: Human Learning and Memory* 6, 174– 215.

Stanovich, K.E. and Siegel, L.S. (1994) Phenotypic performance profiles of children with reading disabilities: A regression-based test of the phonological-core variable difference model. *Journal of Educational Psychology* 86, 24– 53.

Swank, L.K. and Larrivee, L.S. (1998). Phonology, metaphonology, and the development of literacy. In R. Paul (ed.) *Exploring the Speech-Language Connection* (pp. 253– 297). Baltimore: Paul H. Brookes.

Torgesen, J.K., Al Otaiba, S. and Grek, M.L. (2005) Assessment and instruction for phonemic awareness and word recognition skills. In H.W. Catts and A.G. Kamhi (eds) *Language and Reading Disabilities* (2nd edn, pp. 127– 156). Boston, MA: Pearson.

Vygotsky, L.S. (1962) *Thought and Language*. Cambridge, MA: MIT Press.

Chapter 20

Phonetic Descriptions of Speech Production in Bilingual Speakers: Empirical Evidence and Clinical Considerations

FREDERICKA BELL-BERTI

Speech assessment of persons who sound different from the typical speech norms of a community, such as children mispronouncing sounds or words as they develop speech, second-language learners, or persons with acquired speech disorders, has traditionally been done perceptually. That is, assessment essentially has relied on the evaluator's ability to identify the nature of the difference (e.g. substitution, distortion, or omission). The difficulty with this method is that we cannot trust our ears when relying on this approach, in part, because our perception of speech is influenced by our native language, but also because of our tendency to identify the speech we hear categorically (Liberman *et al.*, 1967). As to the first point, even if the speech-language clinician's native language differs from that of the client, the clinician's perception of the client may be tainted by the language the client does not fully have. That is, a person's identification of speech sounds is influenced by the language set in which they are heard (Bohn & Flege, 1993). As to the second point (even when a speaker and listener have all languages in common), the listener's ability even to notice some fairly substantial acoustical differences between speech features is lacking (Lisker & Abramson, 1970).

When acquiring a first (L1) and a second language (L2), learners' mastery of L2 speech depends on many factors (Leather & James, 1996, Piske *et al.*, 2001; also see Centeno, ch. 3, this volume). Of all factors, maturational age-related processes have commonly been implicated as a major constraint (Piske *et al.*, 2001). However, though young learners tend to outperform older individuals in the acquisition of L2 speech skills, this does not mean that accent-free speech is guaranteed for learners before puberty (Yavaş, 1998). Other variables besides age, such as motivation, social acceptance/distance, and perceptual capacities (Leather & James, 1996), similarly contribute to the development of native-like speech production. Yet, in learning a second language that contains phonemes that do not occur in the learners' L1, some persons may substitute – or appear to substitute – sounds of their L1 for those L2 sounds. Thus, for example, the L1 French speaker may appear to substitute the alveolar fricatives /s/ and /z/ (which occur in both French and English) for the English phonemes /θ/and /ð/, and the L1 speaker of Spanish may appear to substitute /i/ for the English phoneme /ɪ/.

However, some apparent substitutions may actually involve distortions of the native production of the L2 phonemes; with the second-language learner trying to approximate the native production but falling short of that goal, and the native listener identifying the production as the phoneme it most closely resembles. It is beyond the length and scope of this chapter to discuss the multiple factors in speech development or issues concerning perception of L2 speakers' production by native listeners, the perception of L2 sounds by the second-language speaker, or how perception may limit L2 speakers' ability to produce those sounds. For a discussion of these issues, see, for example, Flege (1993), Leather and James (1996), and Yavaş (1998).

The purpose of this chapter is to propose some strategies for the objective evaluation of the speech of and intervention for bilingual speakers who acquired English (L2) in the context of successive (sequential) bilingualism; that is, after they had acquired considerable skills in their L1 (see Centeno, ch. 3, this volume). Unlike simultaneous bilinguals (i.e. children acquiring both L1 and L2 at the same time from early in development), successive bilinguals tend to have a stronger L1 effect on their L2 speech (Leather & James, 1996; Yavaş, 1998). Successive bilingual environments are often identified as second language acquisition (SLA), foreign language (FL) learning, or, when English is the target L2, English as a Second Language (ESL).

The approach in this chapter is in contrast to the phonological perspective on young bilingual children who are simultaneously exposed to both languages (see Goldstein, ch. 13, this volume). Throughout this chapter, reference is to the acquisition of English as an L2. Though research in Spanish–English bilinguals will be emphasized, pertinent data and discussions on other bilingual groups will also be included for illustration. Further, the reader is advised to refer to the earlier discussion of phonological contrasts between Spanish and English in this book (i.e. Anderson & Centeno, ch. 1), as that content complements the information in this chapter.

Essentially, this chapter is guided by the premise that clinical analysis and decisions made about speech services are enhanced by both empirical and theoretical bases (see, e.g. Ball & Gibbon, 2002; Yavaş, 1998). Focusing on articulatory (speech production) and acoustic (acoustic nature of produced sounds) phonetic considerations, this chapter surveys speech assessment methods based on research procedures and evidence; methods that should facilitate the *objective analysis* of the ways in which the speech of successive bilingual (i.e. ESL/FL/SLA) speakers differs from that of a native English speaker. This chapter concludes by bringing that information into an applied clinical context, particularly highlighting that successive bilinguals seeking speech services may show *speech differences* (due to L1 effects on L2) and/or *genuine speech disorders* (due to pathological circumstances, such as motoric/muscular complications). Most – but not all – of the methods discussed here offer objective measures of speech, whether of *segmental characteristics* (i.e. measures of features of individual speech sounds) or *suprasegmental characteristics* (i.e. measures of those features that convey prosodic information).

Describing the Speech of Bilingual Speakers: Preliminaries

Speech may be evaluated with subjective and with objective measures, the former involving judgments of speech made by listeners and the latter involving physical measures of the acoustical result of speech articulation. Physiological measures are also possible objective measures, but by their generally invasive nature are not, at this time, generally available for the clinical evaluation of the speech. The most common subjective assessment techniques are the phonetic description of speech by the clinician and judgments of speech by listeners. Among the objective measurements of speech available are spectral analysis (i.e. frequency analysis) components of speech segments (particularly vowels and continuant consonants – fricatives, approximants, nasals), the temporal analysis of speech segments (including, e.g. segment duration and relative timing of acoustical markers), and spectral–temporal analysis of prosodic characteristics (including intonation and syllable stress).

The use of objective evaluation tools by the speech-language clinician should make it possible for the clinician to identify the nature of differences identified auditorily (e.g. why a particular vowel sounds inappropriately produced, as when a native speaker of Spanish is understood to have commented on a baseball game and not the weather when he said 'The [hit] was tremendous'). They should also make it possible to determine that there actually are no differences when differences are expected (e.g. in productions that seem to reflect the use of a single phonological unit where two – or more – are expected, as when a native speaker of Spanish fails to distinguish between *they* and *day* due to phonemic underdifferentiation. In Spanish, /d/ is a phoneme with two conditioned variants: [d] occurs in word-initial position and after /n/, [ð] occurs in intervocalic position, Yavaş, 1998).

Subjective assessment

Native speakers of a language are known to be good detectors of a foreign accent (Flege, 1984), and have been shown to be sensitive to aspects of syllable structure and segmental articulation as well as both phrasal and lexical stress (Magen, 1998; Wayland, 1997). But in order to address accent issues, one must first determine what is actually different about a person's speech. This process most naturally begins with the careful – albeit subjective – phonetic description of the speech by trained observers (e.g. phoneticians or speech-language pathologists). The observer should begin by creating a detailed phonetic transcription of elicited speech samples that have been chosen to allow the determination of the kinds of differences occurring between the prevailing speech pattern and that of the individual whose speech is being considered. Such differences may involve the apparent addition, substitution or distortion, and/or deletion of segments (e.g. a native Spanish speaker, only having /i/ in L1, would say [hit] for /hɪt/; and not having /sp/ structures in the word-initial position would say [ɛspɛl] for /spɛl/), as well as differences in stress and/or intonation pattern (e.g. /ˈɑbˌdʒɛkt/ for /əbˈdʒɛkt/).

Objective assessment

Detailed phonetic transcription, however, is not enough, because phonetic description relies on human perception of speech, and although we can improve our ability to identify many different acoustic events as different, we cannot entirely escape the limitations imposed by our auditory systems and the rules of our native languages. For example, we may not be able to rely on our perception to say whether the vowel in *he's* is qualitatively different from that of *his* (the difference may be quantitative; i.e. temporal – a difference in vowel duration); or that the initial consonant of *thumb* transcribed as *some* is spectrally the same as the first consonant of *summer*. Furthermore, what we might perceive as rising (or yes–no question) intonation may result from the absence of the expected amount of F0 fall, or that what appears to be errors of syllable stress may be no more than vowels whose durations exceed those expected (as may be the case with speakers whose first language is a syllable-timed language, in which all syllables are of approximately equal duration). Examples of observed speech and appropriate acoustic analyses are provided in Table 20.1.

Subjective and objective assessment

It is important to note here that the point is *not* that phonetics is useless; indeed, phonetics is what we hear. In all situations in which we are trying to understand the nature of the difference between the ambient pattern and that of a particular talker, we use our perception to identify the phonetic events we are interested in understanding. Thus, phonetic analysis is a necessary part of acoustic and articulatory studies – the starting point of our examination of speech. Furthermore, all the studies in speech acoustics and articulation are meaningless without reference to

Table 20.1 Examples of phonetic analysis and acoustic analysis that may inform understanding of underlying articulatory events, based on Spanish–English bilinguals as target client group

Phonetic analysis	*Acoustic analysis*
Segmental errors	
Substitutions Perceive: *he's* for *his* and /i/ for /ɪ/ in other contexts *den* for *then* and *tin* for *thin* /dɛn/ instead of /ðɛn/ *Some* for *thumb* and *zen* for *then*	Compare formant frequency and duration measures of *he's* and *his* Compare burst spectra and formant loci of /dɛn/with /ðɛ/dɛ.../ words; /tɪn/ with /θɪ.../ words /sʌm/ with /θʌ.../ words; /zɛn/ with /ðɛ.../ words
Insertions	
Perceive: *quiet* for *quite* /kwaɪɪt/ instead of /kwaɪt/ *estate* for *state* /ɛsteɪt/ instead of /steɪt/	Examine formant patterns for evidence of additional vowel resonances; measure the vowel durations in these and other contexts.
Intonation errors	
Question intonation in statements	Examine intonation (F0) contours
Stress errors	
Inappropriate syllable stress	
Perceive: *eleven* for *elephant* /əˈlɛvɪn/ instead of /ˈɛləfənt/	Compare durations, amplitudes, and F0 of inappropriately stressed syllables with those of (minimally contrastive) appropriately stressed syllables

the actual phonetic events. The points, here, are that what and how we hear speech is influenced by the nature of speech perception and also that our perception of one language may be influenced by our experience with another language. Finally, one may objectify listener judgments by creating situations in which listeners are presented with speech samples in controlled formats with a great reduction in contextual cues.

In the sections below, only a small number of studies are mentioned – this is not intended as an exhaustive review, but rather as a starting point for considering the ways in which we may, most profitably, make use of acoustic analysis techniques to understand what speakers are actually doing and translate those principles into actual clinical situations. Some of the references are to studies of second-language learning; others are to studies of clinical disorders; yet others are to language comparisons – all provide examples of ways in which acoustic analysis is already used to evaluate speech.

Describing the Speech of Bilingual Speakers: Objective Measures

Traditional articulatory phonetics describes speech segments in terms of the amount of vocal tract constriction used in producing sounds and the location of that constriction along the vocal tract. For consonants, these are the features of consonant manner and place of articulation; for vowels these are the features of tongue height (or vowel openness) and tongue advancement. There is an additional feature for each of these two segmental groups: voicing for consonants and lip position for vowels. The following sections provide examples of studies reporting objective measurements of the acoustical signal related to these descriptive dimensions.

Objective measures: Consonants

Consonant voicing, place, and manner of articulation may be evaluated acoustically. Some of these speech characteristics have frequently been examined in the speech of learners in SLA contexts while others have been examined less often. Among the most frequently studied characteristic is the voicing of stop consonants in initial position, examined using the *Voice Onset Time* (VOT) measure reported by Lisker and Abramson (1964) in their landmark paper. Indeed, this measure (of the duration of the interval between the release of stop consonant occlusion and the beginning of the voicing signal) has been one of the most widely used tools for the study of the speech of second-language learners, persons with neurological disorders, and children with developmental language and articulation disorders (e.g. Ackermann & Hertrich, 1997; Bond & Wilson, 1980; Caruso & Burton, 1987). For example, studies of bilingual speakers (e.g. Flege, 1987b; Flege & Eefting, 1987; Hazan & Boulakis, 1993) have shown that speakers' L2 VOT values may be influenced by their L1 VOT values, resulting in a shift of L2 VOT values towards those of the L1, or that bilingual speakers may use L1 VOT values when speaking L2 (Flege & Port, 1981). In addition, VOT research has yielded important evidence on possible maturational influences in bilingual speech acquisition. Flege (1991) showed that bilingual persons who learn L2 as young children may develop VOT categories for L2 that are indistinguishable from those of monolingual speakers. Similarly, Yavaş (1996) reported that, though late Spanish–English bilinguals (i.e. those Spanish speakers who started learning English around 12 years of age) had lower English VOT values than early Spanish–English bilinguals (i.e. those Spanish speakers who started learning English in preschool/school age), English VOT values in the late bilingual learners were still within the native English VOT range. These results suggest that acquisition of native speech qualities may diminish but not be completely lost with age.

Acoustical analysis can also be used to evaluate spectral and temporal characteristics of consonant production unrelated to stop voicing. The results of a study of the English liquid consonants /r/ and /l/ produced by native speakers of Japanese (Flege *et al.*, 1995) challenge the view that adult L2 speakers cannot learn to produce phonetic segments that do not occur in their native language (i.e. learning the phonetic patterns of a language has the same age constraints as learning the semantic and syntactic components – see, e.g. Flege, 1987a). The results of a study of the effectiveness of treatment for /w/ for /r/ substitution revealed changes in F2 frequency and transition rate towards values appropriate for /r/ (Huer, 1989). Furthermore, the changes in F2 frequency and transition rate were not always associated with changes in the clinician's perception, reinforcing the importance of having objective measures of speech. In fact, this latter finding underscores the need of similar studies in which comparisons between clinicians' perception and acoustical (i.e. objective) measures are made.

The influence of L1 phonotactic constraints on L2 productions may also be examined acoustically. For example, Flege and his colleagues (Flege, 1993; Flege *et al.*, 1992) have shown that native speakers of languages that have a stop-voicing contrast in initial but not final position may have difficulty producing the contrast in final position in the L2. Another phonotactic influence may be evident when native speakers of languages that do not allow consonant clusters produce L2 utterances with vowel insertions (e.g. the native Spanish speaker who may produce English *stop* as [ɛstɑp]).

Objective measures: Vowels

Vowels may vary from each other in spectral and/or temporal characteristics. The spectral properties of vowels (including formant frequencies and bandwidths) are determined by the size and shape of the vocal tract (Fant, 1970; Stevens & House, 1955). The sources of intrinsic temporal differences among vowels (of English, at least), however, are very complex, as they involve the interaction of coarticulatory contextual factors (e.g. consonant environment, syllable structure and number: VC, CVC, CVCCVC, etc.), speaking rate (i.e. the faster the speech rate, the shorter the vowel duration), and prosody (e.g. phrase-final lengthening:

lengthening of the last stressable syllable in a major syntactic phrase or clause) (Lisker, 1974; Shriberg & Kent, 1995). Languages differ in the sizes of their vowel inventories; thus, for example, Spanish has five vowels, and American English has at least 15 vowels, including rhotics as well as monophthongal and diphthongal vowels (see Anderson & Centeno, ch. 1, for related discussion).

Understanding the ways in which an L2 speaker's vowels differ from those of native speakers may be gained from comparisons of the formant frequency and duration patterns of the L2 speaker's vowels with those of native speakers. English vowels differ in spectral and temporal characteristics; that is, English does not have vowels that differ only in quality (spectral pattern) or only in quantity (duration). Native English speakers often perceive L2 speakers of English as having substituted one vowel for a spectral neighbor (resulting, e.g. in *hit* being perceived as *heat* or *bet* as *bait*). Flege *et al.* (1997) studied the English vowels of native speakers of four languages, languages with vowel inventories that contrast with that of English in different ways (e.g. languages that do not have some of the vowel quality differences of English – no /i/ versus /ɪ/ contrast, or no /ɛ/ versus /æ/ contrast; or that have vowel quantity contrasts – /i/ versus /iː/). Their results support the notion that L2 speakers' vowel productions are influenced by their L1 vowel systems, their experience with L2, and their perception of L2 vowels. More recent data reported by Lydtin *et al.* (2004) on the vowels of Spanish–English bilingual speakers support the results of Flege *et al.* (1997). Similarly, in a study that reinforces the importance of acoustic analysis to provide a basis for accent modification, Munro (1993) reported that L2 vowel formant frequency measures were correlated with ratings of the speakers' accentedness.

Objective measures: Suprasegmentals

That languages differ in their native prosodic patterns is well known. Indeed, there has been some evidence that some infants learn the melody of their native language before they have produced their first words (Weir, 1966). Thus, the value of research on prosodic characteristics for developing methods for modifying foreign accent – that is, understanding how different languages convey meaning through prosody – is obvious.

Suprasegmental analyses of speech are complicated by the interaction between the segmental units and suprasegmental features, and also by the ways that different speakers realize the suprasegmental features (Harris, 1979). For example, in English different vowels have different intrinsic durations (e.g. Peterson & Lehiste, 1960) and the location of a syllable in an utterance affects its duration (e.g. Klatt, 1976). Also, some speakers increase syllable stress by increasing vowel duration, whereas other speakers may increase syllable stress by increasing vowel intensity (Harris, 1979). Hence, it is difficult to examine the effects of suprasegmental changes on the acoustical characteristics of speech.

In spite of the difficulties, however, some studies have managed to look at the effects of prosodic variations across languages. Swerts *et al.* (2002) compared Dutch and Italian to identify how these languages use accentuation in conveying new information. They found that the accentuation patterns in Italian were not important in distinguishing information status (new versus old information), whereas accentuation was a significant factor in conveying information status in Dutch. In a study of how native Spanish speakers fare with morphophonological alternations associated with shifting stress and vowel reduction (in such word pairs as *apply* and *application*), Flege and Bohn (1989) concluded that speakers learn the stress alternations more easily than vowel reduction, and that they may learn these stress-vowel reduction alternation patterns individually (i.e. word by word). Both of these studies reinforce the idea that, if one wants to help the L2 speaker convey information effectively, one must understand the prosody of the L1 to be able to focus training on those aspects of L2 most likely to be problematic – and also that one must objectively evaluate the speaker's L2 prosody to identify the individual speaker's difficulties.

Conclusion and Applications

This chapter aimed to survey phonetic considerations of speech production that may be used for the objective assessment of speech in ESL/FL/SLA speakers and its differences from the speech of a native English speaker. Most – but not all – of these methods offered objective measures of segmental or suprasegmental characteristics of speech. As was said above, this chapter aimed to point the speech-language clinician in the direction of research on bilingual speakers' speech production that can be used clinically to distinguish speech differences (due to L1 effects on L2) from genuine disorders (due to pathological circumstances, such as motoric/muscular complications). Hence, these principles may be valuable for accurate diagnostic and intervention decisions when addressing clients' needs for accent modification or when, for example, a bilingual client, who had a stroke, may exhibit both phonetic features due to his/her L1 and others that result from acquired neuromuscular conditions (e.g. Gurd *et al.*, 2001; Theron, 2003).

This discussion intended to spark the reader's imagination based on evidence and empirically based observations describing what bilingual speakers are actually doing with their articulators. Such an understanding is critical to the development of more objective and systematic diagnostic and treatment approaches and, in turn, to the resulting improvement in speech production.

Based on the discussed material, the following applications may be implemented:

- One approach that clinicians might use would be to obtain recordings of contrastive minimal word pairs (e.g. *heat* and *hit*, which are contrastive for /i/ and /ɪ/; *think* and *sink* contrastive for /θ/ and /s/; *bet* and *pet* contrastive for /b/ and /p/; *bet* and *bed* contrastive for /t/ and /d/) and subject the recordings to acoustic analysis and perceptual identification. One might also obtain recordings of phrases with minimum suprasegmental contrasts, perhaps using reiterant speech (Liberman & Streeter, 1978) in which the same syllable (e.g. *ma*) is substituted for each syllable in the utterance, thus providing material for the evaluation of prosodic components of speech. Such recordings may then be subjected to acoustical and perceptual analyses, in each case providing the clinician with an indication of communication ability and also allowing the clinician to identify the aspects of articulation to target in treatment. Such research may be done with tape recorders and acoustic analysis software packages available for microcomputers (PC or Macintosh).
- One may examine the ability of the ESL/FL/SLA speaker to produce the vowels of English by comparing formant frequencies and durations of the vowels in minimal pairs like *heat* and *hit* and also have listeners identify the words.
- One may examine the ability of the ESL/FL/SLA speaker to produce the fricatives of English by comparing the amplitude and frequency ranges of the frication in minimal pairs like *think* and *sink* and then also have listeners identify the words.
- One may examine the ability of the ESL/FL/SLA speaker to produce the distinctions between the voiced and voiceless stops of English by comparing the VOT measures of the initial stops in *bet* and *pet* and by comparing vowel durations for *bet* and *bed* and also have listeners identify the words.
- One might examine the ability of the ESL/FL/SLA speaker to produce the prosodic distinctions by measuring the fundamental frequency contours, segment durations, and signal amplitudes of the prosodically contrastive phrases/sentences, and having listeners identify the phrases/sentences and also identify which syllables receive stress.

When used in conjunction with typical speech assessment steps with bilingual speakers (e.g. Yavaş, 1998), it is hoped that the above discussions and suggested applications will be put to the test in clinical practice and serve as models for the development of strategies and ideas for future research. There remains a great paucity of research on L2 speech acquisition with clinical relevance in adult contexts (see Theron, 2003). At this stage, clinical efforts employing available empirical evidence and methodology may lead to improved approaches to assessing and treating speech in unimpaired (speech difference) or impaired (speech disorder) successive bilinguals and, thus, to evaluating clinical uses of collected evidence and to developing more fruitful research programs.

References

Ackermann, H. and Hertrich, I. (1997) Voice onset time in ataxic dysarthria. *Brain and Language* 56, 321–333.

Ball, M. and Gibbon, F.E. (2002) *Vowel Disorders*. Boston: Butterworth-Heinemann.

Bohn, O.-S. and Flege, J.E. (1993) Perceptual switching in Spanish/English bilinguals. *Journal of Phonetics* 21, 267–290.

Bond, Z.S. and Wilson, H.F. (1980) Acquisition of the voicing contrast language-delayed and normal-speaking children. *Journal of Speech and Hearing Research* 23, 152–161.

Caruso, A.J. and Burton, E.K. (1987). Temporal acoustic measures of dysarthria associated with amyotrophic lateral sclerosis. *Journal of Speech and Hearing Research* 30, 80–87.

Fant, C.G.M. (1970) *Acoustic Theory of Speech Production*. The Hague: Mouton.

Flege, J.E. (1984) The detection of French accent by American listeners. *Journal of the Acoustical Society of America* 76, 692–707.

Flege, J.E. (1987a) A critical period for learning how to produce foreign languages? *Applied Linguistics* 8, 163–177.

Flege, J.E. (1987b) Production and perception of English stops by native Spanish speakers. *Journal of Phonetics* 15, 67–83.

Flege, J.E. (1991) Age of learning affects the authenticity of voice-onset time (VOT) in stop consonants produced in a second language. *Journal of the Acoustical Society of America* 89, 395–411.

Flege, J.E. (1993) Production and perception of a novel, second language phonetic contrast. *Journal of the Acoustical Society of America* 93, 1589–1608.

Flege, J.E. and Bohn, O.-S. (1989) An instrumental study of vowel reduction and stress placement in Spanish-accented English. *Studies in Second Language Acquisition* 11, 35–62.

Flege, J.E., Bohn, O.-S. and Jang, S. (1997) Effects of experience on non-native speaker's production and perception of English vowels. *Journal of Phonetics* 25, 437–470.

Flege, J.E. and Eefting, W. (1987) Cross-language switching in stop consonant perception and production by Dutch speakers of English. *Speech Communication* 6, 185–202.

Flege, J.E., Munro, M.J. and Skelton, L. (1992) Production of the word-final English /t/-/d/ contrast by native speakers of English, Mandarin, and Spanish. *Journal of the Acoustical Society of America* 92, 128–142.

Flege, J.E. and Port, R. (1981) Cross-language phonetic interference: Arabic to English. *Language and Speech* 24, 125–246.

Flege, J.E., Tokagi, N. and Mann, V. (1995) Japanese adults can learn to produce English /r/ and /l/ accurately. *Language and Speech* 38, 25–55.

Gurd, J.M., Coleman, J.S., Costello, A. and Marshall, J.C. (2001) Organic or functional? A new case of foreign accent syndrome. *Cortex* 37, 715–718.

Harris, K.S. (1979) Vowel duration change and its underlying physiological mechanisms. *Language and Speech* 21, 354–361.

Hazan, V.L. and Boulakis, G. (1993) Perception and production of a voicing contrast by French–English bilinguals. *Language and Speech* 36, 17–38.

Huer, M.B. (1989) Acoustic tracking of articulation errors: [r]. *Journal of Speech and Hearing Disorders* 54, 530–534.

Klatt, D.H. (1976) Linguistic uses of segmental duration in English: Acoustic and perceptual evidence. *Journal of the Acoustical Society of America* 59, 1208–1221.

Leather, J. and James, A. (1996) Second language speech. In W.C. Ritchie and T.K. Bhatia (eds) *Handbook of Second Language Acquisition* (pp. 269–316). San Diego: Academic Press.

Liberman, A.M., Cooper, F.S., Shankweiler, D.P. and Studdert-Kennedy, M. (1967) Perception of the speech code. *Psychological Review* 74, 431–461.

Liberman, M.Y. and Streeter, L.A. (1978) Use of nonsense-syllable mimicry in the study of prosodic phenomena. *Journal of the Acoustical Society of America* 63, 231–233.

Lisker, L. (1974) On "explaining" vowel duration. *Glossa* 8, 233–246.

Lisker, L. and Abramson, A.S. (1964) A cross-language study of voicing in initial stops: Acoustical measurements. *Word* 20, 384–422.

Lisker, L. and Abramson, A.S. (1970) The voicing dimension: Some experiments in comparative phonetics. In *Proceedings of the Sixth International Congress of Phonetic Sciences, Prague, 1967* (pp. 563–567). Prague: Academia.

Lydtin, K.A., Bell-Berti, F., Jacobson, P.F. and Centeno, J.G. (2004) Relations between native Spanish speakers' perception and production of English vowels. *Journal of the Acoustical Society of America* 116, 2604.

Magen, H.S. (1998) The perception of foreign-accented speech. *Journal of Phonetics* 26, 381–400.

Munro, M.J. (1993) Productions of English vowels by native speakers of Arabic: acoustic measurements and accentedness ratings. *Language and Speech* 36, 39–66.

Peterson, G.E. and Lehiste, I. (1960) Duration of syllable nuclei in English. *Journal of the Acoustical Society of America* 32, 693–703.

Piske, T., MacKay, I.R.A. and Flege, J.E. (2001) Factors affecting degree of foreign accent in an L2: A review. *Journal of Phonetics* 29, 191–215.

Shriberg, L.D. and Kent, R.D. (1995) *Clinical Phonetics*. Boston, MA: Allyn and Bacon.

Stevens, K.N. and House, A.S. (1955) Development of a quantitative description of vowel articulation. *Journal of the Acoustical Society of America* 27, 484–493.

Swerts, M., Krahmer, E. and Avesani, C. (2002) Prosodic marking of information status in Dutch and Italian: A comparative analysis. *Journal of Phonetics* 30, 629–654.

Theron, K. (2003) Temporal aspects of speech production in bilingual speakers with neurogenic speech disorders. PhD thesis, University of Pretoria.

Wayland, R. (1997) Non-native production of Thai: Acoustic measurements and accentedness ratings. *Applied Linguistics* 18, 345–373.

Weir, R. (1966) Some questions on the child's learning of phonology. In F. Smith and G.A. Miller (eds) *The Genesis of Language: A Psycholinguistic Approach* (pp. 153–169). Cambridge: M.I.T. Press.

Yavaş, M. (1996) Differences in voice onset time in early and later Spanish–
    English bilinguals. In J. Jensen and A. Roca (eds) *Spanish in Contact: Issues in
    Bilingualism* (pp. 131–141). Someverville, MA: Cascadilla Press.
Yavaş, M. (1998) *Phonology Development and Disorders*. San Diego: Singular.

Epilogue

LORAINE K. OBLER

Already at the height of the Roman Empire, more than one dialect of Latin had developed (e.g. Herman, 2000). The daily speech would evolve, in Spain, into Spanish, and elsewhere into its sister languages, French, Portuguese, Romanian, and so forth. In medieval Spain, Spanish incorporated useful terms from Arabic, as Muslims, Jews, and Christians lived in culturally rich harmony for a period. Then, Columbus traveled, on behalf of the Spanish royals, to what became, for Europeans, the New World. Though he brought along a Hebrew-speaking translator to speak with those of the ten lost tribes he expected he might find, the native American languages proved many and their speakers vulnerable to much that Europe brought, so Spanish was introduced to the Western hemisphere where it has flourished and evolved over time, spoken as a first or second language throughout Latin America.

Beyond Latin America, the Spanish language and Latin culture continue to blossom widely in the USA, no longer only on the borders with Mexico or in vibrant urban centers, but throughout the country wherever immigrants and their descendants have settled. Demonstrating that one can retain core elements of one's culture of origin and the language that encapsulates them, Spanish-speakers in the USA manage to acculturate to a range of degrees with the mainstream culture, as a number of chapters in this volume remind us (e.g. Centeno & Gingerich, ch. 8; Brozgold & Centeno, ch. 5, this volume). In doing so, they enable us all to appreciate treasures of high culture (e.g. writers from Cervantes to García Márquez, the poet Anzaldúa, the playwright Machado, the composer Osvaldo, to name but a few) and of popular culture (e.g. Latin dancing, reggaetón [i.e. Spanish rap music], bilingual singers like Shakira, among so many others). The ramifications infuse the mainstream as well, as in Leonard Bernstein's *West Side Story*, in plantains in the salad-bars of Manhattan's Korean-owned delis, in burritos and their offspring, wraps, in burgeoning restaurants and chains across the country.

Within Hispanic groups in the USA themselves, bilingualism and biculturalism form an elaborate mosaic. Among Hispanics as in any other group, attitudes toward the value of acculturation vary. Specifically, not all Hispanics in the USA embrace diversity, which is reflected in their contrasting degrees of bilingualism and those of their descendants (see Brozgold & Centeno, ch. 5, this volume). Some will choose, or be obliged by the larger culture, to acculturate to English and mainstream culture at the expense of their Spanish language and heritage; others will manage to maintain both, *codeswitching* bilingually in the appropriate contexts, and by extension, *cultureswitching* as well. There is also a cohort of Hispanic individuals for whom acculturation is very fluid and requires another, more flexible interpretation. In this category, we include people who are very recent immigrants in the country and those who live along the border with Mexico or frequently travel to their country of origin (see Hidalgo, 1993; Matute-Bianchi, 1991).

Linguistically speaking, the result of such acculturative patterns is a mixed population of speakers with different language profiles. While there are those individuals who mostly know and use either Spanish or English, hence technically being monolinguals in one of those languages, there also are individuals who know and use both languages in varying degrees, and, thus, are bilingual. Bilingualism will, hence, easily enrich many, from children, as most children's brains are clearly innately set up to acquire the languages to which they are exposed, to adults, for whom dual-language ability means, for example, more occupational options and marketability.

In clinical communication, both monolingual and bilingual Spanish groups often represent challenges in the absence of in-depth theoretical and empirical bases to guide practice and research. Thus, speech-language clinicians and researchers must be aware of the phenomena addressed in the chapters of this book: the variety of dialects spoken in Hispanics' countries of origin (Goldstein, ch. 13), the contrasting degrees of language and educational opportunities available to Hispanics in their countries of origin, if they are immigrants, and, in the USA, the beliefs about bilingualism and acculturation that link to the sociopolitical reasons for immigration to the USA (Centeno & Gingerich, ch. 8), the ways in which the structures of Spanish and of English differ (Anderson & Centeno, ch. 1), the ways in which the orthography used for Spanish is not altogether transparent, even when it is much more so than that of English (Ijalba & Obler, ch. 18; Iribarren, ch. 17; Weekes, ch. 7), the patterns and consequences of simultaneous, as opposed to sequential bilingual development and of dynamic patterns of living back and forth over the years in predominantly Spanish-speaking locations (e.g. Puerto Rico, Mexico, and the Dominican Republic) and predominantly English-speaking ones, and the influence of manner of learning the second language (in school or by immersion) (Centeno, ch. 3; Kayser & Centeno, ch. 2).

As the authors in this book make clear, relative to other immigrant languages, there is already substantial information available about the Spanish and English language abilities of Hispanics in the USA, and about their schooling achievements and their cultural values. Yet, a dearth of bilingual speech-language pathologists to address the clinical needs of Hispanic children and adults has meant that there are even fewer clinicians who have the time and training to do the research in which sound clinical practice must be grounded.

Recent demographic data underscore the great need for such research to provide bases for current and future practitioners working with Hispanic clients (see Introduction to this volume). Further, because understanding communication abilities in monolingual and bilingual Spanish speakers goes beyond the realm of Linguistics proper, a *multidisciplinary approach* is warranted. Thus, as the chapters in this book remind us, speech-language pathologists, neuropsychologists, applied linguists, and educational psychologists must undertake precisely such research, carried out in culturally appropriate ways (Centeno & Gingerich, ch. 8).

We have predicated this book on the fact that more investigators in clinical communication than ever understand the need for research with Hispanics and are preparing to design it. Such research will inform *evidence-based clinical practices*. Such research will be necessary at all levels from the most applicable (e.g. what specific therapeutic treatment works best for Spanish–English bilingual children or adults with a particular language or speech problem?; how can Hispanic and non-Hispanic researchers best enlist Hispanic participants in their research?) to the most theoretical (e.g. what do we learn about humans' brain organization for language from contrasting how aphasic syntactic impairments manifest differently in Spanish–English bilinguals compared to bilinguals speaking languages that have markedly fewer cognate lexical items or shared syntactic structures?)

Indeed, one of the themes that runs through this book is the important interplay of clinical practice, descriptions of normal development and performance, and theories that link typical and atypical language use. Ostrosky-Solís and her colleagues (ch. 19) provide us with a fine example of a test of evidence-based reading instruction. Bell-Berti (ch. 20) and Anderson and Centeno (ch. 1) provide us with the descriptive information we need to ground our clinical and theoretical work. Moreover, the directionality of influence among clinical practice, normal development, and theory goes both ways. Anderson (ch. 9) gives an example of how evidence from the performance of children with SLI on specific Spanish morphological items can enable us to choose between different models of SLI in any language.

A second major theme that carries across the chapters in this book is that of *diversity*, in the sense of language varieties. Hispanics in Spanish-majority countries vary in the dialects they speak, as Goldstein (ch. 13) reminds us, and in their levels of education, as Ostrosky-Solís and colleagues detail (ch. 19). Hispanic immigrants to the USA differ in those same dialects of origin and preimmigration levels of education, and in their educational and work-related circumstances in the USA. Those whose work keeps them in the home caring for children are more likely to maintain strong L1 skills and develop lower L2 skills than those whose work outside the home requires substantial English.

Diversity in language use is a complex phenomenon that can be studied at many levels, as Anderson and Centeno evidence in their chapter contrasting linguistic phenomena of interest in Spanish as compared to English. Linguists tend to focus on one of these *levels*: phonetic (Bell-Berti, ch. 20) and phonological (Goldstein, ch. 13), morphological (Anderson, ch. 9), syntactic (Reyes, ch. 14), literacy (Kayser & Centeno, ch. 2), and discourse levels (Ansaldo & Marcotte, ch. 16; Pietrosemoli, ch. 15); each provides fascinating patterns even for the monolingual speaker of Spanish as for any language. The complexities at each level are naturally compounded for the bilingual or second-language learner, with diverse resulting *balances of proficiency* in different aspects and modalities of the languages in question.

Language performance, of crucial interest to the clinician asked to evaluate a client and, if necessary, design and carry out therapy, requires considering language less from concepts of language levels and more from those of language tasks. Bell-Berti (ch. 20) invites us to ask whether a client has native-like pronunciation, and if not, precisely why not. Pietrosemoli (ch. 15) considers whether the client is able to follow the rules of cohesive conversation after a stroke. Selecting the appropriate functors (e.g. prepositions, conjunctions, auxiliaries) can also be an indication of impaired or non-native proficiency. Functor selection, we have seen, is reported as a problem for children with SLI (Anderson, ch. 9) and for adults with aphasia (Reyes, ch. 14). It can, thus, be indicative of language difficulties as the result of frank brain damage or minimal brain damage, but it can also result from late L2-acquisition (Gitterman & Datta, ch. 4).

Additional diversity is seen when we consider the most challenging of complex language tasks, reading (Kayser & Centeno, ch. 2; Ijalba & Obler, ch. 18; Iribarren, ch. 17; Ostrosky-Solís *et al.*, ch. 19; Weekes, ch. 7). Depending on whether one learned to read in one language as a child – easily, or with difficulty, depending on precisely what the reading strategies the language one learned to read as a child permitted (Ijalba & Obler, ch. 18) – or, if, indeed, one learned to read as a child (Kayser & Centeno, ch. 2; Ostrosky-Solís *et al.*, ch. 19), one may have different outcomes as an adult. When frank brain damage (from an accident or a stroke) is added to the brain of those who knew how to read premorbidly, the same language-specific and orthography-specific factors that interact in the developmental process now play a role in how the acquired reading problems of alexia manifest (Iribarren, ch. 17; Weekes, ch. 7).

Variability, too, is seen among the brains of humans. Most pertinent for readers of this volume are the differences in abilities to learn a first language generally (as in children with SLI) and, more specifically, differences in learning to read (as in developmental dyslexia). And, even for those children with no apparent difficulties learning a first language, brain-based difficulties may arise in second-language acquisition (Ijalba & Obler, ch. 18). Additionally, special talents may be evident in this skill as well (Gitterman & Datta, ch. 4).

A third theme that arises across numerous chapters in this book is the importance of context. Of course the term *context* has many meanings generally, but it is interesting to consider how many it takes on in this volume. Kohnert and Kan (ch. 12) point out that young bilingual children learning a second language do so in different settings, with different demands; such contextual differences will contribute to these children's current and eventual lexical abilities in both their first and their second languages. For Kayser and Centeno (ch. 2), it is the degree of literacy-richness in one's environment that constitutes the context of interest, that contributes to one's success in learning to read. For Brozgold and Centeno (ch. 5), it is the sociocultural attitudes that clients bring to the clinical setting that must be understood and addressed by the clinician. In Reyes's terms (ch. 14), it is the greater or lesser linguistic context of a task that contributes to aphasics' ease in providing the correct preposition.

In a sociolinguistic sense, context provides both the mainstream base towards which acculturation works itself out for immigrants in a new country, and also the immigrant community's attitudes that contribute to the form acculturation may take. The interaction of class-, education-, and age-based attitudes influence one's willingness to acculturate, as Brozgold and Centeno (ch. 5) describe in this volume. Acculturation may influence one's abilities in the first language as well, if the second language dominates in the environment, and if the first language was not fully mastered before immigration.

One of the most fascinating context-dependent phenomena that bilingualism permits is codeswitching. This being one of the areas about which relatively more is known concerning Spanish–English bilinguals (e.g. Poplack, 1980; Zentella, 1997), Ansaldo and Marcotte (ch. 16) focus here on the neurocognitive underpinnings of the skill, noting how the pragmatic ability to appropriately mix languages may break down in aphasia (or, I would note, in dementia of the Alzheimer's type, as De Santi *et al*., 1990, and Hyltenstam & Stroud, 1989, have reported). Normal bilinguals may select from their two (or more) languages and codeswitch between them exclusively, when appropriate, in bilingual environments. Aphasics, by contrast (especially, I suspect, those with nonfluent or anomic difficulties) will use the translation equivalents of words that are hard for them to produce, even when speaking to an interlocutor who is monolingual. The fact that translation may help such word-finding problems, as Ansaldo and Marcotte demonstrate, means that while aphasics may be inappropriately codemixing when they do so, they have, nevertheless, developed a strategy that may help them find a word they were looking for.

A final theme that is woven throughout this book is how much more we have to learn about Spanish language usage in typically developing children and adults – monolingual as well as bilingual – despite the fact that we already know a fair amount. For example, we know a great deal about some of the types of information crucial to our practice, e.g. about the structural differences between Spanish and English (Anderson & Centeno, ch. 1), about the types of patterns that can be seen in cross-linguistic studies (Anderson, ch. 6), about values and attitudes of Hispanic immigrants to the USA, considered as a group (Brozgold & Centeno, ch. 5; Centeno & Gingerich, ch, 8). Also, about the specific phenomena associated with clinical populations of Spanish speakers, we have some information, with cases and small-group studies presented here (Ansaldo & Marcotte, ch. 16; Iribarren, ch. 17; Pietrosemoli, ch. 15).

One realm of interest that remains untouched with our focus on bilingualism in the current volume is that of some Spanish speakers' *trilingualism* or bilingual interaction between individuals' indigenous languages and Spanish. Such phenomena are of interest both in many Latin American countries and in bilingual immigrants from countries where indigenous languages survive to the USA. For example, as Centeno (personal communication) notes, increasing numbers of Mexican immigrants have been arriving in the New York City area as bilinguals in Mexican Spanish and Mixteco, an indigenous language in Mexico. In fact, among those considered bilingual Spanish–English speakers in this book, a number may actually be *polyglots* who mastered an indigenous language as a mother tongue before Spanish. The field of trilingualism studies is in its infancy, and will surely invite interesting discussions of this phenomenon among Hispanics (e.g. Goral, 2001). In addition, American indigenous languages are structured more differ-ently from either Spanish or English than these latter are from each other. As a result the interactions among the languages – in normals as well as those with language impairment – are numerous and interesting.

A second realm that is only alluded to in the current volume is that of the ramifications of socioeconomic class on language register, language development, access to health care including speech-language pathology services, attitudes towards health care, opportunities for second-lan-guage instruction and tutoring, expectations vis-à-vis education for oneself and one's children, ability to interact effectively with health care and educational institutions, and the like. One aspect of the variation seen among Spanish-speakers in the Americas is their broad range across socioeconomic ranks, and the language effects of this range invite further sociolinguistic study that can then feed clinical and theoretical work (see Oller & Pearson, 2002, for more general development of this topic.)

Clearly, then, more research is called for, especially if one wants to consider the diverse forms of variation among the world's Spanish speakers discussed above. Moreover, because communication skills are not learned in a vacuum and are subject to multiple variables (e.g. cognitive, neurocognitive, sociolinguistic, linguistic, acculturative, and so forth), as illustrated by the various chapters in this book, this research should have a multidisciplinary approach (see also Ball, 2005; Miccio *et al.*, 2002). To that end, we find in this book numerous hints and recommendations about how participants should be selected and encouraged to enroll in a research project (Centeno & Gingerich, ch. 8), what information the researcher should gather and report about them (Anderson, ch. 9), how discourse can be elicited and analyzed (Ansaldo & Marcotte, ch. 16; Pietrosemoli, ch. 15), how utterance length can be measured (Jackson-Maldonado & Conboy, ch. 11; Restrepo & Castilla, ch. 10), how stimuli should be constructed (Anderson, ch. 9) and how tasks should be selected (Reyes, ch. 14). As Institutional Review Boards are coming to understand, ethical research is not just research that *does no harm* and is respectful of participants (see Centeno & Gingerich, ch. 8, in this volume for related discussion); it is also research that is methodologically sound, thus justifying the time and efforts of the participants as well as the investigators. Sound research, furthermore, permits development of sound theories that themselves encourage collection of interpretable data on which to design evidence-based therapy, as the chapter by Ostrosky-Solís *et al.* (ch. 19) exemplifies. Monolingual and bilingual Spanish speakers represent great numbers in our world. We do hope that the contents of this volume and the knowledge that complements it inspire practitioners and researchers in clinical communication to undertake segments of this much-needed research. We, and all our current and future readers, look forward to learning what you find!

References

Ball, M. (ed.) (2005) *Clinical Sociolinguistics*. Malden, MA: Blackwell.

De Santi, S., Obler, L.K., Sabo-Abramson, H. and Goldberger, J. (1990) Discourse abilities and deficits in multilingual dementia. In Y. Joanete and H. Brownell (eds) *Discourse Abilities and Brain Damage: Theoretical and Empirical Perspectives* (pp. 224–235). New York: Springer-Verlag.

Goral, M. (2001) Language processing and language proficiency of trilingual speakers. PhD thesis, The Graduate School and University Center of the City University of New York.

Herman, J. (2000) *Vulgar Latin*. University Park, PA: Pennsylvania State University Press.

Hidalgo, M. (1993) The dialectics of Spanish language loyalty and maintenance on the U.S.–Mexico border: A two-generation study. In A. Roca and J.M. Lipsky (eds) *Spanish in The United States: Linguistic Contact and Diversity* (pp. 47–74). Berlin: Mouton de Gruyter.

Hyltenstam, K., and Stroud, C. (1989) Bilingualism in Alzheimer's dementia: Two case studies. In K. Hyltenstam and L.K. Obler (eds) *Bilingualism Across the Lifespan: Aspects of Acquisition, Maturity, and Loss* (pp. 202–226). Cambridge: Cambridge University Press.

Matute-Bianchi, M. (1991) Situational ethnicity and patterns of school performance among immigrant Mexican-descent students. In M. Gibson and J. Ogbu (eds) *Minority Status and Schooling* (pp. 205–247). New York: Garland.

Miccio, A.W., Hammer, C.S. and Toribio, A.J. (2002) Linguistics and speech-language pathology: Combining research efforts toward improved interventions for bilingual children. In J.E. Alatis, H. Hamilton and A.-H. Tan (eds) *Georgetown University Round Table on Languages and Linguistics 2000 – Linguistics, Language, and the Professions: Education, Journalism, Law, Medicine, and Technology* (pp. 234–250). Washington, DC: Georgetown University Press.

Oller, D.K. and Pearson, B.Z. (2002) Assessing the effects of bilingualism: A background. In D.K. Oller and R.E. Eilers (eds) *Language and Literacy in Bilingual Children* (pp. 3–21). Clevedon, UK: Multilingual Matters.

Poplack, S. (1980) Sometimes I start a sentence in English y termino en español: Toward a typology of code-switching. *Linguistics* 18, 581–618.

Zentella, A.C. (1997) *Growing up Bilingual*. Malden, MA: Blackwell.

Index

Authors

297

Subjects